BIOETHICS: A TEXTBOOK OF ISSUES

George H. Kieffer

University of Illinois

ADDISON-WESLEY PUBLISHING COMPANY

Reading, Massachusetts • Menlo Park, California
London • Amsterdam • Don Mills, Ontario • Sydney

To Craig

He didn't quite have enough time.

ISBN 0-201-03891-9
ABCDEFGHIJK-MA-798

PREFACE

This text grew out of my personal need for teaching materials for bioethics courses, a need I have felt both as a teacher at the University of Illinois and as a course director in the NSF-Chautauqua Short Course College Program. In this latter capacity I was given the opportunity by the American Association for the Advancement of Sciences (AAAS) to prepare a study guide on contemporary problems. This was completed under the title *Ethical Issues in the Life Sciences* (Washington, D.C.: American Association for the Advancement of Science, Study Guide on Contemporary Problems (Test Edition) 1975). Because of the significance and implications of topics included, a more extensive presentation seemed necessary. Hence this text.

Several texts have appeared recently that have focused especially on the ethical questions faced by medical practitioners, and medical schools across the country have developed courses or programs which consider these profession-related issues. The physician-patient relationship, truth telling, death and dignity, abortion, and medical resources and their allocation are a few of the topics commonly included. These books are usually anthologies of readings drawn from the extensive and growing ethics literature. The format includes a short introduction to a topic followed by one or several reprinted articles in which ethicists, theologians, or scientists express their views on that issue. There is much to be gained from this approach, for the student is led to an in-depth study of a particular value question, including a consideration of his or her own position. However, a study which selects one or a few of the better-known papers on a topic is time-consuming and can focus on but a few of the many issues arising from the "new biology." Furthermore, only a limited number of opinions may be revealed. Papers by single writers tend to argue for a particular ethical viewpoint at the expense of alternative positions. For the general student or the nonspecialist or even the medical practitioner, this approach may not provide the kind of overall awareness that can encourage intelligent discussion and involvement with the issues. Easier access to a large number of views on specific value questions can be gotten by a comprehensive summary and synthesis of divergent opinions. The present text endeavors to implement this approach by reviewing the broad spectrum of opinions iterated most frequently in the ethical and scientific literature.

This book is also designed with another consideration in mind. Over the past years, courses on ethical issues in the life sciences have been appearing in colleges and universities at all levels of study with increasing frequency. This is in keeping with the current wave of interest in science-related ethical issues. Often, however, resource materials are difficult to come by, especially in smaller institutions, and availability of references limits the study of these complex problems. Even when resources are near at hand, searching through the vast bioethical literature is a difficult and sometimes arduous task. Interested persons usually cannot devote the time nor do they possess the wherewithal to search out relevant study materials, forcing a reliance on outdated or inferior sources. To gain the degree of general awareness required for decision-making, it is more desirable to examine a variety of current views pertaining to a question. Broader coverage is more likely to uncover the many sides of an issue. The vast nonspecialist audience must have a readable volume which summarizes the issues if they are to participate intelligently in the resolution of biomedical questions. This book is addressed to students comprising that vast nonspecialist audience.

There is yet another objective sought after in this text. At least two meanings can be given to the term bioethics. In a narrow sense, it applies to those issues confined to medical matters. And in many minds it is this perception that predominates. A broader, more encompassing view includes not only the issues of biomedicine but those of a nonmedical nature as well. Examples of the latter are population ethics, environmental ethics, the ethics of scientific research, and so forth. This second definition is the definition adopted in this text, for these issues too must become part of our concern if many of society's vexing problems are to be resolved. Hence, a major goal of this text is to sensitize students to the ethical concerns arising from the whole area of modern biology.

On the face of it, this objective may seem to be presumptuous, for it can be argued that no one can be so well informed on these myriad issues that they can engage in thoughtful debate aimed at resolving them. But we live in a very complex age. Scientific knowledge, including that coming from biological study, is the root of technological changes which are transforming our social and political environment. We have to decide how to deal with them or the decisions will be made by default. And with many of these issues we must decide soon. While this author is acutely aware of his own personal inadequacies as well as the ambitious nature of this task, he labored in the hope that this book will contribute to the preparation of citizens for informed public discussion and to the raising of moral awareness in a way that can be sustained.

The text singles out for detailed study a number of topics under three major subdivisions: (1) preliminary issues; (2) medical issues; and (3) nonmedical issues. A discussion of the topic includes a summary of the relevant biology where appropriate and a discussion of the social and ethical issues raised. At the end of each section there is a list of values that can be used in making an ethical decision on a specific issue. As the student will subsequently learn, the choice of values is critical in the formation of an ethical decision. In fact, the primary concern of ethics is the weighing of respective values, many of which may be conflicting. Unless a purely pragmatic stance is taken, values always provide the foundation on which ethical decisions are based. The reader is encouraged to identify those values that best fit a personal position. The lists of values point out the plurality, the complexity, and sometimes the discordant nature of human judgment. There is no attempt in this text to make choices for the student nor to resolve ethical issues. The goal is to stimulate thought and help clarify personal choices. Extensive referencing is included so that those with a special interest can pursue each topic further. A bibliography is also contained listing references that, although not specially referred to by citation in the text, are applicable to that topic.

This book is intended for the interested nonspecialist with little or no training in philosophy or ethics. A chapter on ethical decision-making is included in Section I, "Preliminary Issues." It is the assumption here that many students using this text have not had a course in ethics; they could gain from a brief review of major ethical theories that are frequently applied in the biomedical–life sciences areas. Although a complete discussion of ethical theory is not possible within the short space of a single chapter, such a review can provide readers with sufficient knowledge of ethical theory that they can apply ethical methodology to the moral problems arising from modern biology. It is also hoped that those trained in the disciplines of ethics and philosophy can derive benefit from a study of this book, especially from the discussions of the many issues arising from the social applications of biological knowledge. There are difficult value choices to be made and social value judgments frequently exceed the decision-making prerogatives of any single profession or discipline. Ethicists and philosophers, natural scientists and physicians, public policy makers and social scientists must all join together with concerned laypeople to work through the many questions before us.

It is evident that not all aspects of any topic can be addressed within the space limitations of this volume. Each by itself has attracted the attention of specialists who have devoted long hours to their studies, written many words examining their ethical connotations, and engaged in heated debate. The issues are complex; difficulties in communication confound and ethical dilemmas bewilder. This text is intended to provide direction to individuals in formulating responses to the issues by pointing up their many ethical and social dimensions.

I express my appreciation to the AAAS for first involving me in the writing of these issues. Without their encouragement and generous assistance, it is doubtful that I would have involved myself in this arduous task. I would also like to express my appreciation to the many students and Chautauqua participants who generated ideas and provided feedback to various portions of this text.* Also, I cite the determination of the typist Mildred Stevens, who probably struggled as much as I in deciphering my hand-written manuscript. Lastly, my deepest appreciation to my wife, Beverly, who sat alone for the many hours required for this project.

Finally, as the single author, it is I who must bear all the responsibility for the errors of omission and commission. But I do this willingly, for it is to the communication of those matters relating biology to human affairs that I have committed

---

* The original work, *Ethical Issues and the Life Sciences* (AAAS, 1975) is presently available through the distribution network of the ERIC Information Analysis Center for Science, Mathematics, and Environmental Education in Columbus, Ohio. The author wishes to thank both the AAAS and ERIC for permission to publish this work in its expanded form.

my professional career. I am convinced that enormous shifts in our ethical thinking will be required if accommodation to the new biomedical knowledge is to be effectual. To those who would join in the search for this "new ethic," I especially dedicate this book.

Urbana, Illinois
November 1978

G. H. K.

CONTENTS

INTRODUCTION

The assertion that we are living in a "biological revolution" comes as no surprise to anyone. It has been emphasized on a number of occasions and from a variety of sources that some of the most significant scientific discoveries in the near and the long term will be in the life science–biomedical areas. Furthermore, some of the major social problems in this and the next century will be biological or will have significant biological components associated with them. The new circumstances of life today coming out of these developments is having and will continue to have enormous implications for ethics. In a very real way, the "new biology" has forced ethicists and theologians back to the drawing board for a reconsideration of the older conceptions of life and death and of what it means to be human. Such developments portend dramatic changes in our ethical thinking and have serious implications for the enactment of public policy.

The fundamental issues in question must not be decided by the educated few if democracy is to work effectively. Our whole society must face the choices formerly reserved for others, or as in previous times more often than not, left to fate. Such questions as these demand attention: Should defective fetuses be aborted? Is parenthood a right or a privilege? Will only persons who can afford life-prolonging and expensive medical care be treated? Can an overmedicated society lose its sense of identity? Do we as a nation of affluence have the right to dictate population policy to less wealthy nations even to the point of refusing aid if they fail to comply with our demands? Does it make any sense to talk about a moral responsibility toward the environment? Do we have moral obligations to those yet unborn? Are there any special responsibilities of scientists doing scientific research, and what is the proper relationship between science and society? These are but a few of the issues requiring response from both individuals and the community. Lawyers, sociologists, philosophers, theologians, and concerned lay-persons have already joined scientists and physicians in examining the present and looking toward the future.

Over the past years, much has been made of the crisis of confidence in science by the public and there is much ambivalence concerning the validity of this charge (see Chapter 13). Modern biology, too, has come under suspicion by that public.

Witness the recent clamor over legislation to regulate recombinant DNA research (see Chapter 4). Orwellian apparitions may be the layperson's perceptions of the "new biology" and much in the popular media conjures up images of far-out consequences: mass cloning of persons; human-ape chimeras; creating people to genetic specification; pre-assignment to an intellectual caste; societal-level control of behavior by chemical or physical manipulations; promises of immortality by various techniques from cryogenic freezing to serial replacement of worn-out body parts; destruction of the nuclear family, and continued erosion of traditional parent-authority relationships. "I think it would be disgusting" was the way a graduate student at a major university responded to an in-class assignment to describe a future composed of physically immortal humans. So often it is conjectured that the consequences of the new biology would inevitably lead to an overthrow of our most highly prized human virtues and destroy democratic society. Little wonder that thoughtful persons become alarmed when futuristic projections like these are made.

These distant events, however, are not the urgencies that demand our inspection, nor are they the ones discussed in this book. Ethical issues raised by the "new biology" are quite different from the sensationalized variety which attracts the public's attention. Scientists and medical practitioners are much less pessimistic about sinister applications of their work than is the nonprofessional laiety. This does not mean that serious ethical concerns do not fall within the present-day uses of biology. On the contrary, the ethical and social questions are numerous, and formulating acceptable solutions to them will be enormously difficult. The point here is that real ethical issues are raised by the "new biology" but these are quite different from the sensational, science-fictionlike ones designed to whet the appetite of the general public. What is needed first of all is a more realistic understanding of the clinical and social applications that have arisen and are likely to arise. Having learned all we can from our specialists, we must then work our way through these complex matters. Social value judgments are properly the prerogative of the citizens.

So what are the urgencies? Some are listed in Table I.*

Even a casual reading of the list suggests that many need attention now. Their human implications can dwarf the conventional issues of everyday life. As Jean Rostrand has stated it, man has learned to play God before he has become a human being. For better or for worse, the present generations—those who now hold power and those still in school—will have to make decisions about options for the future. The central question remains: How should we as a society respond to value-loaded problems when no clear-cut ethical resolutions expose themselves?

Many of these issues extend beyond individual preferences to the greater community, and social policy questions require a community answer. Laypersons, educators, medical professionals, scientists, government leaders, ethicists, and theologians must respond. The fortunes of science, politics, and society are inextricably enmeshed and cooperation between those concerned with the human application of science and the makers of governmental policy must become a working hypothesis.

---

*   George H. Kieffer, "Futures Planning: Biology, Society, and Ethical Education," *The Science Teacher* 42: 8 (1975): 12.

Table 1
Some moral and ethical issues in the new biology*

Bioethics

Modern science and biological man
Modes of ethical reasoning
Philosophical, moral, and ethical foundations for making value judgments

The new genetics

Prospects for genetic intervention: gene therapy, gene screening, genetic counseling, eugenics
Reproductive technologies: artificial insemination, sex predetermination, *in vitro* fertilization, contraception, prenatal diagnosis, abortion
Futuristic questions: cloning, genetic engineering, ectogenesis

Human experimentation

Free and informed consent
Guidelines for human research: research on fetuses, on children, on prisoners, on mentally handicapped
Social and professional control of experimentation

Behavior control

Fact and fallacy of control
Physical control: surgical, electrostimulation of the brain
Institutionalization
Chemical control: psychopharmacology
Psychotherapy

Health care

Concept of health
Delivery of health care
Cost of health care
Allocation of scarce medical resources
Prolongation of life

Death and dying

Euthanasia
New technologies: transplantation therapy, artificial organs

Population control

Right to reproduce
Birth control: contraception, abortion, sterilization
Population policy: incentive programs, relationships between developed and less developed countries

Environmental ethics

Obligations to the unborn
Ethics and ecological issues

Scientific research

Scientific conscience
Limits to research
Regulation versus freedom to investigate (e.g., fetal research, restriction enzymes)
Regulatory agencies
Science and the public good

Miscellaneous issues

Suicide
Biological weapons
Physicians and war
Pharmaceuticals, drug companies, and the public interest
Physician-patient relationships: truth-telling, consent to treatment
Malpractice

* From *Science Teacher* 42 (1975): 12.

The mass involvement of those affected by these new discoveries and techniques will certainly depend on an awareness of the issues. This will require not only an adequate knowledge of science and technology but also an understanding of fundamental aspects of human existence. A study of biology informs us that we humans are still linked to our biological heritage. But we are not exclusively determined by our biological makeup. We humans are guided by ideas of how people *ought* to relate to each other. The choices people make do make a difference. Education for effective participation in these decisions should provide assistance to confront the new problems wisely and to provide direction in finding adequate answers to them. These are central problems in education for the coming decades. It is the objective of this book to contribute toward this awareness by focusing on some of the questions.

Throughout the discussions that follow it is well for the reader to recognize that the approach adopted here is to make statements designed to open up issues, not to solve them. The debates on the problems presented are far from ended. The real purpose is to communicate a sense of the process of ethical reasoning through an uncovering of some of the facts and general principles and relating their near- and far-term consequences to moral positions. We cannot aim here for the specificity sought by policy makers. This must come about by an evolution in our thinking. It has been noted in this regard that we are at present technological giants but ethical infants. Many growing pains must necessarily be experienced. Its beginning form must be an awareness and appraisal of the factors leading to a listing of options. To work through the problems effectively will require an informed citizenry reflecting with scientists upon the moral implications and social uses of biological discovery.

Our future is shrouded with uncertainty. There are difficult value choices to be made that exceed the decision-making prerogatives of any particular expert or discipline. In this democracy, public policy still rests on the choices of the individual voter. The ultimate success of any policy rests on the willingness of voters to explore the principles on which an action may be based. It is both the glory and the burden of democracy that lay citizens must make the final choices. The quality of those choices depends on the quality of the public debate that precedes the decisions.

I

PRELIMINARY ISSUES

1

ETHICS AND EVOLUTIONARY BIOLOGY

INTRODUCTION

For the larger part of their intellectual history, humans have operated with the view that ethics was separate from the natural sciences. The facts of the sciences were presumed to be value-free while ethics involved considerations that went beyond such concepts as organic evolution, genetics, and the behavioral sciences. The sciences concern themselves most often with what people *want*, which in practice is based on very practical matters. In so doing, the sciences and scientists usually ignore the connection between actual wants and what is desirable. The latter requires a good deal more thought. There is a logical distinction between judgments of value and neutral statements of fact—or so it is contended.

Furthermore, much of the literature in the area of value either directly concerns or indirectly mirrors the assumption that ethics or moral philosophy is purely a matter of taste and as such cannot be analyzed using scientific methodology. In some ethical systems, preference may be given to divine command while in others human authors specify the moral life. In this conventional approach, ethics is accepted as readymade; the only intellectual problem is to validate the system of choice either by some rational process or by appealing to a final judge who speaks through revelation. Science certainly can provide little help.

There is a tendency on the part of philosophers to distinguish and hold apart organic evolution on the one hand from cultural change on the other. It is as though humankind somehow emerged as the result of strictly biological processes and when our nature was complete, then culture issued forth. In this model, ethics is restricted entirely to what humans have produced since their biological evolution was completed.

However, this is all starting to change. For a lot of compelling reasons, ignoring man's connections with his own past and with other animals is simply no longer scientifically acceptable. Science has many important things to say to ethics. With increased understanding of human evolution, it is becoming possible to piece together that conversion that changed a genetically selfish animal into a cooperator such as has never been matched in the biological world. The message that is coming through from these studies is that value systems, either in the form of religion or ethics, are an almost inevitable result of the way the brain evolved.

The human brain is an organ of survival honed for its unique function by organic evolution. This biological specialization has enabled the organism to integrate both external and internal sensory information into patterns that enabled it to adapt and remain viable. This magnificent brain empowered a biological species of the common variety to transcend its biological progenitors and become cultural. Human evolution became cultural when social interdependencies emerged as a way of life. It is unlikely that this life-style could ever have been achieved solely on a genetic basis. For instance, the early development of incest taboos and rules of exogamy cannot be explained using genetic mechanisms alone. The selective accumulation of skills, technologies, beliefs, customs, organizational structures, and the like, retained through purely social modes of transmission rather than in the genes, comes to identify this phase of human evolution.

Biological evolution formed the foundation for the development of culture. The development of culture led to the emergence of ethical and moral behavior, independent and sometimes at odds with purely biological responses—for example, in an ethical system cooperation is favored over competition. Teilhard de Chardin, the Jesuit priest-anthropologist, saw this relationship sometime ago when he wrote:

> The ethical principles which hitherto we have regarded as an appendage, superimposed more or less by our own free will upon the laws of biology, are now showing themselves—not metaphorically but literally—to be a condition of survival of the human race. In other words, evolution, in rebounding reflectively upon itself, *acquires morality for the purpose of its further advance.* [1] (Emphasis added.)

Ethics in this view is not simply a matter of taste; moralizing behavior has a utilitarian, evolutionary-adaptive function to perform. The facts and processes of biological evolution which brought into being the human species probably influenced the content of ethics. Exploration of these connections, which no doubt will prove to be an arduous task, is beginning to make the study of ethics at least partially amenable to scientific analysis.

THE IMPORTANCE OF AN EVOLUTIONARY ETHIC

Taking a broad view, an evolutionary ethic provides a new perspective for regarding human values. Human nature, including its potentialities, may be a source from which values can be derived. The argument that there are no universal values and that all values are relative is thus brought into question. It can be argued that there may be some values which are not time- or culture-bound and that these relate to the nature of our species which set the conditions for our long-ago survival and development in the cultural setting. These same or derivative values could prove crucial for accommodating the social change sorely needed in a modern world experiencing more than its share of moral dislocations. Such an ethic most probably will not provide us with all the light we crave but it can provide a fuller understanding of ourselves so that specific moral problems may be resolved in ways that minimize human suffering and maximize the generation of human good-will. Above all, an evolutionary ethic carries with it the expectation of enhanced survival of the human species, including an improvement in the quality of life for the individual and the whole of society.

It thus seems fitting that we start this discussion of ethical issues in the life sciences with a study of the possible relationships between biological evolution and ethics for, in addition to the above-mentioned reasons, other advantages can be gained. Several can be cited.

1   *An evolutionary ethic provides a view of human nature that could serve as a basis for the resolution of the life sciences-ethical dilemma.* At the moment there does not exist a perspective for dealing with the sensitive issues raised by recent advances in the biological sciences. Traditional Western metaphysics and morals have so far been quite unable to resolve the conflict between ethics and the power resulting from new-found biological and medical expertise. With its heavy emphasis on individual freedom including the guarantee under law of free choice, Western culture has produced a great diversity of ethical opinion, much of this not founded upon any full rationale.[2] The ethical premise that one position is as good as another, with no more justification than that a person be sincere, is a principle with very limited serviceability. There is a point beyond which ethical diversity and freedom ceases to be valuable. At least in matters dealing with the public good, it is rarely possible to honor all values simultaneously. Most of us do not find the societal good served by a do-your-own-thing tolerance—e.g., of industrial pollutors, the practice of abortion, government manipulators, genetic experimentation, etc. The confusion surrounding the widely publicized Karen Quinlan case clinches the argument against a do-it-yourself ethics in the biomedical sciences. All too often, different standards of what is good for the individual can result in conflict between patient-physician judgment as well as physician-physician judgment. It is simply not enough to say that the only ethical requirement for the physician is that he act according to his conscience, or that he be allowed to make a free choice. Decisions affecting the lives of others, both in the present and in future time, must be made less capriciously. The search for a new ethic must begin with the proposition that the life sciences-ethical dilemma must be cultural (i.e., societal), not individual. This is what Daniel Callahan of the Institute of Society, Ethics, and the Life Sciences has called for when he stated, "to build a fresh ethic for the life sciences is to build a new culture."

According to Callahan, two of the aspects that have overriding importance in shaping a new culture are these:

a) the nature of man—what he is and what he can become;
b) the extent to which nature, both human and non-human, can and should be manipulated and controlled.[3]

What Callahan and others are saying is that every culture holds a view of human nature which shapes policies and practices of human interaction. A culture requires some image of man on which to hang its hopes, some image of its relationships between personal-self and fellowpersons. This composite view *in toto* represents that culture's "Weltanschauung"—its comprehensive world view and serves as a measure to test proposals to cure, change, or improve upon the human condition. Ervin Lazlo, a systems philosopher, states this relationship quite clearly:

> If one is to make recommendations for adherence to right principles, what is required is a conception of the human animal as embedded in the real world that surrounds him including other men—structured societies. How can we tell what is right and good for man until we know what man is and how he relates to other men?[4]

Moreover, James Drane, a contemporary philosopher has stated, "every ethic is founded in a philosophy of human nature and every philosophy of human nature points toward ethical behavior."[5] Ultimately our primary values must rest on our conception of human nature.

If this is true, then our apparent inability to resolve many of our current and upcoming medical-moral dilemmas stems from the fact that our culture lacks a meaningful view of human nature. A meaningful view would suggest humane moral values to govern our new knowledge. Alternatively, if our values are not consistent with the real world it is to be expected that conflict will result. From the preceding, it is clear that our task, although immense, is to impart into our culture—its religions, its economic systems, its political institutions—a scientifically grounded view of human nature that will not be in ignorance or at variance with biological realities. The problem, then, for humans is to come to understand their own nature and from that nature to extract some guidance for the creation of effective ethical structures.

2 *An evolutionary ethic is consistent with present-day theories of the origin of moral behavior.* In locating the moral components of any situation, it is usually helpful if we know the facts. One of the most exciting problems of our time has become how to explain the mystery of the emergence of a beastly ape into a civilized human being. An increasing number of scientists from many disciplines are working on this problem. Certainly, some kind of history must be admitted that can explain how cooperative behavioral values arose, and that shows these to be tied to the genetically programmed human organism, which is itself a product of evolutionary forces. Callahan expresses the issue this way:

> If there is one crucial problem in the relationship between science and theology in the future, it is going to be the problem of ethics. The basic choice facing us is whether ethics is a kind of an "ex nihilo" creation by human beings simply for the sake of survival, where human beings have to develop moral codes and guidelines to enable them to survive together; or whether, indeed, if there is a nature out there, that nature finally provides some guides for the creation of guidelines, and whether there is something in which to root an ethic other than survival needs.[6]

How could a beast whose genetic programming included selfishness, stinginess, greed, gluttony, perpetuation only of its own line, envy, theft, lust, self-serving dishonesty, rage, and anger emerge as a cooperator par excellence; whose behavior optimized the social organization level even to the point of an occasional self-sacrifice of his body even for nonkinfolk? How could genetic competition ever result in cooperation? This is a fascinating problem for science but, at the same time, it has the potential to offer mighty assistance to the urgent problems facing humankind today where fast-growing scientific knowledge is causing dislocations in moral and religious knowledge. So fast is the onslaught that increasingly individual and institutional psyches are showing signs of approaching breakdown, disintegration, and death. It would, therefore, seem imperative that we seek to develop that knowledge required to provide a true and balanced wisdom for life. The relationship between

biological and social evolution and between knowledge and moral wisdom can provide a scientifically credible approach to understanding and addressing the present
human condition.

3 *The joining of human evolution with the development of ethics is a highly controversial issue in the sciences and the humanities today and has implications in the
realm of social policy.* The proposal that scientific justification can be made for
moral behavior is shocking to many, within both the sciences and the humanities.
Philosophers for several centuries have contended that the proposition is essentially
impossible to establish—that ethics is purely a matter of preference and not accessible to scientific analysis. However, we know quite a lot more facts now than we
did when that bit of "conventional wisdom" was being established. Surely, the intellectual task is not to deny *a priori* the existence of such a relationship but to evaluate
the compatibility of the known facts of biology and evolution with an explanation
of human values.

Social scientists, too, find the suggestions of a relationship revolting for it rein-
troduces notions of natural selection in cultural evolution. Social Darwinism, an
obsolete and repressive myth which was a product of this mistaken relationship, was
thrown out at least by knowledgeable persons a half-century ago. By providing
scientific backing to yet another misconceived interpretation of evolution backing
repressive remedies for healing troubled individuals and societies is a luxury that we
can well forgo. The mere suggestion of some sort of biological determinism, that is,
human social behavior determined by genes, conveys a reactionary political message analogous to Nazi eugenics or doctrines of racial supremacy. Social scientists
have been loath to admit that any of human social behavior is determined by the
genes for it all too easily allows for dangerous political consequences by providing
justification for discrimination and inequalities in the existing social order.

In response, Callahan contends that understanding the philosophical implications of evolution, including that evolution that drove humans in the direction of
forming ethical values, can guide us in developing an effective system today.[7] A
common fault, he suggests, is that we start too late in trying to understand ourselves, that is, after we have emerged as biocultural beings. Students of ethics would
do well to explore as deeply as possible the implications of evolution. Still more
emphatically, the controversial ethologist from Harvard University, E. O. Wilson
(of whom we will have more to say later in this chapter), states with unabashed
brashness, "the question that science is now in a position to answer is the very origin
and meaning of human values from which all ethical pronouncements and much of
political practice flow."[8] Thus, when ethical philosophers try to decipher the canons
of morality, they are consulting the survival values programmed into their own
brains by natural selection. As Wilson and others contend, social progress can only
be enhanced by the deeper investigation of the origins of human nature. Knowledge
humanely acquired and widely shared can replace rumor and folklore; the latter is
perhaps a far greater danger to political freedom. It seems proper, then, that we consider evolution and ethics as an issue in the life sciences.

THE IS-OUGHT DICHOTOMY

The point has been made that there is a relationship between the natural sciences and
human value. It might, therefore, be quickly concluded that science can, in and by

itself, provide the required ethics. But any effort to derive ethical concepts from empirical observations of fact can be challenged on the basis of the so-called "naturalistic fallacy" of David Hume. Hume's law asserts that there is an unbridgeable gulf between fact and value; or, as it is classically portrayed, the conflict between the "is" and the "ought." Science deals with what is—the facts of the physical universe; on the other hand, ethics considers what ought to be—values which can guide human behavior. Now, although it has been disputed by some,[9] according to moral philosophy one cannot derive an "ought" from an "is." Facts are one thing, values another. Statements about what is cannot yield statements about what ought to be for the reason that the transition from the is to the ought cannot be made without inserting a value judgment independent of the fact—the is. When we say science has many important things to say to ethics, science itself does not provide the ethics. In this context, science is knowledge but it is not wisdom. Wisdom is knowledge tempered by judgment. Although wisdom is based on knowledge, the first is not an automatic product of the second. Scientific knowledge can assist in the formulation of what is right or wrong by making us more aware of the facts, but it cannot determine which values are right or wrong.

Now, even though scientific facts do not constitute the values, such facts should be adequately reflected in the values lest the presumed facts be unreal or destructive of the values and the purposes they are intended to serve. When societal ethics are inconsistent with scientific facts, the net effect can be chaos, carrying with it the potential of losing freedom. The search for an effective ethic which can bring together the opportunities for individual and societal good with the fruits of modern science and technology must not ignore the facts of science. To do less, it seems to me, will result in a terribly flimsy structure. Therefore, underneath what follows in this chapter is the assumption that a fuller understanding of the evolution of human nature (the is) can provide a philosophical basis for *promoting* humane moral values to govern our science and technology (the ought).

EVOLUTIONARY TRANSCENDENCE OF MAN

The Darwinian revolution brought humans face to face with a radical change in their view of themselves and their place in nature. The proclamation so shocking and upsetting to Darwin's contemporaries was that humans are a part of nature, descendants of living beings not human, a biological species related to other species of the order primates. So incontrovertible has become the evidence that our species is the product of evolutionary processes, it is by now almost a truism.* The Darwinian image of man seriously challenged the prevailing concept of purpose in a

---

* Evolution is a response of living matter to its environment; it maintains or improves the adaptedness of a living species to its surroundings. Evolutionary changes are not, however, imposed on the organism by the environment. The environment or outside world contains conditions to which organisms may or may not respond by adaptive genetic change. Failure to respond may lead to diminution and eventually extinction. Successful responses allow the species to survive and expand. Genetic change must come *before* environmental change. Evolutionary success is measured by the number of viable (i.e., capable of reproducing) offspring produced by a certain genetic combination.

divinely ordained universe and cast permanent doubt on any notion of an absolute deontology.

The impact of Darwinian biology was threefold:

1   The human species as well as the rest of the universe is in process. Life since its inception on our planet has always been in process, so that what exists now did not exist in the past. This points to the conclusion that there is no finished or perfect life form, including human life.

2   Chance plays a large role in biological change. Two major chance events lead to change—chance genetic variation producing many forms within a population, and environmental change. Natural selection, as an objective force, integrates these to produce biological change. It was, of course, hard to see purpose in chance.

3   There is competition for survival. Nature, far from being benign or an abode watched over by a benevolent God, is depicted as a "struggle" characterized by fierce and deadly intra- and interspecies competition. This concept hit hard at the idea of a loving God who had designed nature.

Proponents of Darwinism were quick to point to its liberating effects: it freed one from the tyranny of traditional metaphysical dogmas, especially the absolutism of a deity who left nothing to chance and controlled all events in every detail. Furthermore, there is no point in involving concepts of purpose or direction to life if it owes its origins to natural and random processes. If there is purpose at all, it must reside somewhere other than in a directive imputed once and for all time by a Creator-god.

Some of the first efforts in the search for purpose tended to focus on the similarities rather than the differences between human and nonhuman forms. This narrowing of the gap between humans and animals was succinctly encapsulated in the slogan "man is nothing but an animal." They are no better or no worse and are subject to all of nature's law. However, failure to accord humans a special position has misled not a few philosophers and ethicists (e.g., naturalism) and has been used by racists as justification for race and class exploitation.

A refinement on this model conceded to humans the ability to reason. Man is not just an animal but, rather, is a rational animal. However, possessing the ability to reason is a quantitative property of behavior and provides little basis for ethical behavior, that is, behavior based on judgments of right and wrong. That humans are rational animals does not at all tell us how to act in rational ways. For this reason, the model must be judged deficient.

Since Darwin's time a variety of attempts have been made to account for the great differences between people and animals and the world has seen a good deal of oscillation. In the words of the biologist Julian Huxley:

> Man's opinion of his own position in relation to the rest of the animals has swung pendulum-wise between too great and too little conceit of himself, fixing now too large a gap between himself and the animals, now too small. . . . The gap between man and animals was here reduced not by exaggerating the human qualities of animals, but by minimizing the human qualities of men. Of late years, however, a new tendency has become apparent.[10]

Let's examine this tendency.

No doubt, humans are subject to nature's biological laws, at least to some of them, but to leave the matter at that does humans a great disservice. We alone in the biological world are subject as well to quite different laws stemming from our cultural evolution. As George Gaylord Simpson says, man is "not just another animal. He is unique in peculiar and extraordinarily significant ways." What are these ways?

Karl Popper, a contemporary philosopher, has proposed that humans alone are capable of being alive in three worlds: (1) the world of matter and energy, which is the material world, both living and nonliving, containing machines and all living forms; (2) the world of conscious experiences, which encompasses perceptual experiences of sight, hearing, touch, hunger, joy, etc., and also memories, imagination, thoughts, and planned action; and (3) the world of objective knowledge, which includes all intellectual effort and theoretical systems[11] (Fig. 1.1).

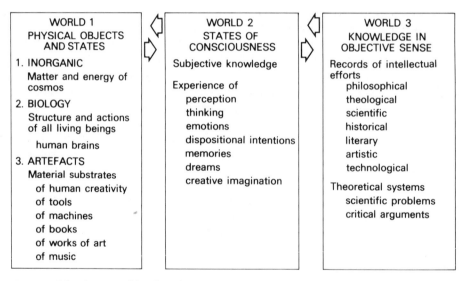

Fig. 1.1 *The three worlds of Karl Popper. (Source: J. C. Eccles, "Cultural Evolution vs. Biological Evolution," Zygon* **8**, *3–4 (1973): 283. Used with permission of the University of Chicago Press.)*

World 3 comprises the world of culture, a product of the genius that is distinctly human. Our species is unique because of its mental abilities. Evolution has conferred upon us the special endowments of educability and plasticity. Our behavior is not fixed but can be modified by experience. Evolution has made us capable of abstract reasoning, of learning, of recording what we have learned and communicating it to our posterity. And lastly, it created in us the ability to discriminate and to choose more or less freely among behavioral options. We are the only beings that live in a cultural as well as a physical world. We alone possess that quality of self-awareness which makes possible a contemplation of our present and future condition. Human evolution transcended biological evolution by bringing into existence a being with mental capacities, differentiating us from all other animals more radically than animals differ from each other. We alone are dwellers of Worlds 2 and 3 while animals live only in physical World 1. What this means is that with the appearance of humankind and the evolution of culture a new dimension or level of being was added to previously existing ones. Although cultural evolution was made possible by biological evolution, the former is not constrained by the latter. Natural selection, acting on genes, can optimize genetic fitness in such a way that those characters which control the capacity for culture can be maximized but the rules for the transmission of genes and culture are most probably quite different. Culture differs from the more ancient genetic way of acquiring and using information. Among the differences are:[12]

1 The timing of transmission: genetic transmission occurs only once, at conception, while enculturation is spread over a longer time, extending up to an entire lifetime. This would imply a greater importance on post-reproductive individuals stressing quite a different life cycle than is found in many, strictly biological species where genetic propagation is the single objective of the cycle and one's usefulness to the species is measured by reproductive potential.

2 Nonphyletic transmission: cultural information may be transferred to nonrelated individuals. The new condition might require that the number of genetic offspring within a social grouping be reduced to enhance cultural transmission. This is contrary to genetic fitness where the time test of adaptability is the number of viable offspring produced.

3 The serial nature of cultural transmission. In genetic transmission, the whole message is given simultaneously; in cultural transmission, the information is passed on in smaller packages with some messages being influenced by previous messages. This requires a complex series of interactions between the various agencies within the culture tending to reinforce its development.

4 Differential contribution of mother and father: unlike strictly biological mechanisms where male and female contributions to the offspring are half-and-half, cultural flow does not automatically prescribe such an equi-partition. One, both, or neither of the parents may contribute so that intragroup cooperation is required and reinforced.

There are undoubtedly other differences between the transmission of genes and culture. These, however, are sufficient to suggest that the kinds of behavior that maximize genetic fitness are not necessarily the same as those that made for an evolution of culture. Clearly, the evolution of culture is postgenetic, being produced by some sort of nongenetic selection of certain brain patterns. Cultural information is stored in the brains of the population where it functions as an integrating mechanism. Three levels of interaction can be discerned:

1 the genotype;

2 the physical environment;

3 the culturetype.[13]

The human societal organism is programmed partly by the human gene pool. Countless numbers of biological changes were required to convert our proto-ape ancestors into the modern human form. For much of the time when the necessary anatomical functional adaptations were evolving, only biological processes were involved. But even at this phase, human evolution assumed a new direction. The special evolutionary endowment that begins to set our forebears apart from all other animals is a large brain with the unique and special property of conceptual thought. This is truly a remarkable phenomenon. By means of conscious reasoning, humans have the potential to short-cut the slow and often wasteful process of biological evolution, substituting new and different standards for living. The enjoyment of beauty, the achievement of efficiency, the enhancement of life and its variety, the accomplishment of extreme sociality, the execution of value judgment—these things humans alone can do because of a magnificent brain.

But all these things could not have happened by purely genetic mechanisms. The brain's activities are structured in two ways. First, from the inside by the genetic code. This code directs the construction of each of the ten billion cells of this organ and specifies the main pathways of the brain. To assemble this fantastic array of millions of neurons with their proper structures requires many interlocking production lines operating with the highest precision during development. Many tightly programmed schedules must be met. This complex organization contains a memory—genetically recorded—of successful ways to live, selected from long experience with past environments. These memory units have been coadapted with one another to serve the organism over a wide range of internal and external environmental circumstances.

The second structuring of the brain comes from the outside—the physical environment—where all the messages received from the surroundings, beginning during its development in the fetus and continuing until death, provide a living record of its existence. This presumably is the physical basis of our educability and plasticity—neuronal structures that can be modified and/or restructured as a result of experience. In no other organism is there such an enormous number of possibilities for internal modification of neuronal pathways. This fantastic organizational complexity of the human brain can account for our concern with science, philosophy, theology, art, and ethics. The special genetic adaptation to receive and process a large block of environmental information converts this organism into a social being. Biological evolution became permanently and profoundly altered with the invention of a new kind of living creature in the environment.

The societal organism is made possible only by the evolution of a complex brain. Ralph Burhoe, research professor of theology and the sciences, calls this brain the new "gonad" of information, serving the function of storehouse for societal structuring and cooperation much like the gonads of biological reproduction store genetic information.[14] And, in fact, the societal organism has no other gonad than the human brain. Without a living brain, a product of the human genotype, no rituals, no myths, nor any printed books are generated, communicated, and responded to.

The viability of a societal organism depends upon the communication of information in such ways that reciprocal gains are experienced by the participating individuals. This portion of the generating information of the societal organism is its culturetype (the analogue of the genotype). A communal coadaptation links the individual phenotype—the product of genotype and the physical environment—to other cooperating phenotypes. In communal organization, life-shaping information is developed and transmitted independently of the human gene pool. The promise of greater benefits from a symbiotic union between a group of genetically diverse societal organisms propels social evolution along its course. Unlike biological organisms, the individual parts—language and technology—making up the social group-ings are readily transplantable from one societal organism to another. Societal organisms are modifiable and can evolve by recombinations of information in a multitude of ways. Richard Dawkins, in his book *The Selfish Gene*, labels these "memes" (as contrasted with genes). Examples of memes are tunes, ideas, catchy phrases, clothes fashion, better ways of building things, and the like.

With culturetype, the societal organism transcends all creatures in the bio-logical kingdom. The emergence of the human brain with a new memory system for phylogenetic information independent of the gene pool and yet coadapted to it in a communal arrangement of mutual benefits between cooperators brings into being human urban social complexity. In the words of John Kendrew:

> We may thus describe three different types of information that are important in bio-logical systems: (1) the genetic information which does not have a feedback from the organisms but is passed on from generation to generation; (2) stored sense data (in the brain) which do have considerable feedback into the storage system of the organisms but are not passed down (like genes) from generation to generation; and finally, (3) communicated data, which do have feedback and are passed down to the next generation. It is the possession of this third kind of information in large amounts that makes *Homo sapiens* unique as a species.[15]

In spite of the amazing accomplishments of this societal organism, Burhoe and others are quick to caution that biological evolution is not over nor is it nonessen-tial. Genetic selection is just as necessary today as it ever was and it must continue to be part of our ethics if we are to continue to survive. Cultural wisdom must satisfy the prior requirements inherent in the variety of genotypes that shape the pheno-types of the societal organisms. Matching genetic with sociocultural information to achieve a viable social organization must be carried out. For example, the new memes can leap from brain to brain and transform persons and culturetype in seconds, as when a new technology is developed. But, errors of mismatch between culturetype and human genotypes within the society can bring about the elimination of part or all of that grouping. The recent concern over genetic research with recom-binant DNA is a case in point. Although opinions vary considerably over the uncer-tainties of direct manipulation of the genetic material, anxiety has been expressed over the possibility of inadvertently creating an "Andromeda strain" of microorga-nism capable of wreaking havoc of epidemic proportions on an evolutionarily unprepared population. The potential of making viable organisms with untoward properties that may escape into the environment is inherent in these researches. The memes are nonharmonious with the genes. The question over whether to proceed in a new area of potentially hazardous research seriously challenges the consideration of matching genotype with culturetype. Anthropologists and historians have noted that there are societies that have failed or have been eliminated because of mismatch between the two.

BRAIN EVOLUTION

The central focus of this discussion has been on the relationship between brain structure and cultural evolution. By now, it is a pretty well-accepted dogma of neurobiology that the main agency of human behavior, feeling, and thinking of all kinds is the brain. A considerable amount of data has been acquired in recent years that traces the development of this remarkable organ from rather inauspicious beginnings to the structure which it has come to be today—the most complex three pounds of matter in the universe.

The localization of nerve cells in the head end of ancient crawlers pulling themselves through primeval environments was the forerunner of complex nervous systems. The tendency to concentrate nerve cells into clumps at the head of an organism makes good sense since this is the part that leads the way through water, through mud, and through the air, communicating environmental information backward to the rest of the body trailing behind. Increasing centralization of the nervous tissue in the head can be followed up through the invertebrate and vertebrate groups. In vertebrates, from the fishes through dinosaurs, most animals have been guided by their noses. It is, of course, our enlarged cerebrum that sets humans off from the rest of the biological world. It is thought that the cerebrum came into being largely as an overgrowth of the ancient smell centers.

The evolution of the vertebrate brain is thought to have occurred in several waves or surges with each addition being superimposed on previously evolved structures (Fig. 1.2). Reptiles have little brain matter in excess of the necessary minimum for the preservation of life. Their tiny brains persuade them to eat, to reproduce, and to defend themselves. But there is room for little else to take place inside their skulls. The reptilian brain, according to Paul D. MacLean (Chief of the Laboratory of Brain Evolution and Behavior, National Institute of Mental Health), persists in the higher vertebrates, including humans.[16] Being the first part of the mammalian brain to arise in evolutionary time, it continues to function as the basic brain, located at the top of the brain stem; succeeding layers of nervous tissue are stacked upon it. In higher animals, the reptilian brain is basic for the behavior of social communication that is involved in self-preservation as well as the preservation of the species. MacLean theorizes that the reptilian brain may be important to many species as an organizer of such basic behavior as the selection and preparation of a homesite, the establishment of territory, routine daily activities such as foraging,

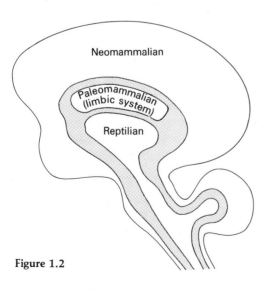

Neomammalian

Paleomammalian (limbic system)

Reptilian

The evolution of the brain occurred as a series of surges or waves with succeeding levels superimposed on existing structures.

Figure 1.2

hunting, greeting, grooming, breeding, and migration; in short, life's instinctive behaviors. However, it is not very adaptable. Nerve connections within its various parts and between it and other brain regions allow for few behavioral options.

About 150 million years ago, an early mammal, *Triconodon*, living among the dinosaurs, began to show the first evidences that a better brain was possible. This was the first animal known to have a significantly encephalized brain. Encephalization refers to the special process wherein the brain expands more rapidly than the rest of the body. The big evolutionary contribution of *Triconodon* was the expansion of the primitive cerebrum which came to overlie the reptilian brain. It is found today in an area called the limbic region that surrounds the so-called brain stem or reptilian brain. MacLean calls it the paleomammalian brain and believes that it is the center for rational control over the basic instincts originating in the reptilian brain. Not only was there a physical impositioning of the paleomammalian brain over the reptilian brain but the two became functionally related as well, with many neural fibers being established between them. The paleomammalian brain provided for emotion, for exploring the novel, and for loosening the bonds of genetic determinism so that more behavioral options were opened up. Behavior became less stereotyped and more refined. For these reasons, the limbic region or paleomammalian brain has been referred to as the "social brain." One example of this is demonstrated in the care of the young. Most reptiles have no regard for their young. They lay their eggs and never see their offspring again. Mammals, on the other hand, nurture their young if the species is to prosper. The appropriate feelings for doing this are somehow built into the paleomammalian brain.

For the next 100 million years, natural selection exerted little pressure to improve upon this arrangement. Until about 50 million years ago, early mammals showed about the same degree of encephalization. But then, some mammalian brains once again began to encephalize. The neomammalian brain or neocortex started to overgrow the paleomammalian brain. With this, the cerebrum proper initiated its development. Some of the highly encephalized mammals—for example, the whales and the dolphins—reached their present level some 20 million years ago. At about that time, the process once again stopped. But in other vertebrates, especially the primates, encephalization continued so that in the comparatively recent history of the past 3 million years, one group of primates, humans, carried encephalization the furthest. The fossil evidence indicates that *Homo sapiens* reached its present brain size about 250,000 years ago and that it had tripled in size in the 3-million-year period preceding that time. The brain of modern humans, notably the cerebrum, surpasses several times over the average of other living mammals. (See Fig. 1.3.)

The enlargement of the neomammalian brain enhances the capacity of the individual to sense, store, and integrate information. The quantum leap from biological to cultural development in human evolution was initiated by this most recent addition to the mammalian brain. The use of abstract symbols to create a complex language is considered to be one of the key developments in human evolution. The brainpower for speech resides largely within the neomammalian brain. The remarkable ability of vocalization with the attendant capacity for cognition, as well as the capabilities of abstract thought and increased intellectual capacities, were all made possible by this third wave of encephalization. As has been said, humans no longer live in the physical world but in a symbolic one.

Consciousness revolution	Time from 1976	Brain
7. Homo sapiens	−40,000	
6. Homo erectus	−162,000	
5. Homo habilis Australopithecus	−651,000	Neomammalian
4. Hominidea	−2,207,000	
3. Primates	−8,428,000	
	−33,315,000	Paleomammalian (basic social)
2. Mammalia	−132,850,000	
1. Reptilia	−531,010,000	Reptilian

Evolution of consciousness and the brain.

(Note: the time references in the right-hand column are not drawn to scale.)

Figure 1.3

As the cerebrum got progressively larger, greater and greater plasticity of activity and increased educability became possible. In humans, the cerebrum comes to dominate almost everything the body does. The skilled activities of the concert pianist, the cabinet maker, the artist, the craftsman, all attest to this evolutionary achievement. The capacity to expertly manipulate our environment has given us an unmatched advantage over every other form of life. Animals with brains functioning like this are distinguished by their capacity to gather more information from their environment, to act upon it, to think abstractly, and to communicate among themselves. That unique specialty of action upon rather than reaction to the environment is bestowed on the owners of such big brains.

And so it is seen that the three levels of brain evolution under proper direction of the neocortex results in harmonious hierarchical operations of behaviors, feelings, and capacities for rational thought. Genetic selection has given us our reptilian brain which produces automatic behavior designed to maintain life at the basic level. We generally are not conscious of much of this behavior. The paleomammalian brain, superimposed on the first, directs the behavior of the tightly prescribed responses provided by the reptilian brain. At this brain level, integration of information from inside the organism with information from outside the organism takes place so that alternative courses of action can be chosen. Moral responses between what is right and wrong presumably are the outcomes of this activity as well as the essential feelings of individuality and personal identity. The third level, the neocortex, is genetically structured so that a still more generalized control of behavior is possible. Because of the neocortex, linguistic symbolization integrating the outside world with the inner one is effected. On the basis of a culturally developed program, the symbols can be manipulated to relate current happenings to future potentials, and, insofar as the brain allows it, we can bring future states into our present decisions; as we shall see, this is a matter of great importance to ethical evolution. Linguistic communication makes possible a new level of social transmission of culturally evolved and inherited information that has greatly enriched the human heritage. It is the evolution of this outer layer, the neocortex, that explains how humans emerged as a new life form above that of all other creatures and why humans alone were able to motivate social cooperation over genetic competition. It is consistent with evolutionary biology to suggest that this third level provides us with the capacity to carry on ethical reasoning.

THE EVOLUTION OF ETHICS

The problem that interests us now is the evolutionary origins of ethics and values. Has the bioevolutionary development which made humans possible in the first instance endowed humankind with some particular ethics? Or has it made members of the species capable of being taught various kinds of ethics and morality? Further, can evolutionary ethics provide logical grounds for moral norms? These are difficult questions to answer.

To begin with, the problem of explaining or tracing in detail the evolution of ethical and moral capacity is not an easy one for the obvious reason that there are no fossil records to which one might turn; and the dissection of genes to locate the DNA code for ethical behavior, if such a material base indeed exists, is still far from possible. Studies of modern human behavior or comparative morphology provide few insights into this perplexing problem. Even the very problem of defining moral or ethical behavior itself is a difficult one on which to obtain agreement.

For purposes of this discussion let us accept, at the least, the assertion that ethical and/or moral behavior involves acting for the sake of some nonbiological end; that is, such behavior is not concerned with reproduction or self-maintenance. Acting in the interest of another or in the interest of group welfare, even though it may go against individual welfare, might be considered one feature of this kind of behavior. To simplify matters somewhat, let us dismiss from our thinking this form of behavior as it is sometimes thought to occur in some nonhuman organisms. Group social behavior as found, for instance, in baboons differs in its level of sophistication quite dramatically from that practiced by humans. Urban humanity in its ancient and modern forms is far more social, and achieves more complex social interdependence, than any of the other vertebrates. Even the social insects, with their high degree of division of labor and social class achieved on a genetic basis alone, do not demonstrate the high degree of cooperative behavioral dispositions and achievement of humans. Humankind, by almost any measure one would use, has become by far the single most successful form of life evolution ever produced.

However, the observation of moral behavior in nonhuman forms has profound evolutionary significance in that it suggests that such behavior can, in fact, arise by natural processes. Its occurrence in simpler forms in organisms not considered human, and its gaining greater degrees of refinement as *Homo sapiens* is approached, lends credence to the proposition that ethical behavior can arise through natural means in response to environmental pressures. The degree of sociability and altruism achieved by some primates (e.g., baboons, monkeys), as well as other vertebrate groups (e.g., California woodpeckers, turkeys), may represent evolutionary experiments with social coordination and altruism on the genetic level. Treating these as having evolutionary adaptive value provides a case for believing that rudiments of something like a moral sense may be present in non-human organisms.

Edward O. Wilson, a Harvard biologist, has developed the theme of sociality in nonhuman forms to a high level in his work *Sociobiology: The New Synthesis*. According to Wilson, some of our noblest sentiments may derive from behavior selected because of their basic survival value. The emotional control centers of the brain—hate, guilt, and fear—as well as forms of altruism, have evolved by natural selection. If this be the case, then somehow the survival of those species in which social behavior occurs is promoted. Whether or not traces or rudiments of moral behavior are found in animal species other than humans need not concern us here. As our earlier discussion has emphasized, the appearance of man brought into existence a being which, in terms of its capacities, differs from all other animals in ways radically different than from animal to animal. In this sense, human evolution has transcended biological evolution. The transcendence, however, is to be interpreted here as emerging from biological evolution and not the interposition of some supernatural or metaphysical force.

Can evolutionary ethics provide logical grounds for imperative moral norms? The response to this question is probably no. Systems of ethics are the products of human wisdom and the experience of humans living together and not of the expression of human genes. In this regard, it is well to emphasize that evolutionary change as a natural process has in itself no moral worth. Whether species X or species Y, in competition for the same ecological niche, momentarily wins the evolutionary prize of survival carries no implication beyond that of the continuation of life on this planet. In this sense, mountain lions and human beings are of equal value. It is difficult to get clear answers as to why this or that species ought to go on, and here evolution teaches an ambiguous lesson. The vast majority of species haven't survived, while a few have survived for millions of years, for example, the cockroach. There is no point in considering that the changes wrought by natural processes are good, or bad, or a mixture of the two; in other words, it is pointless to consider biological survival in value terms. So we see that, though a rational system of ethics cannot be independent of evolution, neither can a system of ethics be derived directly from evolution.

The prevailing view of those who have studied the question is that, although the potential for developing an ethical system is the outcome of evolutionary processes, meaning and values are culturally determined. This analysis was presented by the well-known contemporary evolutionary biologist George Gaylord Simpson when he wrote:

There are no ethics but human ethics, and a search that ignores the necessity that ethics be human, is bound to fail . . . the means to gaining right ends involve both organic evolution and cultural evolution, but human choice as to what *are* the right ends must be based on human evolution. It is futile to search for an absolute ethical criterion retroactively in what occurred before ethics themselves evolved. The best human ethical standard must be relative and particular to man and is to be sought in the new evolution peculiar to man, rather than in the old, universal to all organisms. The old evolution was and is essentially amoral. The new evolution involves knowledge, including the knowledge of good and evil.[17]

Humans, then, are born with a capacity to become ethicizing beings, much like we are born with the capacity to learn a language. Human genes evidently enable us to speak but have nothing to do with what particular language we will speak. According to C. H. Waddington, humans are "born with a certain innate capacity to acquire ethical beliefs but without any specific beliefs in particular."[18] Here we might borrow Simpson's criteria for practicing ethical behavior:

1   there are alternative modes of action;

2   humans are capable of judging the alternatives in ethical terms, that is, decisions involving that which is judged to be good;

3   we are free to choose what we judge to be good.[19]

In evolutionary models, behavior, no less than anatomy and physiology, is shaped by natural selection. It is therefore not inconceivable that humans had the proclivity for ethicizing built into their genetic constitution during evolution. If ethicizing, that aspect of behavior relating to moral behavior or the principles of duty, is a feature finding its highest expression in *Homo sapiens*, and if it is universally distributed in the species, there must be some evolutionary reason for its inclusion. In other words, the character demonstrates evolutionary fitness; it has survival value for that group of organisms that possesses it.

Various cultures, past and present, have exhorted their members to live up to moral and ethical standards, frequently deriving from them the laws of social organization. Individual behavior for optimizing collective goals promoted and reinforced a social organizational level of evolution over selfish and potentially destructive self-interest. In this way, ethical behavior has contributed mightily to the survival of the species. The universality of ethical behavior can be demonstrated in several ways. The first of these is respect for the individual. In most, if not all human societies, it is right and good to be honest, generous, kind, and brave. Human life, including that of a stranger, is sacred—except in war. Life is to be preserved. On the contrary, it is wrong to steal, rob, injure, or kill—especially members of one's own group—even if doing so is profitable or the misdeed is undetected and no vengeance or retribution is feared. Another universal value is basic honesty in human relations. All ethical systems appear to condemn deception, dishonesty, and trickery. These values are not simply the preferences of values propounded by religious leaders or philosophers. They derive from the experiences of humans living together with other humans in society. Without the observance of these values or their implementation at least at some minimal level, society probably could not have survived. Respect for life, in some degree and in some situations, is necessary for the survival of the species. The infant requires someone to provide it a minimal degree of caring or love for its sheer physical survival. The individual needs a minimum of caring and loving from others in order to become a person or develop a self. If there is not a minimal level of honesty in society, a basic trust in others, the social order would collapse. There have no doubt been certain times and certain (small) groups wherein these values have been absent, and of course there have been individuals who ignore or fail to subscribe to them, but the values described here appear to be endorsed by major religions and philosophies of all times and cultures. The summit of these ethics, according to Dobzhansky, is the commandments of universal love, service to others, and nonresistance to evil.[20]

Paleontological evidence reveals that mutual cooperation and altruism, often going so far as self-sacrifice, have long been practiced. One of the first Neanderthalian skeletons discovered was that of a man approximately 50 years old who had suffered from extensive arthritis. His disease was so severe that he must have been unable to hunt or even to engage in strenuous activity. He had, therefore, to depend upon the care of his clan for his survival. Many prehistoric finds suggest similar attitudes of affection. A Stone Age tomb contains the body of a woman holding a young child in her arms. Whether or not the words altruism and love were in the Stone Age language we do not know, but the social behavior which denoted them did exist.

The view reiterated here emphasizes that the function of ethics is to mediate the progress of human evolution; further, that natural selection has provided us not with ethics and values, per se, but with a capacity to acquire them. It can be argued that the direction of human evolution from earliest times favored flexibility derived mainly from increased learning potentials. As primitive humans viewed a problem, alternatives were suggested. This raised the necessity of choice requiring foresight and prediction, since the results of an option selected and the consequent responsibility or outcome for the action had to be judged in future terms. It bears repeating that the evolutionary development of ethics depended upon the human capacity to predict the results of one's action. This unique ability is directly correlated with cerebral function and of necessity awaited the evolutionary refinement of that organ before futurizing was possible. As primitive peoples organized into human societies this adaptation was carried out in a cooperative social environment. Our ancestors thus learned from both their fellows and their own experience to consider some actions right and some wrong; with continuing evolution and new capabilities, some things became more right or more wrong. The product of this potential eventually takes the form of ethical systems, subject to alteration or rejection as dictated by local conditions and social change. In this fashion, biological evolution has created a species capable of entertaining ethical beliefs. The biological function of ethics seems to be to promote human evolution, especially in the cultural-sociological mode.

In this regard, we might conceive of the evolution of ethics as an inverted pyramid. According to Fig. 1.4, ethical concepts grew over time to embrace larger and larger groups. We might conjecture the following: For thousands of years ethics applied to very small groups, possibly only to individual behavior. Under the pressure to survive, a person might even cannibalize his own offspring or mate. Then an expansion of ethics occurred to include the family. More time passed and the ethical province expanded to the tribe. In this state, for example, the daughter of a fellow tribesman was protected by tribal ethics, but if one encountered a woman from

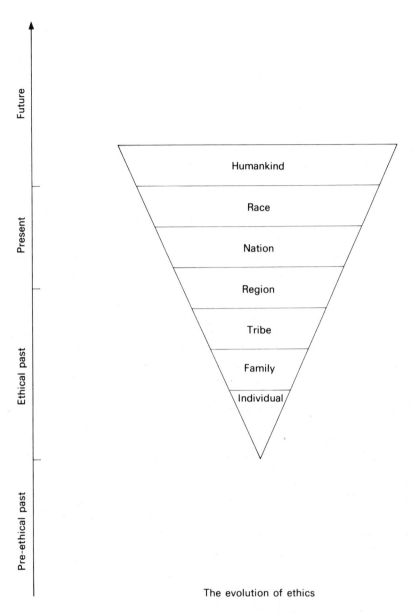

Future

Present

Ethical past

Pre-ethical past

Humankind

Race

Nation

Region

Tribe

Family

Individual

The evolution of ethics

Fig. 1.4 *(Adapted from Nash, Reference 21. Used with permission.)*

another tribe on a forest path, she might be claimed instantly. Right or wrong did not apply to her, only to one's own group. Continuing on, time brought the extension of ethics to everyone in a region and then a nation. Today, we may be in the midst of another ethical leap, a widening of the ethical circle to include all of humankind. Some promising moves are seen occurring in this direction in the form of assistance programs for people in distant lands. The oft-heard "family of man" appeals have as their base the concept that all members of the human species should be loved as children or as brothers and sisters. Here then, is the commandment of universal love.[21] In times of wars, however, restraints observed by soldiers in regard to their own families, neighbors, and countrymen do not apply to people outside the group.

Dobzhansky conceptualizes how this may have occurred when he distinguishes between two kinds of ethics: family ethics and group ethics. He describes family ethics as *genetically* determined, the products of natural selection. These are exemplified as altruistic behavior toward members of one's own group, especially the family group. Altruism is defined as behavior which benefits others but may harm or place at a disadvantage the practitioner. Filial activities such as the care of children, where the individual willingly denies some advantage to herself or to himself for the welfare of the offspring, or the communal defense response even to the point of mortal self-sacrifice, might be representative behaviors. Family ethics are shared by humans with at least some animals; for example, distraction displays of ground-nesting birds when a predator approaches or the feeding and care of young by parents even at enormous cost to themselves.

Group ethics, on the other hand, are products not of biological but of *cultural* evolution and they also confer no advantage and may be disadvantageous to individuals who practice them. However, they are indispensible to human societies, for group living could not endure without them. Group ethics, because they are culture-based, differ from culture to culture. Such examples as variations in child-rearing techniques, parental love, self-sacrificial devotion, aggressive behavior, and sexual mores argue for the cultural preference of these ethics.[22]

The basic behaviors included in the category of family ethics have probably been shaped in humans by natural selection much like homologous behavior patterns have been selected in many nonhuman animals. However, as Dobzhansky goes on to point out, natural selection also favors egotism, hedonism, cowardice—except in defense of one's own children or family—and cheating, and exploitation of nonfamilial individuals. Yet in most human societies one finds rules, either implicitly understood or codified in some formal fashion, that specify intragroup cooperation. The design of such group ethics could well have been to counteract the anticooperative behaviors and, in fact, glorify their opposites: kindness, generosity, and even self-sacrifice for the good of others, especially one's tribe. The establishment of more-or-less permanent settlements and the domestication of plants and animals required that property rights be protected and that duties and responsibilities to the widening community be ordered. It thus appears that extending family behavior to group relationships promoted complex social interdependences contributing mightily to human social and cultural evolution.

According to this model, natural selection in humans by favoring educability and plasticity substituted a culturally determined altruism for a genetically fixed one. This becomes a dominant directive agency in human behavior. Love and dedication to the welfare of one's own children and other close relatives becomes extended in cultural evolution to include wider and wider circles of people. Parenthetically, this ethical expansion could conceivably someday be extended to all of humankind.

Because of its fundamental contribution to survival, it has been postulated that ethical behavior may have as its first cause specific genes located within individual genomes. For example, J. B. S. Haldane, a British biologist, some time ago (1932) postulated that the *genes* for altruism may have appeared when humankind began gathering in social groups. Small tribes containing individuals with altruistic genes may have gained an advantage over other groups through the willingness of some of its members to sacrifice themselves in defense of the tribe; hence, the groups possessing these genes and spreading them by interbreeding may have multiplied while those who conducted their affairs on the principle of individual self-interest were eliminated.

More recently, the concept of kin selection has been advanced as an evolutionary mechanism for promoting altruistic social behavior. Here, too, a genetic base is imputed to the behavior. The term *kin selection* is used to distinguish a kind of natural selection in which genetically related individuals more willingly cooperate with one another for survival than they will with nonkinfolk. Kin selection accounts for within-family altruism; the closer the relationship, the stronger the selection. Mathematical calculations may be used to compute the genetic relatedness between any two individuals, indicating thereby the willingness to cooperate. For example, individuals contain 100 percent (or 1.0) of their genes in their own body. A son or daughter would contain one-half of any one individual's genes; a grandchild, only one-fourth; and so on. Full brothers and sisters each carry one-half, while identical twins are a special case having a relatedness of 1. Uncles and aunts, nephews and nieces, grandparents and grandchildren, and half-brothers and half-sisters are intermediate with a relatedness of one-fourth.

The goal of kin selection (teleologically speaking) is to promote the shared genotypes in the next generation. Hence, the willingness to cooperate is predicated on the assumption that personally owned genotypes are the most desirable in the next generation. Saving five nonkinfolk through altruistic self-sacrifice would not be as evolutionarily desirable as saving five brothers or ten cousins. The former has no genetic relationship with the altruistic donor while brothers are more closely related than cousins. Hence, the genes for altruistic self-sacrifice for nonkinfolk are not as likely to spread in the next generation as are the latter. According to this view, genes have different loyalties to different bodies. In this respect, parental care or suicidal self-sacrifice for members of one's own group are special cases of kin altruism. Such genes tend to live on in the bodies of enough individuals saved by the behavior to compensate even for the death of the altruist himself or herself.

The previously mentioned Harvard biologist, Edward O. Wilson, in his controversial book *Sociobiology: The New Synthesis* applies the concept of kin selection to a study of the evolution of sociality.[23] Slime molds, ants, and apes belong to the three groups of species among which sociality evolved in nature. In the text, he develops the thesis that social behavior among these nonhuman groups is mostly or wholly determined by genes. Only in the last chapter of this lengthy tome does he speculate on the species that occupies nature's fourth social pinnacle—humans. The issue that Wilson raises and around which a good deal of contention has been stirred is how much of human social behavior is genetically determined?[24] His position is that while in nonhuman organisms this behavior is thoroughly deterministic, in humans "the genes have given away most of their sovereignty." Subsequently, he has theorized that maybe 10 percent of social behavior has a genetic basis.[25] In other provocative suggestions in the last chapter of his book, Wilson speaks about the evolution of ethics. The emotional control centers of the brain—of hate, love, guilt, fear—have evolved by natural selection. Some of what we regard as our noblest sentiments of social behavior may derive from ancient times when these actions were absolute requisites for basic survival. Forms of altruism, such as sacrificing one's life for the sake of the family or group, may be programmed into us by natural selection because they favor the representation of those genes in future generations. Science, he contends, is now in a position to approach the "very origin and meaning of human values, from which all ethical pronouncements and much of political practice flow. Only by interpreting the activity of the emotive centers as a biological adaptation can the meaning of our canons of morality be deciphered. Since philosophers have not traditionally explored this problem, it is time for ethics to be removed temporarily from the hands of the philosophers and biologicized."[26]

With a fuller understanding of the human brain, according to this view, we may arrive at new levels of disenchantment with ourselves.

> In completing the Darwinian revolution we are likely to see some of our most exalted feelings explained in terms of traits which evolved. Human beings see themselves in transcendental terms. But we may find out that this is an overestimate of the nature of our deepest yearnings. We tend to be very respectful of these emotions, as we should be, because they are very human qualities, but we may discover that they have very humble origins.[27]

Wilson is not without his detractors. He has been attacked especially on the claim of biological determinism, that is, saying that behavior is genetically preprogrammed. Although it will not serve our purposes to investigate this charge (see, for example, *New York Review of Books*, Nov. 13, 1975, or "Sociobiology— Another Biological Determinism," *Bioscience* 26:3), the other side of the coin submits that there is no direct scientific evidence to suppose that any of human social behavior is determined by the genes. Human social behavior being entirely learned is infinitely malleable. Critiques see Wilson's thesis as part of the historic debate concealing a reactionary political message: The contention that present human social arrangements are either unchangeable or, if altered, will demand conscious social regulation because changed conditions will be "unnatural" alarms many.

Returning to the subject at hand, George Pugh, principal scientist at General Research Corporation, McLean, Virginia, has developed a theme somewhat analogous to Wilson's in his book *On the Origins of Human Values* (Basic Books). He starts with the proposition that the human brain is a "value-driven decision system" with evolution playing the part of system designer. He distinguishes two kinds of values: primary and secondary values. The primary values provide the system with its ultimate criteria for evaluating decisions and are built into the hardware of the brain itself. Hence, the primary values are innate or instinctive. They cannot be deduced by rational thought. Manifestations of our primary values are our subjective sensations such as the unpleasantness of pain and hunger, the pleasant taste of good food, or the pleasure of a sexual encounter. These innate primary values are reflected in both the emotions and the traditional biological drives. Being built into the modern brain, they are almost exactly as they evolved during our primitive prehuman past. These are so much a part of our reality that we seldom perceive them as values.

Human beings also make use of secondary values. Whereas pain and hunger are the manifestations of primary values, our moral, ethical, and social principles are examples of secondary values. These are the products of personal and cultural experiences with the physical environment and with the primary human values. They are the products of rational thought.

Actual human behavior is affected by both sets of values with secondary values normally reflecting the primary values. For example, the hunger sensation is an innate response to an environmental deficiency, a sensation demanding satisfaction, while the wherewithal for appeasing this sensation reflects secondary values. Thus, we may work to obtain the deficient commodity, we may cooperate with others to obtain it, or we may even steal if that be our value. In this model, the behavior that is manifested is the product of both the primary value system and the mental perception of the world environment. Personal and social experiences with that environment condition the perception. According to Pugh, this perspective on decision-making may provide a method for scientifically understanding and evaluating our social and ethical values.[28]

The Pugh model of the origin of human values is highly reminiscent of the newly proposed concept of structural ethics. Structuralism admits to the possibility of innate knowledge not derived from direct experience. The mind constructs reality from experience by the use of innate perceptions. Behavior is generated from the functioning mind. The innate perceptions are designated as deep structures and are inaccessible to direct observation. Mental deep structures, like Pugh's primary values, provide us with the ultimate criteria for evaluating decisions. Structuralism starts from the premise that certain human conceptions which we regard as the finest human sentiments are universal; all nonpathological members of the species are believed to possess them; they are inborn, being part of the a priori knowledge all human beings possess; and they are not arbitrary. Examples of mental deep structures might be the concept of the objective good, or the intrinsic value of human life, or the obligation we feel to obey moral principles. Theologians, ethicists, moral philosophers, and prophets have through the ages tried to define empirical truths such as these or to understand the human motivations for honoring them. Structuralism would submit that they are not explainable; they are unanalyzable. It is not possible to validate these universal propositions by any rational process or direct observation in the manner in which other theories can be validated. They constitute one of humankind's "givens."

Structuralism may provide some illumination into the meta-ethical question of how morals are possible at all. Covert or hidden deep structures motivate overt behavior, called surface structures, through a process of transformation. In transformation, the abstract ethical deep structure gives rise to the concrete moral code of the surface structure. The premise of structural ethics is that moral judgments arise by transformational operations on subconscious mental deep structures. Differences in extant moral codes are attributable to the particular way individuals or societies carry out the deep-to-surface transformational processes. Thus, according to structuralist concepts, moral systems all share certain fundamental commonalities rooted in the universal deep structures—a quality of the species, not of individuals or culture—for example, the Golden Rule.

Guenther Stent, a molecular biologist lately turned philosopher, at the University of California, Berkeley, provides a biological basis for understanding deep structures. Again, by postulating the phylogenetic development of the brain through evolutionary history, it can be argued that individuals can know something of the world innately, without the independent acquisition of any personal experiences with it. Knowledge could be passed between generations through genes that determine the organization and function of the nervous system. The genetic specifications for the construction of a particular kind of brain came into being through the process of natural selection operating on our remote ancestors. Although there may be no specific genes for meanings and values, the human genetic endowment codes these virtues as deep structures in the architecture of the brain. The refinement of these instructions may have been guided by the creature responses to adaptations necessary for successful living in stages of an evolutionary past. From the vantage point of evolution it is not difficult to conjecture that the basic pattern for a social-organizational lifestyle could be articulated and transmitted by the structuring of the human brain in a certain way and reaching ever higher levels of attainment with succeeding generations. In other words, the *a priori* knowledge or deep structure on which moral behavior is predicated is fully compatible with present mainstream evolutionary thought.[29]

Recently, a controversial new paradigm was introduced into the literature under the title of genetic self-interest.[30] Whereas in the earlier models, reference was made to the genes for altruism, the new idea speaks about "selfish genes." Richard Dawkins in his book *The Selfish Gene* examines the proposal that the predominant quality of any successful gene is "ruthless selfishness."[31] And this must be so according to a number of modern evolutionary biologists since, in their opinion, pure altruistic behavior is self-limiting. The argument goes as follows: A self-sacrificing altruistic trait benefits the whole group, including those who lack it. Individuals with the trait, however, lose more than they gain if self-sacrifice results, since their genes are not as likely to be passed on to succeeding generations. For those lacking the trait, the benefits are enjoyed without the costs. These will experience a net gain in procreational opportunities and the proportion of altruistic genes must be diminished in subsequent generations. There is, therefore, no way for pure altruism to pass the test of natural selection if strictly biological mechanisms are to be employed. "Good guys," as a well-known baseball manager once said, "always finish last."

But there is a way out. If the cost of participation returns a greater gain to the cooperator than what is invested, barring an occasional fatality, then it may be advantageous to be a joiner. If animals live together in groups, they must get more benefits out of the association than they put in. Most aspects of animal sociality—including human culture—are beneficial to the cooperating individual. To the casual observer, the selfishness being selected *appears* to be altruistic behavior for it includes many of the traits that we normally think require some self-sacrifice. For example, warning cries of birds probably have a net advantage for the bird sounding the alarm in spite of the increased risks to it of predator attack. Dawkins provides several possible explanations. One he calls the "never break ranks" theory. One starts with the assumption that there must be important advantages in flocking behavior in birds; otherwise they would not use this behavior. The individual bird who leaves the flock ahead of the others will forfeit some or all of that advantage. If it must not break ranks, what is the bird who first observes a dangerous intruder to do? If it does nothing and carries on normal activity, relying on the protection of flock membership, it, along with the others, is vulnerable to attack. If it would simply fly off by itself without warning the other members, it no longer has the protection of the flock. The best policy is to fly off but to make sure first that everybody else does too. The uttering of a warning call is thus seen to have a purely selfish advantage. That which formerly was interpreted as a self-sacrificing altruism is really a behavior designed for doing whatever is best to keep alive.

Explanations based on selfishness have provided another interpretation of altruism—the concept of reciprocal altruism. As the term implies, the participant in this strategy performs altruistic acts only insofar as he expects something in return. Mutual grooming behavior is a very common example of reciprocal altruism found in both birds and mammals.

Dawkins suggests that reciprocal altruism probably played an important part in human evolution, since a long memory and the capacity for individual recognition are well developed in our species. "Doing unto others as you would have them do unto you" means that someday I may need you to return a favor done earlier. It is best that I build up a supply of credits in advance so that my future is protected. Robert Trivers, an ethologist, acknowledges that many of our psychological characteristics—envy, greed, gratitude, sympathy, and the like—have been shaped by reciprocal altruism. He argues that humans alone have the conscious foresight whereby, through advanced planning, they can assure their own personal future interests. This can be done by entering into pacts or conspiracies with others; but every individual bargains so that the terms of the agreement are to his/her advantage. One's best interests are served by obeying the rules of the pact.

The evolutionary objective of the selfish gene is to survive. Whereas the lifespan of a chromosome is one generation, a gene is nearly immortal if it can form enough copies of itself and distribute them in successive individuals. In this model, the gene becomes the basic unit of selfishness and it will do what it can to maximize its own survival, including future survival. One strategy is to build an organism—a survival machine—whose behavior the genes can control and thereby optimize their own longevity. The best behavior in this strategy is to program the body in such a way as to insure its survival, and in doing so protect the genes, and to also reproduce large numbers of itself. Therefore, do whatever is best to keep alive and propagate yourself. Indeed, the control of the survival machine by the genes is indirect, but it may still be very powerful.

A second maneuver might be to assist replicas of one's genes situated in other bodies. If one survival machine assists another that has a related genetic copy, then the first genome, in effect, is promoting its own longevity. The earlier described kinship selection would set the rules for this behavior. Cooperative behavior is directly proportional to relatedness. Again, the behavior that is seen here appears as individual altruism, but it would be brought about by gene selfishness.

The third strategy of reciprocal altruism could account for altruistic behavior toward unrelated individuals. Gene survival and group cooperation are intimately linked in social organisms. The literature of ethology provides numerous examples of this symbiosis.

In the case of human evolution, a new kind of survival machine was created: an organism which can escape the tyranny of selfish genes. The ability of the human brain to ponder the future has given rise to culture, and through the workings of culture, emancipation from the dictates of individual selfishness has been realized. However, Dawkins warns that since individual genetic self-interest still exists, altruism must be taught. Altruism is possible, but only culturally acquired altruism. It is not in the genes. But the old evolution, based on genes, by making brains has provided the wherewithal to see through the designs of selfish genes. Memes, the complex thoughts and ideas of the brain in action, propagate themselves in the cultural environment. But leaping from brain to brain, memes can be duplicated millions of times, changing in a very short time individual persons and whole societies the world over. In his closing words, Dawkins leaves with us this qualified optimism:

> We are built as gene machines and cultured as meme machines, but we have the power to turn against our creators. We, alone on earth, can rebel against the tyranny of the selfish replicators.[32]

Over and over again, these discussions have pointed to the essential role of the brain as a value-driven decision system. R. W. Sperry, professor of psychobiology at the California Institute of Technology and one of the leading scientists in the field of brain research, is a vigorous advocate of a scientific approach to the problem of human values in which the brain plays a crucial role. He, like so many others, recognizes that human values originate in the basic design of that brain. He contends that when human values were recognized as an essential part of nature's design for the brain, they became a subject for scientific study. Sperry states his case with these words:

> I tend to rate the problems of human values Number One for science in the 1970's, above the more concrete crisis problems like poverty, population, energy, or pollution on the following grounds: First, all these crisis conditions are man-made and very largely products of human values. Further, they are not correctable on any long-term basis without first changing the underlying human value priorities involved. And finally, the more strategic way to remedy these conditions is to go after the social value priorities directly in advance, rather than waiting for the value changes to be forced by changing conditions. Otherwise we are doomed from here on to live always on the margins of intolerability, for it is not until things get rather intolerable that the voting majority gets around to changing its established values. It is apparent, further, that other approaches in our crisis problems already receive plenty of attention. It is the human value factor that has been selectively neglected and even considered, in principle, to be "off limits" to science.[33]

The central question of providing an adequate explanation of how human evolution overcame the prohibition of cooperation over competition was approached in still another way. To repeat an earlier premise, it is generally accepted that biogenetic evolution by itself cannot produce self-sacrificing behavior that benefits other individuals who are in genetic competition (nonkinfolk). Except for close kin, each individual is competing genetically with others within the society. How, then, was the genetic competitor changed into a social cooperator?

Donald T. Campbell, in his presidential address to the American Psychological Association in 1975, finds this resource in religion.[34] If the stability and complexity of society requires a certain amount of altruistic, self-sacrificing behavior, the extinction of these virtues, as would be the case if genetic factors alone were involved, will gradually lead to the collapse of society; that is, unless social evolution retains some other mechanism than enlightened self-interest for the enculturation of values. According to Campbell, religions have evolved to transmit those values and motivations in their adhering populations considered necessary to suppress the usual consequences of genetic competition. He makes the following argument: (1) complex societies of the past independently but regularly evolved inhibitory moral traditions, in other words, religion; (2) the moral norms of these traditions and transcendent beliefs systems were remarkably similar to one another; (3) the moral norms probably possessed adaptive functions, particularly the curbing of some aspects of human nature in order to achieve complex social coordination and promote collective purpose.[35] In Campbell's words, "committing oneself to living for a transcendent good purpose, not one's own, is a commitment to optimize the social system rather than the individual system."[36] Inhibitory moral traditions act to set limits upon individual selfish tendencies. The traditional list of sins— including selfishness, stinginess, greed, gluttony, cowardice, envy, theft, lust, rage, anger, dishonesty, blasphemy, and promiscuity—all related to biological optimization of self and children, are kept in check by religious ethical codes with their heavy emphasis on societal altruism. These highly idealistic, abstract, inhibitory codes can more easily maintain direct interactional overseeing of large and complex urban societies than face-to-face methods of personal admonition, such as scolding or gossip, typical of simple social groups. Burhoe insists that we cannot do without the religious prophets and priests as the perceivers of sin and evil.[37] The whole system for social and ethical motivation of individual persons requires that there be a set of communal requirements that serve as the central value for societal organisms. Religious beliefs prompting a person to optimize social behavior, including compensatory rewards for deprivations in this life, would promote social-system functioning. Social groups effectively indoctrinating such individual altruistic commitment might well possess a social-evolutionary advantage and in doing so they might discover a functional, adaptive truth. Lacking the purely genetic supports for altruistic behavior, ethical systems, especially codes that encourage strong altruism, were invented. Mutual benefits, accruing to both the individual and the larger social group, spur its evolution onward.

The power of religion to motivate behavior comes from its intimate association with our most basic genetic nature: ritual communication encoded in the reptilian brain. Intraspecies signaling and adaptive display evolved at first in order to signal forms of behavior, for example, reproductive display. This communication was mediated by the reptilian brain. Birds and mammals carry this a step further by adding cultural transmission to cultural patterns. An example might be the imitation of a territorial bird song learned from other members of the species. The phylogenetic sequence continues in humans with the inclusion of further embellishments to the rituals and oral myths tied to these rituals by our human ancestors who by that time had a brain which bestowed the capacity of linguistic communication. Consciously created logical explanations of the myths-theologies arose only in the past few thousand years, after the emergence of writing and extensive refinement of linguistic symbols. Note again that the brain functions as the coordinating center. Religion, then, is an almost inevitable result of the way the brain has developed.[38]

Hence religions have evolved, promising long-term salvation of the soul beyond the death of the body to those who would cooperate. Religion in the form of rituals, myths, and theologies became the memes in the evolution of the human culture type. Presumably such belief systems have evolved independently and many times. Belief in the afterlife as the reward of the cooperator, for instance, is reflected in the burial customs of antiquity the world over. Neanderthalian graves reveal the care and concern accorded this part of the belief system. What seems to be a deliberate waste of useful tools and other adornments buried with the corpse is outweighed by the social gains, namely, the optimization of the social system.

Examination of the anthropological data indicates that all sociocultural systems possessed inhibitory moral codes and transcendent belief systems. In general, they all function to control and coordinate behavior in a cultural setting. Moral norms, oughts and ought nots, act to set the limits upon individual selfish tendencies in all sociocultural systems. The implicit assumption of sharedness is the mainspring which propels the refinement of moral norms in the culture type.[39]

In this model, religion from early times gave correct recognition to the true nature of man—carnal and guilty of the "original sin" of self-centeredness. The evolutionary scientific view of man concurs with this conclusion: His covert desires and overt behaviors are motivated by genetic self-interest. In whatever perspective we consider him, inhibitory moral codes are necessary as a means of checking these egoistic tendencies. It seems clear, then, that in order to remain and prosper, humans themselves must consciously elect to cooperate actively in creative evolution.

The Jesuit Father Pierre Teilhard de Chardin, as a paleontologist, attempted a synthesis of the main features of the Darwinian view of man and Christian theology. Building on the model that evolution is a continuum of "progressive transcendencies," he considered human life as a part of the evolution of the universe moving in the direction of greater and greater levels of refinement.

He perceived the planet as a series of successive layers or envelopes. The lithosphere is the solid part of the globe and contains on its surface the hydrosphere and atmosphere, portions of which combined together constitute the biosphere. Life, arising and evolving in the biosphere, becomes aware of itself with the formation of man. A further and yet unfilled step projects a growth in awareness through "association with other men" finally to achieve the megasynthesis: in the noosphere, or thinking envelope (Fig. 1.5). This process, which he terms planetization, is the mark of supreme progress. The planetization of humankind in his view is made inevitable by the swiftly increasing facility of communication as well as by increasing knowledge. Teilhard makes love the main agent in evolution, and it is through love that one ultimately achieves transcendence and self-fulfillment. The eventual consumma-

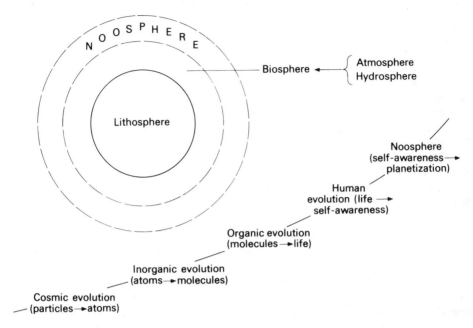

Fig. 1.5 *The Teilhardian view of progressive transcendencies.*

tion of all evolution in the megasynthesis as envisioned by him is the convergence in the Omega (Jesus Christ), the "spiritual renovation of the earth." The point he stresses again and again is that humans are not to be passive witnesses but, rather, active participants in this unfolding process.

Teilhard's position that unselfish love has its origin in our evolutionary past where it served important biological and psychological functions can be supported by the symbiosis model of social development. Although the behavior per se is not programmed by any gene pool, the kind of harmony in a world community Teilhard would have is accessible through conscious activity of the human brain.

It is interesting to note that an everincreasing body of evidence procured from a variety of sciences demonstrates the revitalizing and enobling power of unselfish love. For example, studies have shown that love is a factor which seems to increase the duration of life; that a minimum of love is absolutely necessary for survival of newborn babies and for their healthy growth; and that love has the power to mitigate interhuman hatred and eliminate interhuman strife. What future studies of human behavior may find difficult to explain is why we so long ignored love as a basis for human behavior, concentrating instead on hunger, thirst, and similar physiological drives. What appears demonstrated here is a tremendous force for human cohesion capable of finding application at every level of interaction from the personal to the international. This force, so universal in its demonstration, could well have arisen as a means to promote the welfare and survival of our species. A new and nobler social order can be ours if this power of creative unselfish love can be effectively tapped.[40]

The evolutionary image projects a dual image of man: one operating by natural selection acting on genes to maximize the individual, and the second, escaping the direct control of natural selection, to optimize sociality. Understanding of the mechanisms for sociocultural evolution are still at a primitive level but it seems reasonable to conjecture that the development did progress through various levels of refinement, passing from the simple to the complex. It might, therefore, be instructive at this point to investigate whether individual moral orientation can change over time; if so, this might suggest a crude approximation of the evolution of moral behavior toward higher levels of attainment. Comparative studies of this kind, in which modern living forms are studied in an effort to gain understanding of evolutionary events, is a strategy frequently used in science. Some common examples are comparative anatomy or comparative behavior. The approach derives its validity from the recapitulation hypothesis which asserts that much of what is observed in the present has evolutionary antecedents in less highly evolved organisms or in the ontogony (that is, the life history) of the same organism.

Dwight Boyd and Lawrence Kohlberg, social psychologists at the Harvard University Laboratory of Human Development, investigated the development of moral behavior in humans. They exposed experimental subjects to situations designed to induce moral conflict and require moral deliberations for resolution. Their study found that, in spite of significant age differences between the subjects tested, as well as socioeconomic level or ethnic background, a common set of moral categories were observed. Further, the moral orientation of individuals passed through a series of stages or levels roughly correlated with age. With developing maturity, a higher moral stage was demonstrated. The Boyd/Kohlberg stages of moral orientation are given:

I. Premoral Level

At this level the individual is responsive to cultural rules and labels of good and bad, right and wrong, but interprets these labels in terms of either the physical or the hedonistic consequences of action—e.g., punishment, reward, exchange of favors—or in terms of the physical power of those who enunciate the rules and labels. This is generally the level of the young child. The level is divided into the following two stages:

Stage 1. The Punishment and Obedience Orientation. The physical consequences of action determine its goodness or badness regardless of the human meaning or value of these consequences. Avoidance of punishment and unquestioning deference to power are valued in their own right, not in terms of respect for the underlying moral order supported by punishment and authority.

Stage 2. The Instrumental-Relativist Orientation. Right action consists of that which instrumentally satisfies one's own needs and occasionally the needs of others. Human relations are viewed in terms like those of the marketplace. Elements of fairness, of reciprocity, and of equal sharing are present, but they are always interpreted in a physical, pragmatic way. Reciprocity is a matter of "you scratch my back and I'll scratch yours"; not of loyalty, gratitude, or justice.

II. Conventional Role-Conformity Level

At this level, maintaining the expectation of the individual's family, group, or nation is perceived as valuable in its own right, regardless of immediate and obvious consequences. The attitude is not only one of conformity to personal expectations and social order, but of loyalty to it, of actively maintaining, supporting, and justifying the order, and of identifying with the persons or groups involved in it. At this level, there are the following two stages:

Stage 3. The Interpersonal Concordance of "Good Boy–Nice Girl" Orientation. Good behavior is that which pleases or helps others and is approved by them. There is much conformity to stereotypical images of what is the majority or "natural" behavior. Behavior is frequently judged by intention—"he means well" becomes important for the first time. One earns approval by being "nice."

Stage 4. The Law and Order Orientation. This orientation is toward authority, fixed rules, and the maintenance of the social order. Right behavior consists of doing one's duty, showing respect for authority, and maintaining the given social order for its own sake; "my country, right or wrong."

III. Postconventional or Principled Level

At this level, there is a clear effort to define moral values and principles which have validity and application apart from the authority of the groups or persons holding these principles, and apart from the individual's own identification with these groups. This level has two stages.

Stage 5. The Social Contract Legalistic Orientation. Right action tends to be defined in terms of general individual rights and standards which have been critically examined and agreed upon by the whole society. There is a clear awareness of the relativism of personal values and opinions and a corresponding emphasis upon procedural rules for reaching consensus. Aside from what is constitutionally and democratically agreed upon, the right is a matter of personal "values" and "opinions." The result is an emphasis upon the "legal point of view" but with an emphasis upon the possibility of changing law in terms of rational considerations of social utility rather than freezing it as in Stage 4 where "law and order" are uppermost. Outside the legal realm, free agreement and contract are the binding elements of obligation. This is the "official" morality of the American government and Constitution.

Stage 6. The Universal Ethical Principle Orientation. Right is defined by the decision of conscience in accord with self-chosen ethical principles appealing to logical comprehensiveness, universality, and consistency. These principles are abstract and ethical (e.g., the Golden Rule); they are not concrete moral rules like the Ten Commandments. Essentially, these are the universal principles of justice, of humane reciprocity, of equality, and of respect for the dignity of human beings as individual persons.[41]

This scheme assesses moral development as a sequence of stages in which the individual moves from the egocentric self to a more generalized moral-consciousness world view. Boyd and Kohlberg emphasize that the sequence is not invariant among individuals; the order listed is not necessarily the order followed in every case. It is perhaps even a dangerous thing to assert that one is better than the other. It is apparent that many otherwise mature individuals function at surprisingly unsophisticated levels of moral reasoning. It would thus seem that all people do not pass invariably through all six stages; nor must all six stages be passed through in the sequence described. Some persons or whole societies might be permanently stalled at one of the lower levels. In fact, it may be an oversimplification of a very complex process. At the very least, what this model represents is that (1) moral orientation can change over time, and (2) the change is from an egocentric viewpoint toward one of increasing human concern based on values.

THE MEANING OF AN EVOLUTIONARY ETHIC

It is becoming increasingly clear that what humans choose to do will be the sole agent for future evolution on this planet. Here we reach what appears to be the most significant aspect of this study of evolution and ethics, namely, that it is open-ended with creative possibilities for the future. By making our thinking evolution-oriented, we can plan with assurance that our long evolutionary rise has made possible our present spectacular but precarious success; the evolutionary imperative can give us hope by pointing to the time that lies ahead of our species if we do not destroy ourselves or damage our own chances; the evolutionary model can remind us of the vast store of human potentialities—of intelligence, imagination, and cooperative good will—which still remain to be developed to even greater levels of fulfillment; and above all, our evolutionary rise as a social organism teaches us that progress and survival in the evolutionary sense mean progress and survival at the community level. All of humankind—black, white, oriental, Frenchman, American, Indian, New Caledonian, Vietnamese, Congolese, Biafran—we together comprise that community and as the community goes, so goes the individual.

On a more practical side, the formidable challenge in selecting ethical codes to guide our future comes down to the question: To what extent should the motivators in the emotive centers of the brain be obeyed? Given that these controls affect our moral decisions, how faithfully must they be consulted? The answer to this question still evades us for to begin with, although the suspicion is well founded that these innate motivators do influence our moral decisions, their exact definition has not yet been assayed. But, we cannot follow them blindly. At some time in the future it will be necessary for us to decide where we would like the human condition to be. This will require that we consciously pick and choose from among the emotional guides we have inherited and the axioms which have come down to us. If the function of ethics is to promote human evolution, then the resolution of specific moral problems must be done in ways that maximize the survival of the human community while at the same time insuring that the individual is not eliminated. In doing so, the two sides of our nature can be accommodated—the socially cooperative and self-denying side required of all social organisms, and the biological side which insists on calling attention to our own individual existence and promotion of self-interests.

Growing out of this dual image of human nature comes a pair of complementary ethics—the one emphasizing the oneness of the human community and the other placing the highest value on the development of selfhood. The two ethics are complementary, not contradictory. Together they encourage both cooperation and wholesome competition, both love and individuality. Each serves to check the excesses and misapplications of the other.[42]

Human nature itself, then, can provide the starting place for deriving values in roughly the following way:

1 Whatever is necessary to meet the needs of human survival becomes of value.

2 Whatever is necessary to meet the psychological needs for individual human fulfillment becomes of value.

The first goes beyond just sheer physical survival of individuals but includes love and concern for others within the community of other persons. We became human through interactions with other humans; we retain our humanity in the same way. On the second, clearly we do not have agreement as to what is required to promote individual human fulfillment. Here we are addressing the questions of the quality of life. As a tentative beginning, one could submit that it is inherent to strive for happiness and productivity. These may be only two manifestations of a single drive—to preserve and enhance self, made up of the physical body and the psychological potential. These are the identifying features of what humanistic psychology refers to as the self-actualizing person—the person who has a positive self-image and one who accepts others.

To return to an earlier assertion, there may be at least two basic values which transcend time and culture. The first of these is respect for the individual. In its ultimate form it is respect for human life, including a concern for others, a caring and compassion. In its broader form it is taken to mean respect for the human person. Aspects of this respect include the rights of the individual, freedom of choice, and freedom to act within the context of the rights of others.

The second value is a basic honesty in human relations. As we have said, all ethical systems include a condemnation of deception, dishonesty, and trickery. If there were not a minimal level of honesty in a society, a basic trust in others, the social order would collapse.[43]

These values may not simply be the product of preferences or of utterances of religious leaders or philosophers. They could be the products of humans living together in society. Without the observance of these values, or at least some minimum implementation of them, society could not survive. A society which chooses to frustrate them annihilates itself.

If society collectively could agree on the nature of human nature and, in collaboration with the sciences and the humanities, decide how human we wish to be, at least two important goals would be realized:

1   We could have a set of values which would be anchored in the biological and cultural nature of the species;

2   These could function as criteria against which we could measure desirability or acceptability of human behavior toward other humans.

In terms of our present concerns, specific moral problems will be resolved in such ways as to minimize human suffering and maximize those human values that will enhance the survival of the human community, the quality of life for the whole society, and the enhancement of human potential for each individual. The pertinent question in this process is not "should we play God," but "how should we play Human?"

A FINAL WORD

The relationship of science to human values has been shown to be a very complex one. From one point of view at least, values are outside of science, but science can provide us with some leads as to their origins and meanings. Our understanding of the relationships is very primitive indeed, and the data available in support of an evolutionary hypothesis of ethical behavior is highly conjectural. We have made just the barest of beginnings in this study.

This chapter exposed the reader to a great deal of current thinking in the matter of values as they relate to genes and culture. Much more could have been included. The literature is vast and growing steadily. The treatment here has not done justice to the ideas introduced; much of the supporting analysis and data necessarily are omitted. Rigorous documentation would be too laborious. The objective of this text is to expose issues for study and discussion—not to analyze or validate them. The interested reader is encouraged to study the references if clarification is desired. I hope I have convinced you that there are important matters here. Scientific reasons exist for believing that there is profound wisdom that went into the social system we presently have and that, when understood more exactly, can be employed in the ongoing process of building a "better society."

REFERENCES

1 Pierre Teilhard de Chardin, *The Phenomenon of Man* (New York: Cathedral Press, Harper & Row, 1959) quoted in Dobzhansky, "Ethics and values in biological and cultural evolution," *Zygon* 8 (1973): 262.

2 Daniel Callahan, "Normative ethics and public morality in the life sciences," *The Humanist* 32, 5 (1972): 5-7.

3 Daniel Callahan, "Living with the new biology," *The Center Magazine* 5, 4 (1972): 4-12.

4 Ervin Lazlo, "The purpose of mankind," *Zygon* 8, 3-4 (1973): 310-324.

5 James Drane, quoted in James E. Trosko, "Philosophical basis for moral decisions in modern technological culture," *Science, Technology, Public Policy and Society News*, 30 (October 1975): 1.

6 Daniel Callahan, "Science and ethics" in E. Gingerich (ed.), *The Nature of Scientific Discovery* (Smithsonian Press, 1975), p. 441.

7 Daniel Callahan (in Reference 6), p. 442.

8 Nicholas Wade, "Sociobiology: Troubled birth for new discipline," *Science* 191 (March 19, 1976): 1153.

9 Charles Fay, "Ethical naturalism and biocultural evolution," *Zygon* 9, 4 (1969): 24-32.

10 Julian Huxley, quoted in Theodosius Dobzhansky, "Ethics and values in biological and cultural evolution," *Zygon* 8, 3-4 (1973): 262.

11 Karl Popper, cited in J. C. Eccles, "Cultural evolution vs. biological evolution," *Zygon* 8 (1973): 283.

12 Robert Boyd and Peter J. Richerson, "A simple dual inheritance model of the conflict between social and biological evolution," *Zygon* 11, 3 (1976): 258.

13 Ralph Wendell Burhoe, "The source of civilization in the natural selection of coadapted information in genes and culture," *Zygon* 11, 3 (1976): 281.

14 Ralph Wendell Burhoe (in Reference 13), p. 287.

15 John Kendrew quoted in Burhoe (Reference 13), p. 290.

16 Paul D. MacLean, "Our cerebral heritage," *Mosaic* (March/April 1976): 3-10.

17 George Gaylord Simpson, *The Meaning of Evolution* (New York: New American Library, Mentor Books, 1951), pp. 153-156.

18 C. H. Waddington, *The Ethical Animal* (Chicago and London: University of Chicago Press, 1967), p. 26.

19 George Gaylord Simpson quoted in Dobzhansky (Reference 10), p. 265.

20   Theodosius Dobzhansky (Reference 10), p. 271.
21   Roderick Nash, "Can government meet environmental needs?" *Transactions of the 36th North American Wildlife and Natural Resources Conference* (Washington, D.C., National Wildlife Management Institute, 1971).
22   Theodosius Dobzhansky (Reference 10), p. 271.
23   E. O. Wilson, *Sociobiology: The New Synthesis* (Cambridge: Howard University Press, 1975).
24   E. O. Wilson, "Sociobiology—another biological determinism," *Bioscience* **26**, 3 (1976): 182, 187–190.
25   Nicholas Wade (Reference 8), p. 1152.
26   E. O. Wilson, "Academic vigilantism and the political significance of sociobiology," *Bioscience* **26**, 3 (1976): 183–186.
27   Nicholas Wade (Reference 8), p. 1153.
28   George Edgin Pugh, "Human values, free will, and the conscious mind," *Zygon* **11**, 1 (1976): 2–24.
29   Guenther S. Stent, "The promise of structural ethics," *The Hastings Center Report* **6**, 6 (1976): 32–40.
30   Scott Morris, "The new science of genetic self-interest," *Psychology Today* (February 1977): 42–51, 84–88.
31   Richard Dawkins, *The Selfish Gene* (New York and Oxford: Oxford University Press, 1976).
32   Richard Dawkins (in Reference 31), see especially Chapters 2 and 3.
33   R. W. Sperry quoted in Pugh (Reference 28), p. 6.
34   Donald T. Campbell, "On the conflicts between biological and social evolution and between psychology and moral tradition," *Zygon* **11** (1976): 167–208.
35   Robert L. Munroe and Ruth H. Munroe, "Altruistic ethics," *Zygon* **11**, 3 (1976): 212.
36   Donald T. Campbell (Reference 34), p. 192.
37   Ralph Wendell Burhoe (Reference 13), p. 292.
38   Ralph Wendell Burhoe (Reference 13), p. 295.
39   Robert L. and Ruth H. Munroe (Reference 35), p. 212.
40   Pitirim A. Sorokin, "The powers of creative unselfish love," in Abraham H. Maslow (ed.), *New Knowledge in Human Values* (New York: Harper & Row, 1959).
41   Dwight Boyd and Lawrence Kohlberg, "The is-ought problem: a development perspective," *Zygon* **8**, 3–4 (1973): 363–364. Used with permission of the University of Chicago Press.
42   Willis W. Harman, "The coming transformation," *The Futurist* **11**:2 (1977).
43   C. H. Patterson, "Humanistic concerns and behavior modification," paper presented at a conference on "Moral and Ethic Implications of Behavior Modification," University of Wisconsin, Madison, March 20–21, 1975.

BIBLIOGRAPHY

Bronowski, Jacob, *Science and Human Values* (New York, Evanston, Harper & Row, Perennial Library, 1965).
Bronowski, Jacob, *The Ascent of Man* (Boston and Toronto: Little, Brown, 1973).
Dubos, René, *So Human an Animal* (New York: Scribner's, 1968).
Dubos, René, *A God Within* (New York: Scribner's, 1972).
Hardin, Garrett, *Nature and Man's Fate* (New York: Mentor, 1959).

Lancaster, Jane B., "Carrying and sharing in human evolution," *Human Nature* (February 1978): 82–90.

Matson, Floyd W., *The Idea of Man* (New York: Delacorte Press, 1976).

Otto, Max, *Science and the Moral Life* (New York: Mentor, 1949).

Rensch, Bernard, *Biophilosophy,* (New York and London: Columbia University Press, 1971).

Simpson, George Gaylord, *This View of Life* (New York: Harcourt, Brace, 1964).

2

ETHICAL
DECISION-MAKING

THE PROBLEM OF ETHICAL UNCERTAINTY

We began this discussion by noting that at the moment there does not exist an ethical perspective for dealing with the profusion of issues thrust upon us by the recent advances in the biological and medical sciences. In instance after instance, modern Western society has been unable to implement the products of scientific and technological developments effectively. On a more serious level, it is even becoming difficult to judge whether a particular scientific or technological advance is good or bad. A recent example is the controversy surrounding recombinant DNA research (see Chapter 4, Should Genes be Tampered With?) An ever-widening gap is growing between the powers of science to change the human condition and the prescriptions needed to apply the new powers wisely. The two-sided problem of how to live the good life without destroying it or greatly reducing its quality can easily lead to a kind of social paralysis where things are randomly allowed to happen. Whether our social structure can withstand the strain of haphazard application when fundamental values are meddled with is very much at issue. The current abortion issue bears testimony to the discrepancy between what is being done and what ought to be done. Our society lacks a moral consensus from which we may draw.

Depending on experts—whether they be physicians, scientists, moralists, or theologians—is no solution either. As subsequent discussions will show, ethical orientation between and among individuals varies over a wide range. The Karen Quinlan case is a concrete and tragic instance of conflict between what properly constituted the best interests of the patient. Even within the context of a single religion (e.g., Christianity), directives are sufficiently vague as to be subject to quite different interpretations.

Settling ethical issues by flipping coins is less than acceptable either. This approach admits to a kind of ethical pluralism whereby any choice is as good as any other and it is simply a matter of preference whether this or that value is selected. In the end, of course, all ethical views are up to the individual, but to allow a moral free-for-all is simply incompatible with a well-ordered society. When pressed to its limit, complete ethical freedom carries with it the potential of its own destruction. If there is any lesson at all in the earlier discussion of evolution, values, and culture, it is that a total concern for oneself is an unacceptable behavior.

Clearly, we are in need of an ethic that can clarify moral dilemmas and resolve conflicts. It should be clearly understood at the outset that a transition from the "is" to the "ought" cannot be made without inserting a value judgment independent of the fact—the "is." It would seem that we need to engage in ethical theorizing that is responsive to current needs. Whatever our role may be—concerned lay citizen, medical practitioner, scientific researcher, patient—we need some principles to help us resolve the perplexing ethical problems that are thrust upon us in this rapidly advancing technological society.

The thesis proposed here is this: Humans develop their ethics by the method of public discussion leading to public acceptance of what appears to be right and good and a rejection of that which is judged to be wrong or bad. Further, our conception of what is ethical, right, and good changes in the light of new knowledge and continuing debate. Using these tactics, societies can develop effective ways of sanctioning the uses of new knowledge and technology even when these uses initially conflict with existing societal or individual legal, moral, or religious codes.[1] The touchstone of ethical choices is the judgment of humans as to whether something is right and good.

In practice, these ethics can serve as standards for clarifying moral choices for individuals. The "what ought I to do" in a specific situation can be more easily and rationally decided if the issues have been thought through in advance. The present efforts in several states to legalize the Living Will is representative of the movement to present persons with live options before a crisis is encountered. Also, these ethics can assist directly in formulating public policy, often in the form of legislation. And, in this regard, the urgency of the search for a new ethic can be expressed no more poignantly than the words of Chief Justice Burger on the occasion of the public announcement of the Supreme Court's abortion decision of 1973:

> The law always lags behind the most advanced thinking in these areas. It must wait until the theologians and the moral leaders and events have created some common ground, some consensus.

In taking on the challenge of shaping public ethics, we must accept the fact that ethical decision-making is difficult at best. It has been described as the art of drawing sufficient conclusions from insufficient premises. Any ethical decision is a bet on the future. It is based on a prediction that some future world will come about if we take a certain action and that we will value that possible future world in a certain way. Since no one can operate from a position of perfect knowledge about the future, it is impossible to avoid some uncertainty whenever an ethical choice is made. It is simply beyond human capabilities to perceive all alternatives or all the consequences.

The decision-making process is further complicated by the observation that very few ethical problems present genuine choices of unquestionable good over unquestionable evil. More frequently than not, the choice is between good and good or evil and evil. It can be expected then that many issues requiring resolution are morally controversial. Mistakes are inevitable; there will be false starts and blind alleys. We must accept them. Overcoming obstacles will be required of generations to come but a beginning must be made now.

To begin with, ethics deals with the good, and ethical decisions are designed to promote the good. Ethics is a branch of the philosophic sciences. It is a branch of philosophy because it treats the ultimate principles governing right conduct. Accordingly, ethics asks and tries to answer problems about what is right or what ought to be done. Ethics is philosophy for the added reason that it bases its conclusions on reason alone. Whatever ethical position one assumes, it is supported by unaided reason, not by revelation. Since it is reason alone that determines an ethical position, there must be some mental process that one goes through in establishing an ethical position. Ethical decision-making, then, must follow some rather definitive rules or steps. We will refer to this procedure of decision-making as ethical methodology. A rough definition for ethical methodology is the reasoning procedure one goes through to arrive at a decision based on the weighing of different values. Like anything else, ethical decision-making can improve with practice if rational methodology rather than haphazard or intuitive approaches is used to arrive at judgments.

THE CONCEPT OF VALUE

The definition of ethical methodology introduced a new concept, the concept of value. A decision based on values implies a preference. The following are examples of values expressing a preference: All abortions are wrong; or abortion is an exercise of a fundamental right of women to the privacy of their own bodies. Values reveal personal viewpoints and interpretations which have an ethical connotation and express the preferences of the individual. Within the context of this definition, there cannot be any absolute values. However, all values are not equally valid. Ethical methodology is the procedure of evaluating discordant values to arrive at the best course of action in the face of conflicting choices. Stated in ethical terms, this is the *ought* behavior.

Characteristics of values are these:

1   They indicate what is judged to be "the good."
2   They imply preference.
3   They are supported by rational justification.
4   They countenance strong feelings or intense attitudes.
5   They specify a course of action.

In order to qualify as a value, all of these qualifications must be met. This requirement differentiates a value statement from purely technical statements. A very common type of the latter is an empirical statement. Empirical statements assert that a certain condition does or does not exist. By any or all of the five criteria given, an empirical statement does not qualify as a value. The same is true for command statements, for although these fit some of the criteria, they do not allow for preferences. The Ten Commandments are, therefore, not values in and of themselves but may express values if their statements are refined to allow for these qualifications.

We can make the following generalizations about ethical decisions:

1   Every decision involves human beings as the decision-makers and these persons must live with the consequences of the decision.
2   Most decisions involve choices between different outcomes and humans are likely to place different values on the different outcomes.

All decisions, therefore, involving biomedical issues are ethical decisions or have an ethical component associated with them in addition to a scientific or a clinical one. For example, taken literally the practice of medicine is an art, not a science, because inherent to its practice is decision-making linked to human values. It involves *both* facts and values. A number of ethical judgments must be handled along the way as the physician ministers to the needs of the patient.

Ethical versus moral

This brings up yet another distinction in ethics. The terms ethical and moral are frequently used, both within and without the literature, as interchangeable terms. To this point, this author has approximately equivocated the two. There is, however, a difference between them. Each connotes a different level of activity. Moral is the more fundamental level and identifies a way of being based upon rules—moral rules. The question, What *must* I do? characterizes moral behavior. There are few or no choices here. One need not go through any formal reasoning process to determine what is moral. The rules may take the form of revelation or they may be of secular origin. Ethical, on the other hand, is a way of doing. Ethical behavior is right conduct relating human acts to the attainment of the good. The question, What *ought* I to do? identifies ethical behavior. It carries with it choice as dictated by value preferences.

One can be moral without being ethical—the rules simply determine the conduct and no reasoning is required—but one cannot be ethical without also being moral.

Moral rules function as ethical guides, as for example, the Ten Commandments, ecclesiastical law, or some other ultimate or first principle. To some, these starting points may be absolute moral maxims—e.g. "Thou Shalt Not Kill." To others they may be relative, as, "it is permissible to kill in some instances." Much of the discussion of evolution and ethics centered on rules of secular-biologic origins—e.g., communal love. The relationship between ethics and morals is thus seen to be a reciprocal one—the moral rule judges the ethical behavior—and the two together should form a coherent system. The moral rules and the ethical behavior must be consistent with one another. (We will return to this point later in this chapter.)

Henry Aiken, an ethical philosopher, has developed a useful scheme for categorizing levels of moral activity, each of which involves a higher level of reasoning than the one preceding it.[2] Aiken's four levels of moral discourse illustrated by a sample statement on euthanasia are these:

Level	Example
Expressive level	I don't believe in euthanasia.
Level of moral rule	Euthanasia is murder.
Level of ethical principles	Killing the innocent under permissible conditions is conducive to killing the innocent under nonpermissible conditions.
Postethical level	The supreme value is life itself and every life has some worth. No human can presume to know who deserves to live or to die.

At the expressive level, gut feeling determines response to a value question. There is little or no reasoning involved; emotion guides the judgment. The levels of moral rules and ethical principles have previously been discussed. At the postethical level, we move out of ethics to a worldview where commitment to certain principles is universally practiced. An example of the postethical level is the Teilhardian Noosphere discussed in Chapter 1. Needless to say, the world community has not yet attained the postethical level of moral activity.

Most of one's daily decisions are on the first two levels. And this is acceptable providing there is no conflict. Society and individuals can comfortably operate on the expressive level or the level of moral rules if there is general agreement. For instance, most of us agree that public nudity is not allowable in a well-ordered society. There is little or no argument against legislating this behavior. When, however, accord is not forthcoming, then we move to the next level—the level of ethical reasoning—and it is precisely at this level that the issues in the life sciences are at. What should be the individual and societal responses to the matters of genetic engineering, abortion, euthanasia, behavior control, the delivery of medical care, and the like? Thus, although value decisions must be made repeatedly in our daily activities, it is not always necessary that ethical reasoning be used. But, the ethical person or the ethical society is prepared to use the process when decisions require formal justification.

Metaethics and normative ethics

Earlier it was mentioned that moral rules frequently are the bases for making ethical decisions. Moral rightness and moral wrongness lie at the heart of all ethical speculation for the great problem of ethics is what differentiates between the right act and the wrong act. This relationship is suggestive of yet another aspect of ethics, namely, that part which asks and tries to answer questions like the following: What is the meaning of the expressions "morally right" or "good"? How can ethical and value judgments be established or justified? What is the nature of morality? What is the distinction between the moral and the nonmoral? Why should I lead a moral life? Questions of this kind belong in that branch of ethics labeled metaethics and are concerned with epistemological, or semantic, or logical matters that are related to right conduct. The seemingly simple question, What is meant by "the good"? has eluded moral philosphers for centuries and to this day there is no general accord as to its meaning. The history of metaethical thought fills many volumes and a goodly amount of ethical study is concerned with these questions.

The second major branch of ethics is called normative ethics. Normative ethics deals with developing sets of principles that tell us what acts are right or wrong, good or bad, obligatory, permissible, or forbidden. Ideally, these general principles embody some core of values which provide the foundations for important decisions. Hence, normative ethics are guides for directing correct or ought behavior. To have a normative ethics is to be prepared to do something; the more developed the normative ethics, the more forceful and systematic will be the course of action. This is the kind of ethics required for making a proper response to the issues in the life sciences; consequently, it is the kind that will concern us in this study. For the most part, metaethics will not be part of our purview for much more work needs to be directed to that study than we can devote in the short space of this book. Recognize, however, at this juncture that one's normative theory cannot be entirely satisfied until metaethical questions are addressed. Metaethics validates normative principles. A bit more will be said concerning this at the conclusion of this chapter.

Posing ethical issues

One way of posing an ethical problem is the following:

1 Perceive that an ethical problem exists by stating it in plain language.
2 List all perceived alternative courses of action.
3 State values and consequences of all courses of action, both immediate and long-range.
4 Rank order the analyses of values in preferential scale from the most desirable to the least desirable.
5 Make a selection on the basis of the analysis.

The objective (and the usefulness) of this approach is first, to insist that a choice be made and second, to see that the choice is validated in ethical terms.

The recognition of an ethical problem is not always easy. To be effective, ethical methodology requires that the identification of the problem be as clear as possible in order to reduce uncertainty and ambiguity. To gain practice in specifying what the problem is, the student will find it helpful to write it out as a question. Posing the issue in question form is a convenient way to encourage problem analysis for several reasons: There is a clearly stated question that must be answered, and a series of steps should be followed leading to a resolution. We will label the statement of the ethical problem in the form of a question the *value object*—that object about which a value decision must be made. A value object may be a call for action requiring a value choice, it may be a person, or it may be a place or a thing. The term value object will not be found in the ethical literature; it is used here as a way to direct attention to the ethical problem under study. Giving it a special name emphasizes that it has a distinct role to play in ethical reasoning. Again, it should be written with great care to preclude any but a single interpretation.

The following is an example of a value object based on an authentic case study. The case study*:

Can convicts consent to castration?
Two California prisoners
seek freedom by their request.

In 1973, two forty-five-year-old men—Joseph A. Kenner and Paul R. de la Haye—both pleaded guilty to sex offenses involving minors. Having had prior histories of such behavior, both were committed to California's Atascadero State Mental Hospital. After two years of treatment, however, hospital officials reported that the two convicted child molesters had failed to respond to psychotherapy and had remained "dangerous to society" with little or no prospect of improvement. The men were released and returned to county jail to await sentencing.

---

*   Robert M. Veatch, "Case 536, Can Convicts, Consent to Castration?" Reprinted by permission from the *Hastings Center Report*, 5, 5 (1975): 17. © Institute of Society, Ethics and The Life Sciences, 360 Broadway, Hastings-on-Hudson, N.Y. 10706.

On grounds of the hospital's negative prognosis, the judge indicated in court that he would sentence the men to indeterminate terms, with a good likelihood that they would pass the remainder of their days within the confines of the prison walls. Given so bleak a life prospect, the two men signed requests for castration along with waivers releasing their lawyers, the court-approved surgeon, and the judge from any liability. The surgery, known as a bilateral orchidectomy (castration), was to constitute part of a rehabilitation program which might contribute to a possible grant of probation.

The judge delayed the sentencing pending further review. Such operations, formerly common practice under judicial orders in California, had generally been opposed by the courts since the American Civil Liberties Union brought suit five years previously against a San Diego judge and a surgeon involved in a similar "free will" operation.

The difficulties were compounded when Dr. Alan H. Walther, who had originally consented to perform the operation, withdrew his agreement after consultation with his medical colleagues, members of the San Diego County Urological Society and the Malpractice and Ethics Committee of the San Diego Medical Society. Perhaps the most persuasive argument was offered by the medical society officials who informed him that although the Society's group insurance covered him against any malpractice claims, he might still be liable—without insurance protection—to a lawsuit for mayhem or assault and battery, regardless of the waivers.

The *value object* in this case might be: Can convicts voluntarily consent to castration as a condition for parole from jail?

The next step in this procedure is a listing of all the possible courses of action. A common error here is to restrict the choices to as few as possible which usually means either–or. The human mind, it seems, prefers to minimize complexity by reducing the choices to manageable numbers. In the sample case study, the courses of action might be these:

The prisoners should be allowed the castration as a condition for parole from jail providing a physician can be found who will perform the surgery.

The prisoners should be allowed the castration as a condition for parole from jail, and the court should order a physician to perform the surgery, if necessary.

The prisoners should be allowed the castration only if they legally disclaim all future legal rights to bring malpractice suit against the attending physician and/or civil suit for damages against the judicial system.

The prisoners should not be allowed the castration as a condition for parole from jail, but continued efforts should be made to rehabilitate them.

The prisoners should not be allowed the castration, and their incarceration for an indefinite term should be continued without any further special efforts at rehabilitation.

After we have identified all the possible courses of action, the more difficult procedure of comparing one option with another is next. To do this, using ethical methodology, we must list all of the conceivable values that bear some relationship to the case. A caution here: The values should have direct application to the case under study. The obvious problem encountered here is to include all possible values to be considered. Again, as with identifying the value object, values are best indicated by writing them out as simple declarative sentences. Also, a comparison and ranking of values is facilitated if one statement incorporates only one value. Some examples of values in the case study are these [*Note:* this is not intended as a comprehensive catalogue, only as an example of value listing; the values listed are not in any priority order.]:

Individuals should have access to the therapies they voluntarily seek.

The relinquishing of some freedom (e.g., sexual behavior) to gain other freedoms is to be desired.

The prisoners were not capable of giving free and informed consent.

Castration is cruel and unusual punishment.

Castration infringes on the right to privacy as guaranteed in the U.S. Constitution.

A surgical procedure to correct a behavioral disorder is not the proper use of medical therapy.

Surgical removal of an organ when there is no pathological lesion is an unethical use of the healing arts.

It is in the economic best interests of society to grant parole rather than incarcerating prisoners.

Society should protect an individual from those actions which may prove harmful to that person.

If the operation is allowed upon those who consent, it may lead to a coercion of the operation on others who do not consent.

Castration is (or is not) to be preferred over life-long confinement.

Individuals of sound mind, after being fully informed of the consequences, have the right to make decisions about their own personal destiny.

The use of castration for the rehabilitation of sex offenders is (or is not) an effective treatment.

The county medical society did (or did not) act appropriately by addressing the malpractice issue and not the ethical implications of the case.

The consequences of the various courses of action should now become part of our analysis. If the first option is selected, the prisoners would be paroled if a physician could be found who was willing to perform the surgery. There are several uncertainties here: The efficacy of orchidectomy on aggressive sexual behavior is highly questionable and the possibility exists that either or both of the parolees will perpetuate the same act again and be returned to prison. This time, though, they would have sacrificed some body part for their brief foray in the free world. Alternatively, as free men they may make a satisfactory adjustment to life and never return to jail.

Once on the outside, there is the constitutional question of rights to privacy. As indicated in the case, some legal precedent exists wherein a person initially consented to something under one circumstance and then later, under other conditions, changed his mind and won a judgment against the alleged offending party or parties. The circumstances in this case are sufficiently similar to warrant concern.

Another legal precedent seriously challenges the concept of free and informed consent when persons are held involuntarily, as in instances of incarceration. Further, assuming that successful adjustment is made to outside life, the parolees are returned to society with an organic deficiency stemming directly from their imprisonment.

Taking the other point of view, the uncertainty of the surgical procedure makes continued incarceration the preferred alternative. Since they were in possession of their mental faculties, other behavior modifications might be tried which at some future time might prove successful. Also, a spontaneous correction of their difficulties is not to be ruled out. In either case, the persons will be restored or rehabilitated to society, but in full possession of their body organs.

Space does not allow for a continuation of this analysis, but enough has been said to demonstrate how one might go about an assessment of the various options, coupling them with the values that have been identified.

The most difficult part of the entire procedure is the rank-ordering of the values listed. Since values differ even between two people, applying this methodology could conceivably result in two completely different conclusions. This is perhaps the most bothersome aspect of ethical reasoning. Are there any ways one can evaluate the variety of values given so that some reasonable consensus for action can be obtained? The unfortunate response is no. There is no unmistakable set of rules which once and for all time settles ethical questions. But the situation is not hopeless. There are some criteria that one can use so that although no one value can be the sole claimant of ethical validity, there may well be a *few* good answers. Expressive or gut-level responses can be eliminated and ethical relativism with its insistence that any choice is as good as any other choice can be minimized. What are some of these criteria?

EVALUATING ETHICAL POSITIONS

One formula for evaluating the rightness of an action is to compare the consequences with one's own set of values by asking the simple question, "Could I live with this?" If the answer is yes, it can be assumed that the selected action is consistent with one's own value set. This procedure is nothing more than placing oneself in another's shoes—as difficult as that might be—and conjecturing whether or not the behavior is acceptable if you had to experience the consequences. There is a principle in moral philosophy called the Principle of Fraternal Charity which states the proposition this way: Under a similar set of circumstances would I want the same action performed on me? If the answer is yes, it can be assumed that the act is consistent with the decision-maker's own set of values and the action is ethically valid. On the other hand, if there is emotional discomfort, then one need ask the question, "Why does this action bother me?" A reconsideration of the values is then in order to search for and perhaps remove the bothersome element. This may lead to an entirely new ethical statement of action.

Another form of this approach for evaluating ethical decisions is called contractual theory. In contractual theory one should always act as if she/he will come out at a disadvantage. As a variation of putting yourself in the other person's shoes, here the contract is made between two bargaining parties after which the positions are reversed. In this sort of worst-case scenario, the question "Can I live with the action?" becomes more urgent, for now you as decision-maker may be worse off than you originally bargained for. Although contractual theory may be limited in the number of situations to which it can be applied, there probably are circumstances where it may be useful.

As a hypothetical example, consider the position of the United States in sending surplus grain to a needy foreign nation. Coupled with aid, there are certain stringencies attached such that in order to qualify for the aid some specified raw material, plentiful in the recipient country but scarce in the U.S., must be delivered. The price of that commodity on the world market is less than the food aid to be delivered. It would thus seem that both parties in the contract would benefit. However, if the raw material was processed, the price of the product would double that of the cost of the food aid. The acceptor nation, though, lacks the technological capacity to process the resource. Now, the recipient country is relinquishing a longer-term advantage for a short-term gain. Contractual theory would have the U.S. put itself in the position of the foreign country and then ask, Would it be satisfied with the terms of the agreement? If the behavior would be predicated on contractual theory, the ethical position of the U.S. should be not to pose a bargain of this kind for it stands to gain more than it is giving up.

Another method for testing the validity of an ethical choice is the more general principle of *universalizability*. An ethical position, by specifying the right conduct, implies by its ought, that in theory it applies to all people in similar circumstances. The ethical statement, the U.S. government ought not to provide food aid to a country in need when that country is not in a position to protect its own best interests, implies that no country should provide food aid when that country is in an unfavorable bargaining position. Simply deciding to do a thing carries no ethical weight because at a later time and under exactly the same conditions I might decide to do something else. Ethical behavior according to the principle of universalizability has far broader implications. Having decided that behavior X is the correct ethical choice, then what is meant is that anyone like me, under the same circumstances, ought also to do X. This poses the next question: What would be the results if everyone did that? This means more than just the short-term consequences of my own act but both the short- and long-term outcomes if everyone in my position did the same thing.

A frequently used example of universalizability concerns the matter of truth-telling. Suppose we have made a promise we would now rather not keep because it is no longer convenient for us to do so. We ponder breaking the promise. Would this be acceptable? The moral test for the action according to this principle asks, Can we, as rational persons, accept the state of affairs in which anyone may break promises whenever it is found to be inconvenient to keep them? According to the principle of universalizability, the answer would be no, for such an action would result in massive distrust and end up in social chaos. The principle of universalizability is a key way for testing validity of ethical positions.

The two approaches for evaluating an ethical position described above are parts of two major ethical theories that have currency on the contemporary scene: Consequentialist Theory and Deontological Theory. These are two main sorts of normative ethics.

Consequentialist theory, sometimes also called utilitarian or teleological ethics, asserts that the rightness or the wrongness of an action is determined solely by the results of the action. Thus to determine whether an action is ethically right, we should examine the probable consequences of that action compared with the probable outcome of other available actions, to determine if the choice in question would produce a greater balance of good over evil than any of the other alternatives. The heart of consequentialist ethics is "the greatest general good principle." Several schools of teleological theory have arisen primarily concerned with what is meant by the "general good." One form, ethical hedonism, denies the existence of a perfect good. According to Jeremy Bentham (1748–1832) and John Stuart Mill (1806–1873), the founders of utilitarianism, "pleasure is . . . the only good; pain . . . the only evil."[3] Thus, an action is right insofar as it tends to produce happiness and wrong as it tends to produce unhappiness. An objection to ethical egoism says that it demeans human beings by encouraging hedonism since pleasure and pain are the sole determinants for ethical decisions.

The ideal utilitarian takes the position described earlier, namely, that the ultimate end is the greatest good as measured by a greater balance of good over evil. This interpretation does not entail any particular theory of value but instead submits that promoting the greater good is an obligation. The greater good may apply to a certain group—one's family, class, nation, or race—or the universe as a whole. A pure ideal utilitarian might even contend that the right act or rule is the one that most promotes the good of other people.

A number of difficulties can be identified when utilitarianism ethics are applied to specific problems:

1 The concepts of happiness or greater good are so unclear as to make them unworkable.

2 We can never be sure that our actions will result in the greatest good or the greatest happiness.

3 In order to maximize one person's happiness or the group good, it may be necessary to infringe on the happiness of another individual or group.

4 Utilitarianism alone does not provide a basis for our moral attitudes and presuppositions and, in fact, may yield behaviors that are in conflict with fundamental moral beliefs.

To each of these objections, utilitarians have a response. It will not serve our purpose to review what these are; the interested reader is encouraged to refer for a discussion of these arguments to a text on ethics such as William K. Frankena, *Ethics* (Prentice-Hall, 1973). Essentially, utilitarianism sees the endpoint of morality as being an increase in happiness and the alleviation of suffering.

A quite different ethical position with a markedly distinct orientation is deontological or formalist theory. Briefly put, deontological theories hold that one can determine the rightness of an action independent of the consequences of the proposed act. The term *deontological* comes from the Greek word *deon* which means "that which is binding duty." Hence, deontological ethics emphasizes that it is the principle upon which an agent acts that is the morally decisive factor.

One of the most prominent deontological theories was formulated by Immanuel Kant (1724–1804). For Kant, one central feature of human rationality is that the principles derived from reason are universal; they apply to all people at all times and in all places. For example, the laws of logic are not different at different times and places. The human mind works in generally the same way no matter who you are or where you are, or when you lived. Accordingly, Kant proposes, as the basic principle of morality, a principle that combines universality with duty: Act always so that the principle guiding your action can be willed to be universal law. This is the expression of his famous "categorical imperative." The categorical imperative gives no direct guidance as to what to do, nor does it define any basic moral rules. It categorically covers all situations where ethical reasoning is involved. It is applicable in all situations where we are considering what action is the right one.

The previous example of truth-telling illustrates its practical suitability. It is not the consequences of an act that provides us with the transforming principle; it is the principle (or, in Kant's word, the maxim) guiding the act that establishes its moral worth. In this case, the principle of truth-telling is morally more valid than a maxim that allows for falsehood.

For Kant, the truly moral person is one whose actions are made for the sake of doing the moral thing—made from a respect for duty, not merely in accord with duty. It is the motive or the principle behind the action, not the consequences of the act that determine our judgment of the morality of the action. And the central motive is what he calls "good will." By this he means to act on the basis of a sense of duty, as opposed to acting on the basis of consequences or inclination. Finally, the supreme test for determining moral duty is the categorical imperative. This test of right is considered so important that many ethical philosophers hold that a person deserves respect as a moral person only if that person is willing to universalize his or her moral judgments.[4]

There is another way of formulating the categorical imperative. "Act always in such a way that you should always treat people, whether in your own person or in the person of any other, never simply as a means but always at the same time as an end."[5] Kant's view here is that we must recognize each person as a moral being deserving of respect and never use anyone merely as a means to some end. This, too, is part of the categorical imperative, namely, the principle of the moral equality of all persons. Universal right action is predicated on the equality of all human beings and this right must not be violated. Kant sees persons as having an absolute, or unconditional, value because they are capable of making rational choices. Our dignity derives from this capability and this dignity is violated whenever a person is treated merely as an end—as a thing and not a person.

This conception of the categorical imperative finds a number of direct applications in biomedical issues. Several examples are the use of humans as experimental subjects, involuntary sterilization of welfare mothers, or the patient under a physician's care. We will have frequent recourse to this principle in subsequent discussions.

The theories and points of view introduced here do not constitute an exhaustive list of possible ethical theories. To carry these discussions further would take us far afield from the matter at hand, that is, ethical issues in the life sciences. Again, the interested student is encouraged to seek out a more thorough presentation of ethical theory by referring to textbooks in ethics. Several are listed in the bibliography. These theories were chosen since they seem to embody a number of central notions that are important in ethical decision-making. The consequentialist concept of the greatest good or the greatest happiness seems to be humane and realistic when we face some kinds of ethical issues in biomedicine. The Kantian notion of universalizability, or of never treating a person as a means, could be a fruitful way of resolving other kinds of issues. At times, though, the two positions seem to issue contradictory directives in particular cases; for example, in the matter of human experimentation, especially where there is a high risk of inflicting harm on the participant. On the one hand, Kantian deontology admonishes us never to use people as a means. On the other, consequentialism submits that if such experimentation would yield a cure for a disease that would benefit a number of patients later, then the greater good is realized and the experiment can be justified on the grounds of social utility. Perhaps what is required is a more thorough analysis which could resolve some of the conflicts. For instance, one might be able to achieve a synthesis of consequentialism and Kantianism that would retain the best elements of both views. Some philosophers are sympathetic to the view that a mix of the two, if it is possible, could provide society with a working set of principles. Another possible course of action might be that since neither theory is entirely adequate, we could devise some principles by which we could determine when it would be appropriate to use one theory and when the other.

Further, let us not suppose that the final word is in as far as ethical theory is concerned. As is the case with all other branches of learning, new knowledge, or at least different syntheses, can be anticipated in the future.

APPLICATIONS OF ETHICAL THEORY

Moving from the theoretical to the practical, at least three major bioethical positions can be described which represent application of the theories discussed above. These are the Proportionate Good School, the Prohibitionist School, and a third based on John Rawls' theory of justice.

Joseph Fletcher, a Christian ethicist and professor of medical ethics at the University of Virginia School of Medicine, is a leading proponent of the "proportionate-good" position. He is the author of several books on ethics, the most well-known of which is *Situation Ethics*.[6] He holds that an act "acquires its value because it happens to help persons (thus being good), or to hurt persons (thus being bad)." Situations are examined and relative choices are made on the basis of what we judge to offer the most good. This view is easily recognized as consequentialist ethics. According to Fletcher, most of us in our daily lives decide for or against something on the principle of the proportionate good. In medical practice this widely used approach is known as the clinical model, where any therapeutic procedure that is likely to result in an improvement in patient well-being is positively good and is positively the right thing to do.

The heart of a responsible ethics is this question: "What of what can be done, should be done; what of what should be done can we afford; and what of what we can afford are we prepared to pay?"[7] What this means, according to Fletcher, is that the means *may* at times and in certain instances justify the end sought. Enough moral flexibility is required so that acts of necessity which achieve the most good possible can be performed. In the example of surgery, the flesh must necessarily be hurt if the greater good is to be realized. The "do no harm" maxim of medicine really means, "do no harm unless the end justifies the means." An *a priori* insistence that end never justifies the means is inconsistent not only with modern technology but conflicts with moral theory as well since adamant insistence will preclude the doing of certain things that can relieve or reduce suffering in the world. A compassion for people may require that in times of need we override the negative prohibition of absolutism. This does not mean, insists Fletcher, that any end will justify any means regardless of the proportionate good. We assume that the decision-maker is rational and a person of good will (see the earlier discussion of good will).

Fletcher provides us with the ultimate directive in decision-making in the following:

> The only possible moral test of rival views lies in their consequences. When beliefs of nonempirical opinions, neither of them being falsifiable, contradict or clash with each other, the only possible way to choose between them morally is in terms of their consequences if they are followed out logically in practice. The one that results in greater good for people is the correct one.[8]

On this basis there are no absolute ethics, no open and shut authority to which we can turn. The inflexibility of absolutism is a view that can help very little in deciding the variety of real-life situations. We cannot accept as workable a position that says that what is right or wrong can be settled dogmatically in advance of the facts. Sometimes certain actions are right, sometimes they are wrong; sometimes they are good, sometimes they are not. This holds true for abortion, egg transfers, *in vitro* conceptions, sterilization, gamete storage banks, cloning, nonmarital sex, environmental concerns, and population problems.

Fletcher's six guidelines for making ethical decisions are these:

1. compassion for people as human beings;
2. consideration of consequences;
3. proportionate good;
4. the priority of actual needs over the ideal or potential;
5. a desire to enlarge choice and reduce chance;
6. a courageous acceptance of our responsibility to make decisions and a courageous acceptance of the outcome of our decisions.[9]

Proportionate-good decision-makers emphasize over and over again that human needs validate rights, not the other way around. The first court of appeal is human need. In practice, anything that promotes overall welfare is to be encouraged; anything that sets up absolutes and uncrossable boundaries is to be discouraged.

Paul Kurtz, a humanist-philosopher, suggests a humanist ethic which is in all essential respects similar to the proportionate-good model. His guidelines for evaluating a moral issue are these:

1. persistent inquiring into the facts of a case;
2. explicit delineations of existing values and principles in a situation;
3. regard for basic human needs;
4. exploration of new or alternative means for resolution;
5. examination of consequences, short-range and long-term;
6. inclusion of sufficient plasticity to modify and reconstruct values in the light of continuing inquiry;
7. provision for alternative forms of morality so that individuals are left free to respond according to dictates of conscience. [10]

In the position of both Fletcher and Kurtz, it is suggested that even though the best decision may not be made for all concerned, at least the worst can be avoided. Here, then, are examples of the newer thinking, illuminating the earlier suggestion that all of ethical theory has not yet been expressed.

The prohibitionist viewpoint, as exemplified by the Princeton Christian theologian-ethicist Paul Ramsey, takes a contrary position. He submits that there are things that can be done that should not be done; there are things that can be known that should not be known. An example of the first is fetal experimentation, of the latter, knowledge of genetic manipulation. One empirical defense for the prohibitionist position rests on the assumption that there are certain kinds of information or technologies which pose serious and profound ethical problems which society and/or individuals will simply be unable to resolve; more seriously, the acquisition of such knowledge or application of dangerous technology could place humankind in a deeper ethical quagmire than at the start. In his book, *The Ethics of Fetal Research*, [11] Ramsey insists that to carry out research using fetal material merely compounds error with error—the first error is the nontherapeutic abortion (to which he is opposed on moral grounds), the second, experimentation on a human being (i.e., the fetus) who has not given valid consent to the experimenters. As a moralist, he argues that social and moral prices unavoidably linked to the total case of fetal research, such as the "corruption or hardening of the lifesaving professions and the skewing of medical ethics," are not acceptable. In addition, the aim to develop prenatal treatments and to save premature babies will lead "to the possibility of complete extracorporeal gestation and to gene change of every sort." In his words, "anyone who thinks seriously about the morality of fetal research should sort out the 'benefits' and then count the cost" and, according to his tabulations, the debit side wins out.

Not only in the area of fetal research but in others as well—for example, euthanasia, genetic research, and human experimentation—Ramsey cautions concern, for the potential for moral outrages attendant with many of these procedures is far too real to be easily dismissed or disregarded in favor of the "greater good."

The writings of Paul Ramsey reflect the Kantian concern for the moral dignity of the person. In another of his works, *The Patient as Person*, [12] Ramsey forcefully affirms the "sacred" character of human life in the face of an increasingly technological society. The wholesale violation of human rights can be averted only by observing man's "sacredness." One who so regards human beings will insist upon an ethical theory that opts for faithfulness and fairness and rejects arbitrary treatment of individuals even if such treatment results in the greater public good. It is this concern for sacredness, for instance, that validates his position on human or fetal experimentation. The consent requirement insists that research subjects be first fully and effectively informed about the probable consequences of the experiment (see Chapter 7, Human Experimentation). Failure to inform subjects—either because we deliberately choose not to, as when the experiment is potentially hazardous, or when it is impossible to do so, as with a fetus—is a clear abridgment of the sacredness principle. The subject's status as a moral being has been violated.

Treating others as responsible human beings has implication in other relationships, too. The physician-patient one is characterized by Ramsey as a covenant relationship which sets up demands that differ markedly from basing actions on consequences only. As Ramsey puts it, "justice, fairness, faithfulness, canons of loyalty, the sanctity of life, hesed, agape, or charity are some of the names given to the moral quality of attitude and of action owed to all men by any man who steps into a covenant with another man."[13] In a covenant relationship, both parties are bound by certain moral obligations and each has a duty to honor the freedom and dignity of the other. Although attaining the terms of this relationship in everyday events may be exceedingly difficult at times, the struggle for its achievement is well worth the ideals it embodies, such as mutuality, freedom, and shared responsibility.

John Rawls, a Harvard political philosopher, in his widely acclaimed book *A Theory of Justice*,[14] develops a mix of Kantian deontological theory and Fletcher's consequentialism. The idea of a covenant, or contract, between moral agents is fundamental to his theory of justice. The contract is a social contract wherein free and rational persons choose principles of justice from an original or starting position of equality. In this theoretical original condition, all parties are equal in every respect—social, economic, and political—and are able to freely choose principles of justice. The principles of justice which govern such a well-ordered society are designed to advance the good of its members. In practice, these principles provide a way of assigning rights as well as an appropriating of the distribution of benefits and burdens to society. It is especially this latter point that attracts our attention because here, the several principles introduced by Rawls for the allocation and/or distribution of goods and services when there are competing claims has application to the life-sciences moral dilemma.

The major principles of the theory are these:

First Principle. Each person is to have an equal right to the most extensive total system of equal basic liberties compatible with a similar system of liberty for all.

Second Principle. Social and economic inequalities are to be arranged so that they are to the greatest benefit of the least advantaged.

Priority Rules. Restriction of liberty is permissible if:
a) less extensive liberty strengthens the total system of liberty shared by all;
b) a less than equal liberty is acceptable to those with lesser liberty.

Inequalities or differences are permissible if:
a) an inequality enhances the opportunity of those with less;
b) they mitigate the burden of those bearing the hardship.

The first principle is designed to secure basic liberties for all persons. He argues:

> Each person possesses an inviolability founded on justice that even the welfare of society as a whole cannot override. For this reason justice denies that the loss of freedom for some is made right by a greater good shared by others . . . the rights secured by justice are not subject to political bargaining or to the calculus of social interests.[15]

This is decidedly Kantian for it insists that no person be discriminated against or exploited so that others may gain thereby. The primary concern is with justice and the right, as well as the moral equality of all persons, and these cannot be bargained away.

The second principle regulates the distribution of wealth, income, and other social assets, such as medical care and education. Note that the second principle does not strictly insist that all goods be distributed equally. However, if there is to be an unequal distribution, then these differences must increase the benefit of all concerned. This is reminiscent of the proportionate-good concept of Fletcher. It makes sense, for instance, for a society to raise everybody's standard of living even if in doing so, certain inequalities are allowed. Alternatively improving the status of some at the expense of others is specifically prohibited.

Let's take a hypothetical example. Suppose society must decide on one of three conflicting public policies. For example, should it spend one million dollars to buy two hyperbaric chambers which will save few lives; should it carry out a lead screening project in a poor section of town; or should it modernize an existing public-health facility? It has the funds to implement only one of these. The following scheme may be used:

| Decision | Circumstances and Outcome | | | Net total benefits |
	C_1	C_2	C_3	
d_1	−7	8	12	13
d_2	−8	6	14	12
d_3	5	7	8	20

d = decision
C = social class
Benefits = relative benefit in theoretical units

In this simple instance, if C_1 and C_2 represent the lowest on the social ladder, the decision of choice would be d_3. Here, the lowest on the scale would be maximized and all social classes would benefit by the decision. To be sure, an ideal circumstance is depicted in this theoretical example. Much remains to be worked out, as, for instance, how does society quantitatively evaluate the relative merits of each decision? It is of interest to note that social scientists are presently developing approaches to this very difficult problem.[16] Although the general goal that all social primary goods—liberty and opportunity, income and wealth, and the basis of self-respect—are to be distributed equally unless an unequal distribution of any or all of these is to the advantage of the least favored is still a long way from reaching fulfillment in our society. John Rawls' principles of justice could provide us with guidelines for working through some of the complex problems arising from the new biology.

EPISTEMOLOGICAL BASIS FOR ETHICAL THEORY

Earlier it was contended that the basis for any ethical theory must ultimately derive from some particular theory of value. Endeavoring to arrive at acceptable principles and obligations to guide conduct or general judgments of value, the question is put: Is there any way our basic ethical judgments can be justified? We have examined several theories of ethical decision-making, and in the forms in which they have been stated, each is open to strong objections. The thoughtful reader may well be confused for it would seem that it makes no difference what we choose, morality is a personal matter, and one theory is as good, or as bad, as another. What has been demonstrated, of course, is that there is no general rule or directive that has the same status in ethics as a rule of induction has for an empirical science. No one viewpoint is normative, that is, commands general agreement.

The major reason for this wide incongruity is that ethical interests are *second-order* interests inasmuch as they have no object in the absence of higher motivations. Moral inquiry can never occur detached from the context of meanings and presuppositions. Many of our questions themselves arise from concerns that presuppose some values—the value of life, the inequities of social distribution, the mutual respect for individual freedom, and the like. Recall Ramsey's "sacredness" principle as an example of a higher presupposition on which to base an ethic. Moral judgments always commit one to a theory of man or a theory of the universe, or, in other words, a metaphysics.

Metaphysics poses the perplexing question: What is the ultimately defining context for our maxims or principles of behavior? Much depends on our properly seizing the impact of this question for it launches us into that matter which underlies moral judgment. To the question, What is the nature of things?, the answer can take at least three forms: They are revealed either by empirical inquiry, by metaethical construction, or by divine revelation. In sorting through this problem, we are dealing with *first-order* interests.

The question harks back to the dispute in Protagoras: Are humans the measure of all things or are there gods? If humans set the conditions within which they will define themselves, if they set the goal and plan of the *humanum*, then they make themselves the measure of all things—the fixed point in terms of which everything else must be related. Such a position lacks that measure of absolute confidence to defend itself from counter-claims that, while humans may be the measure, some are more of a measure than others; or that the universe is a cosmic accident and humankind's appearance on it is perilously conditioned by uncertainty. On the other hand, if, as Socrates suspected, the gods set the measure, then our lot is more secure. The belief that there is a plan, both for the person and the world, provides for some the ultimate reference for any moral and/or ethical code.

Again, the further pursuit of this topic would lead us far astray, for as is well-known, finding a generally acceptable metaphysics on which to ground our values has eluded our species ever since the question of ultimate concern was first put. The decision of a metaphysics is entirely, or at least primarily, an individual concern. It is probably for this reason that there are so many religious beliefs in the world today. Also, in this regard, one might recall the earlier discussion of evolution and ethics (Chapter 1), which asked the somewhat Kantian question: Are there some universal maxims that provide higher motivations for human behavior and that have as their origin the biological and social evolution of the species? It is of interest to note here that once a metaphysics or world view is established and recognized, it permeates all the other things that human beings find engrossing. It is the authority, and to some the only authority, that can define the content of an ethical choice. Whether hidden or expressed, every ethical decision ultimately derives from a metaphysical perspective. As long as this remains largely presupposed or intuitively assumed, one can pronounce on right and wrong action spontaneously and with ease; taken seriously, one is involved in the furious and agonizing search for a foundation that does justice to the complexities and reckons with the conflicts of everyday questions. As a first-order interest, it seems expedient that one's personal worldview be articulated prior to or at least simultaneously with ethical decision-making.

VALUES IN ETHICS

The association of metaphysics and ethics emphasizes the crucial nature of values in decision-making. Every theory of ethics has as its basis some principles or set of values which are intended as directives for guiding subsequent behavior. We will adopt part of this strategy. Following each topic in this book, a partial list of values will be included which identify some of the ethical positions on issues raised. The list is not intended to be all-inclusive but is designed to initiate thinking in the matter of value clarification. You are encouraged to add to these lists as your study proceeds and you grow in your ability to delineate value positions.

Historically, moral philosophers and theologians have developed a list of ethical propositions that express some universal values. These frequently provide starting points for making moral judgments in perplexing and conflicting cases. Consistent with the aim of including a list of values with each study in this text, the following ethical propositions are added here. No discussion is given for most of them since the terms themselves define each rather well.

Principle of honesty.

Principle of truth-telling.

Principle of self-restraint.

Principle of love.

Principle of responsible action.

Principle of benevolence.

Principle of individual rights and personal inviolability.

Principle of distributive justice—the burdens and benefits of social institutions are to be distributed in accordance with standards of equity.

Principle of equality—all individuals are to be treated as equals; special justification is required if priority is to be assigned.

Reduction of pain and suffering in the world (often stated: it is unethical to bring about an increase in pain and suffering in the world).

Principle of double effect—if a procedure has both good and evil effects, then the following priority should be employed:

a) the course chosen must be good or at least morally indifferent;
b) good must not be obtained by means of evil in such a way that good flows from evil;
c) evil must never be intended but merely tolerated as casually connected with the good intended;
d) there must be a reasonable proportion between good and evil effects.

Principle of fraternal charity—one may do for one's neighbor whatever one may morally do for oneself (the Golden Rule).

A FINAL CONSIDERATION

One last matter remains unresolved in this chapter: the case study that was begun earlier. As you recall, two convicts had requested castration as a condition for release from an indeterminate jail sentence. Our analysis had carried it to the value identification stage. Armed with the information contained in this chapter, continue the analysis to arrive at an ethical decision. Remember that an ethical judgment is more than a mere choice based on preference or inclination. It is a decision which reflects principles designed to promote good and has rational justification on its side. Once we realize this, we must go on to ask whether the choice selected is the best one. At that point, we are also engaged in thinking seriously about our still more basic principles—first order-considerations. As Plato said:

> For no light matter is at stake; the question concerns the very manner in which life is to be lived.[17]

REFERENCES

1 Tracy M. Sonneborn, "Ethical issues arising from the possible uses of genetic knowledge," in Bruce Hilton, Daniel Callahan, Maureen Harris, Peter Condliffe, and Burton Berkley (eds.), *Ethical Issues in Human Genetics* (New York: Plenum Press, 1973), p. 5.

2 Henry D. Aiken, *Reason and Conduct: New Bearings in Moral Philosophy* (New York: Alfred A. Knopf, 1962), Chapter 4, Levels of Ethical Discourse.

3 Thomas Higgins, S.J., *Basic Ethics* (Milwaukee: Bruce Publishing Company, 1968), p. 57.

4 William K. Frankena, *Ethics*, 2nd ed. (Englewood Cliffs, N.J.: Prentice-Hall, 1973), pp. 113–114.

5 Robert Hunt and John Arras, *Ethical Issues in Modern Medicine* (Palo Alto: Mayfield Publishing Company, 1977), p. 31.

6 Joseph Fletcher, *Situation Ethics* (Philadelphia: Westminster Press, 1966).

7 Joseph Fletcher, *The Ethics of Genetic Control* (Garden City, N.Y.: Doubleday, Anchor Press, 1974), p. 121.

8 Joseph Fletcher (Reference 7), p. 138.

9 Joseph Fletcher (Reference 7), p. 118.

10 Paul Kurtz, "The uses and abuses of science," *The Humanist* 32, 5 (1972): 7–9.

11   Paul Ramsey, *The Ethics of Fetal Research* (New Haven: Yale University Press, 1975).

12   Paul Ramsey, *The Patient as Person* (New Haven: Yale University Press, 1975).

13   Paul Ramsey (Reference 12), pp. xii–xiii.

14   John Rawls, *A Theory of Justice* (Cambridge: The Belknapp Press of Harvard University Press, 1971).

15   John Rawls (Reference 14), pp. 3–4.

16   U.S. Department of HEW, *Toward a Social Report* (Washington: Government Printing Office, 1969) or Bertram M. Gross (ed.), *Social Intelligence for America's Future* (Boston: Allyn and Bacon, 1969).

17   Robert Hunt and John Arras (Reference 5), p. 45.

BIBLIOGRAPHY

General Ethics Texts

Brandt, Richard B., *Ethical Theory* (Englewood Cliffs, N.J.: Prentice-Hall, 1959).

Warnock, G. J., *Contemporary Moral Philosophy* (New York: MacMillan, Saint Martin's Press, 1967).

Warnock, Mary, *Ethics Since 1900*, 2nd ed. (New York: Oxford University Press, 1966).

William, Bernard, *Morality: An Introduction to Ethics* (New York & Evanston: Harper & Row, 1972).

Texts Relating Specifically to Ethical Issues in the Life Sciences

Brody, Howard, *Ethical Decisions in Medicine* (Boston: Little, Brown, 1976).

Gorovity, Samuel, Andrew L. Jameton; Ruth Macklin; John M. O'Connor; Eugene V. Perrin; Beverly Page St. Clair; and Susan Sherwin (eds.), *Moral Problems in Medicine* (Englewood Cliffs, N.J.: Prentice-Hall, 1976).

II

MEDICAL ISSUES

3

NEW BEGINNINGS OF LIFE: GENETICS AND DEVELOPMENT

INTRODUCTION

One of the most fascinating areas of biological research—and one of the most unpredictable in terms of application of knowledge learned—studies the events and processes of heredity and development. New-found insights are tumbling from research laboratories the world over regarding the nature of the genetic material and its directing role in the development of organisms from egg to maturity. Indeed, it has been said that one of the most significant discoveries in the sciences for all time has been the elucidation of the chemical make-up of the gene, the alphabet and sentence structure of DNA, RNA, and protein as a remarkable information system. Therein is coded the blueprints of all life forms from the simplest virus to the complex human. So important are these processes to life that they have been christened the "holy trinity" of modern biology—from DNA to RNA to protein! Included in this triad is the study of those many processes required to bring the developing embryo to full term, although at present knowledge is far from complete.

This understanding has suggested ways to manipulate these fundamental life processes directing them along preselected pathways, making possible the direct interposition of human will into the very basis of life itself. This new knowledge and its application raises the question: Can or should the human species control its own biological evolution? In the past, we have not tampered with our own biological evolution. However, with our plants and animals we have done just that. By substituting artificial and selective breeding for the very slow processes of natural selection, we have produced a vast number of new plants and animals which, at least from our standpoint, have many desirable qualities. From the animal or plant point of view, however, these changes may not be so good because in competition with so-called wild types (i.e., the natural forms), the manufactured versions are usually destined to extinction. It is only through the constant care of their human creators that these artificial varieties are able to survive at all.

Humans have, on the other hand, been reluctant to practice this same sort of thing on themselves. Disapproval was voiced on ethical, and moral, and religious grounds arguing that this was not quite the right thing to do. However, more often than not the major reason for not doing it was simply ignorance—ignorance of how one could selectively breed for desirable human characteristics without at the same time doing irreparable harm. Now, or at least in the foreseeable future, the obstacle of ignorance will be overcome. In the short span of about 20 years, the dramatic discoveries in genetics and development have revolutionized our former understandings. We may soon have the capabilities to become something quite different than we are right now. The epoch of "participatory evolution" is coming upon us. It all began with artificial insemination and promises to end with bioengineered or bio-designed parahumans or modified humans. It seems the better part of wisdom that an effective response to these challenges requires advanced preparation.

Before considering the major questions of morality, the sanctity of life, the worth of the individual, and the social and legal implications these methods will present, let's review a bit of this story as background. It is not science fiction we are dealing with here but the fact that real understanding is being procured relative to the "creation" of human life according to plan.

STATE-OF-THE-ART IN GENETICS AND DEVELOPMENT

Developmental engineering. We know of eight different ways to make babies.[1] Some of these are accomplished facts; others only await the working out of technical details. The eight methods are: (1) the coital-gestational way; (2) artificial insemination of a wife with her husband's sperm (AIH); (3) artificial insemination of a wife with a donor's sperm (AID); (4) artificial insemination of a woman's ovum by her husband's sperm and then implantation into her own uterus; (5) egg transfer from a donor to a woman's womb before fertilization; (6) embryo transfer from a donor to a recipient's womb (prenatal adoption); (7) an artificial placenta for development outside of the uterus, also called ectogenesis; (8) cloning, or nuclear transplantation. There is still a ninth method, practiced routinely in nature by some organisms but a long way off in humans, called parthenogenesis or monogenesis, in which a whole organism is generated from a single sex cell without fertilization from a member of the opposite sex. Let's examine a few of the developments relative to these methods more closely.

Some of the pioneering work in the area of developmental engineering was done by R. Briggs and T. King, two experimental embryologists working at the Carnegie Institute in Washington. In 1952, they devised the elegant experimental technique of transferring a nucleus with its full complement of genetic information from one cell to another, a technically difficult operation. They transferred nuclei from different developmental stages of frog embryos into unfertilized and enucleated frog eggs. Enucleated eggs have had the original nucleus removed, but the remainder of the egg, the cytoplasm and yolk, is intact. They found that the younger the donor nucleus (that is, the less specialized), the greater the chances a fully developed frog tadpole would develop; late-stage transfers resulted in abnormal growth or no growth at all. (See Fig. 3.1.)

Their research was designed to investigate the process of cellular differentiation during embryogenesis. But another implication of this work is that it demonstrated the feasibility of transplanting a foreign nucleus into a recipient cell and obtaining normal growth; in other words, the technique of nuclear transplantation is experimentally quite possible.

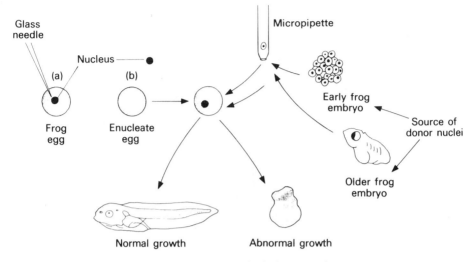

Fig. 3.1 *The Briggs and King experiment in which donor nuclei were transplanted into enucleated eggs.*

Following up on this research, John Gurdon, an English embryologist, in 1964 transplanted an adult intestinal cell nucleus, or skin cell nucleus, from a mature toad into a toad egg. As mature adult cells, they had completed their developmental history and had taken on differentiated function. Although many of his transplants failed to survive, a few did. They became fully formed adult toads, quite normal in every respect (Fig. 3.2). They were normal in every respect except one and that is they had no father or mother in a biological sense. For reasons which are not yet understood, the egg with its transplanted adult nucleus developed as if it had been fertilized, and in some cases gave rise to a normal adult organism. Since almost all of the hereditary material of a cell is contained within the nucleus, the recipient renucleated egg develops into an individual which is genetically identical to the organism which was the nuclear donor. Thus, the origin of the new individual is not the chance union of egg and sperm, with the new generation possessing a new genetic constitution; rather, the new organism is a continued individual, a copy of an already existing genotype. Biologists call genetically similar organisms clones; the donor toad and the asexually reproduced offspring are members of the same clone— they are genetically identical. Gurdon's work demonstrated the feasibility of artificial cloning in vertebrate animals. To a nonbiologist, experimenting with frogs and toads may seem to be trivial pastime, having little if any relationship at all to humans. However, a judgment of this kind should be made with caution. First, biologists operate on the principle of the universality of life processes. That is, organisms share in common a general biology of function, the affinity being a direct reflection of evolutionary kinship (i.e., common ancestry). Hence, extrapolation between organisms is a routine and scientifically valid procedure. And, in fact, the closer the phylogenetic relationship, the greater the commonality. Second, frog and toad eggs have been the embryologist's favorite research tool not because there exists any "prince" or "princess" fixation but for the quite simple reason that they are easily manipulated. Their large size facilitates experimentation and also being non-

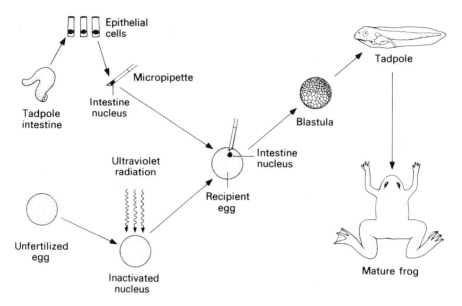

Fig. 3.2 *The Gurdon experiment where differentiated nuclei were transplanted to enucleated eggs to produce clones.*

placental (the young are not nourished inside of the female parent), they are easily cultured in the laboratory. These latter two advantages, of course, are not to be had with mammalian (e.g., human) eggs.

F. C. Stewart, a botanist working at Cornell University, homogenized mature carrot plants to obtain individual cells of the carrot. Again, the cells of the mature carrot are adult cells, fully differentiated. By carefully controlling the environment, Stewart was able to cause these single, isolated adult cells to go back through the entire developmental history of carrots and grow fully formed, adult carrots (Fig. 3.3). His work, like Gurdon's, showed that all the genetic information was present in an adult cell, but more importantly, that this genetic blueprint could be induced to translate once more in its entirety all the genetic information needed to form a mature individual, this time in plants. From these and other experiments, it was concluded that the cloning capability is not limited to a few lesser organisms like frogs, toads, or fruit flies, but seems to be a phenomenon universally present in the biological world, possibly including humans. However, to consider cloning possibilities in humans, we need still more information.

P. C. Steptoe and R. G. Edwards, two scientists working in England, studied and presumably solved the problem of inducing fertilization in human females who could not conceive a child in the normal fashion. Some women have healthy ovaries and a uterus but cannot conceive children because their oviducts are blocked or defective. Crude estimates place the number so affected at about one percent of all women. Blocked or abnormal oviducts account for perhaps 20 percent of all cases of female infertility. To overcome this difficulty, Dr. Edwards and his obstetrician colleague, Dr. Steptoe, have devised a surgical method known as laparoscopy to obtain mature human eggs directly from the follicles of the human ovary just before

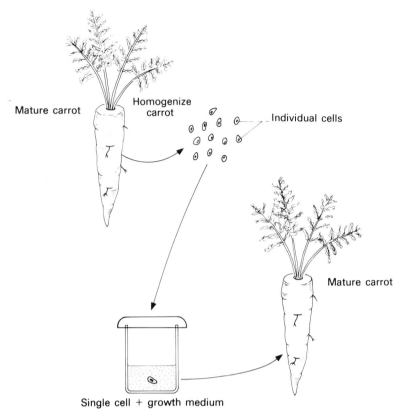

Fig. 3.3 *Stewart's experiment in which single carrot cells were regrown into fully formed whole carrot plants.*

ovulation (Fig. 3.4). Before the operation, the female subject is given reproductive hormones in order to stimulate the reproductive cycle. Several eggs are thus caused to ripen simultaneously in the ovary. Just a few hours before ovulation would occur, a laparoscopy is performed. A small incision is made in the lower abdomen just below the navel, and the laparascope is inserted and directed to a position over each of the ovaries. Under direct visualization of the ovary by means of a slender telescope passed through a second abdominal incision, the thinned walls of the bulging follicles can be visualized. These are then punctured and the contents collected by means of a vacuum aspirator. As many as three or four eggs can be recovered in a single operation. These eggs are placed in a nutrient solution resembling that found in the oviduct. The incision is then sutured closed with one or two stitches and little or no evidence in the form of a scar is visible a few weeks after the procedure.

Upon addition of sperm (which has first been activated in the process called capacitation) to the nutrient containing the eggs, *in vitro* (in glass) fertilization occurs; that is, fertilization outside of the living organism. Kept in the culture medium, the fertilized eggs begin to divide, one of the telltale signs that fertilization has been effected and embryonic development has begun. A few of the artificially fertilized eggs may continue through the early division stages—2-cell stage, 4-cell

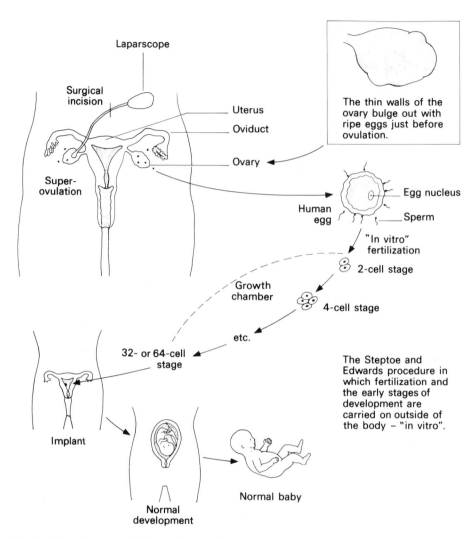

Fig. 3.4 *The Steptoe and Edwards procedure in which fertilization and the early stages of development are carried on outside of the body—in vitro (upper right). The thin walls of the ovary bulge out with ripe eggs just before ovulation.*

stage, etc.—until they reach the stage when the embryo normally implants in the uterine wall of the female. This usually occurs between the 32- and 64-cell stage. Just preceding this time, the embryo is introduced into the hormonally prepared female uterus. If implantation is successful, the embryo will be carried to full term with quite normal fetal development along the way. Successful implantation of laboratory-grown embryos resulting in live and normal organisms is routinely done in rabbits and mice. In the summer of 1974 it was announced that a British scientist-physician, Dr. Douglas Bevis of Leeds University, had succeeded in using this procedure with human subjects. Three children were born, the products of *in vitro* fertilization and artificial implantation. They were, in short, the world's first "test-tube babies." None of the three children born showed any abnormalities. Dr. Bevis emphasized that success was his not because of any medical breakthrough but largely because of luck. A large but unspecific number of similar procedures were attempted in other women without success. In humans, the problem seems to be one of timing of the transfer since the lining of the uterus is receptive to implantation only for a short time and the embryo itself must be at a critical stage before it can implant. It would seem, though, that these difficulties are technical problems. There is no theoretical reason to believe that these cannot be overcome and that successful implantation followed by normal development can be routinely practiced in women desiring it. *

It is worth mentioning that the female who carries the embryo to full term does not necessarily have to be the natural mother; a surrogate mother will do as well. True virgin birth could be realized! This, according to some, could give rise to a new profession, advertised under the title "wombs for rent." Women with uterine abnormalities which prevent normal pregnancy may well seek out surrogate mothers, as may mothers who don't want to go through the rigors of pregnancy but do want natural children. There are certainly enough women available to form a caste of childbearers, especially if the pay was right. One prominent English biologist suggested a fee of $4800 for full term which calculates out to about $500 a month. Recently, a Michigan couple (1977) advertised a fee of $5000, including expenses, as pay to someone who would bear a child for them. (The female partner in this case was physically unable to bear a child.) In November 1977, an unemployed nurse offered to bear a child for a California couple for $10,000, so that she could take herself and her young daughter off welfare. Defending her action quite boldly she asserted, "my whole point is to make some money."

The possibility of egg donation is made a reality by this procedure, too. This may be the case in which an individual has some superior or other desirable genetic characteristic or in which a female friend or relative is unable to ovulate. What the consequences of womb-lending or egg-donation may be is, of course, still an open question. Figure 3.5 pictures a surrogate relationship in cattle, demonstrating quite simply that it can and is being done, at least in nonhuman organisms.

Another possible application of this technique is prenatal adoption, adoption in which the parents adopt an embryo from some other mating and the adopting female carries it to full term in her own body. A variation of this, paleogenesis—life from two sex cells obtained at different points in time but stored in some sort of egg bank ten, twenty, or maybe even a hundred years—may someday be possible. Such cryobanking of genetic material might provide man with a method for influencing the genetic quality of the species. By carefully selecting donors, these banks would make a wide range of genetic material available for selection. The late biologist Herman Muller, a proponent of the idea, suggested that the "most truly outstanding and eminently worthy personalities known" be chosen as donors.[2] There is, of course, the very real problem of determining what human qualities are "desirable," especially with regard to future generations.

---

* The work of Dr. Bevis was not accepted by the scientific community because it lacked rigorous documentation pertaining to experimental method and control. The first authenticated instance of a test-tube fertilization followed by successful birth of the implanted embryo was reported in the summer of 1978 by Drs. Edwards and Steptoe.

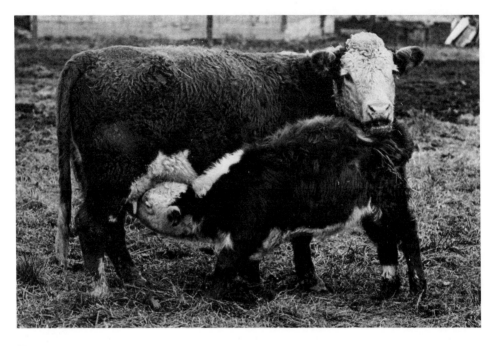

Figure 3.5

The banking of human sperm (and ova) may become an important part of future reproductive technologies. Already many human babies have been conceived, using sperm that has been stored frozen, since sperm banks got their start in 1953. Published reports have documented over 500 normal births resulting from clinical use of frozen semen. The success figure for normal births is well above the general population. It has been found that the fertilizing capacity of sperm frozen and stored in liquid nitrogen at $-196.5°C$ is approximately two-thirds of that expected if fresh semen is used. There are some reservations, though. The American Public Health Association has warned against significant and unanticipated biological and social consequences (see Frankel, "Human-Semen Banking: Social and Public Policy Issues"[3]). Most fertility clinics presently use only fresh semen since there are still some questions concerning the use of frozen sperm. For the most part, these reservations may be more technical than biological, and we can expect that these problems are solvable. However, as Frankel points out, the policy issues in cryobanking may overlap to some extent with those related to the aims and methods of genetic engineering. Hence, it is important and germane that society be alert to applications of cryobanking technology.

Returning to the problem of cloning humans, what are the probabilities? To clone, the following are required:

1 acquisition of mature human eggs;
2 removal of the egg nucleus;
3 insertion of a donor nucleus;

4 transfer and implantation of the renucleated egg into the uterus of a physiologically prepared female.

As a result of Steptoe and Edwards' work, as reported in the summer of 1978, the first and fourth problems have been mostly solved. Regarding the second, recent experiments have shown that chemical methods can be used to remove the nucleus from a mammalian egg. Irradiation can accomplish the same thing but it is also more capable of damaging the egg. The only remaining serious difficulty is the introduction of a donor nucleus into the enucleate egg. (See Fig. 3.6.) This is not to suggest that this is a trivial or minor problem. The transplantation of donor nuclei into enucleate eggs has not met with much success yet except in the case of immature amphibians as previously noted. Apparently the chemical switch that controls gene messages during development prevents the expression of full genetic potential if the donor cell is already fully mature. In like fashion, a donor cell taken from an adult human and transplanted into an enucleate egg is unable to retrace the entire developmental history of humans to result in a duplicate adult genetic copy.

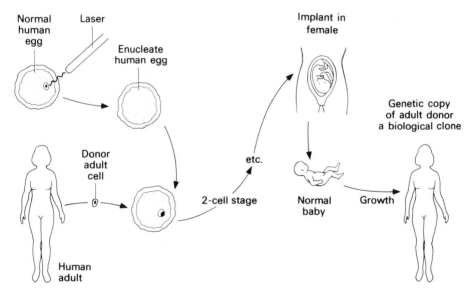

Fig. 3.6 *A theoretical method for cloning humans.*

However, several newer techniques are being pioneered whereby it may be possible that livestock as well as humans could be cloned at some future time. Dr. Peter Hoppe of Jackson Laboratory in Bar Harbor, Maine, is experimenting with an approach that mimics sexual reproduction in certain ways. Using mice as experimental animals, eggs are removed from the female within a few hours after they have been fertilized by male sperm. Under natural conditions the sperm fuses with the egg nucleus to form the full chromosomal complement required to build a new mouse. Working with microscopes and very fine instruments, the father's genetic message is removed from inside these eggs before fusion takes place. Only the mother's chromosomes remain. The eggs are then treated with a special chemical (cytochalasin B) which prevents the eggs from dividing but causes the mother's chromosomes to duplicate themselves. The normal number of chromosomes is then present but instead of one half coming from the father and the other half from the mother, the genetically altered eggs contain two identical halves from the mother.

Implanted into the uterus of an adult mouse, the eggs undergo normal development to result in mature mice. The mouse pups, of course, are not true clones since their genetic codes are not identical to that of the mother. But this can be accomplished by adding another step. Taking the half-cloned mice produced previously, the process is repeated. The eggs are again impregnated with male sperm to trigger embryonic activity, removed from the female, and the male genes removed. Chemical treatment will again result in a doubling of the female's chromosomes. The offspring born in this second step will be true clones because they will be exact copies of their mother's genetic code (but not their grandmother's). Laser irradiation of the father's genes to inactivate them after they have entered the egg has also proven effective in some experiments. The catch to this technique of replicating only the female genetic material contained within the egg is that it is possible to clone only females.

Another experimental approach for cloning which may circumvent this latter obstacle considers using cancer cells. According to some theories, cancer cells are not switched down to selectively shut off the genetic information as in the case of normal cells. Using cancer cell nuclei as donors, this roadblock to development may be breached. The results of successful implantation could be startling if not unpredictable. Further experimentation may provide some insights here.

Methods for introducing donor nuclei into enucleate eggs have been developed in a number of laboratories. Cellular fusion is now a routine laboratory procedure facilitated by inactivated virus, such as Sendai virus, and by some chemical agents, especially PEG, polyethylene glycol. Somatic cell geneticists regularly employ this method to study human chromosome mapping. In this procedure, human somatic cells are fused with cells of another species, for example, mouse or rabbit cells. Cell fusion techniques have also succeeded in pairing together enucleate mouse egg cells with adult mouse cells. The fused cells go through several stages of development. It seems reasonable to expect that within the next few years, fusion of an enucleate mammalian egg with an adult cell from the same species will be accomplished. If the combination proves to be viable such that the complete genetic catalogue can be read-out, and successful implantation into a prepared uterus is accomplished, cloned mammals can be produced in single steps and quite easily.

By whatever technique the first mammalian clones are produced, it is almost certain to be followed by a rush to clone a variety of animals, especially livestock. Champion breeds could be propagated in perpetuity for their meat or milk production without running the risk of losing a prized genome in the randomness of sexual recombination.

Dr. Clement Markert, a Yale University biologist who was an early pioneer in the area of cloning, is educating university veterinary faculties in cloning purebreed livestock. Scientists thus will be able to pick and choose different kinds of genetic traits and create the animals they want almost overnight, a process that now takes many years through selective breeding. It is also interesting to note that a recent scientific report discussed attempts to reproduce superior Douglas fir trees from single cells. The experiments seek to develop a method that will bypass growth of trees from seeds and instead produce them from living cells of desirable strains that are resistant to disease and insects, and that grow rapidly. The step to the first clonal human might require a few additional years but could occur within our lifetime, as early as the 1980s, if the technical problems can be solved and society has the will to proceed with the necessary research.

Such research can and has been proceeding at a rapid rate with little public attention. In June of 1976, three scientists reported the successful birth of a baboon infant produced by embryo transfer.[4] An embryo was recovered surgically from an inseminated female baboon and transferred to a nonmated synchronous female. After a normal gestation time of 174 days, a male baboon was born. Recall that baboons are primates, the order to which humans also belong.

Perhaps as a portent of things to come was the shocking revelation in newspapers across the country that a human was cloned; its birth reportedly took place in December, 1976. Author David Rorvik, in a book entitled *In His Image* (Lippincott, 1978), detailed the presumed creation of a boy from the single cell of a wealthy unidentified man somewhere outside the United States in a land "beyond Hawaii." The method supposedly used was the one set forth earlier in this chapter, namely, the insertion of a donor adult human cell into an enucleated human egg subsequently carried to full term by a surrogate mother. However, because of the apparent barriers to development with this technique, as previously explained, most scientists were extremely skeptical of the report.

The furor over the alleged baby clone brought to the public's attention concern over the possible ramifications if such an event does in fact occur. A movement spearheaded by a group of concerned scientists and Congressman Paul G. Richards (D–Fla.) called for an open hearing to lay the issue out before the Congress and the public. The urgency of the issue was voiced by Jeremy Rifkin, spokesperson for the Washington-based People Business Commission, in these words: "we're worried that we're too close to cloning for comfort; even if the book is a hoax, all our values would be upset if we could xerox life." We will pursue this issue further in a subsequent chapter (see Chapter 5h, Cloning).

One might inquire why anyone would want to clone humans. We list a few of the reasons:

1　Replication of individuals of great genius or beauty to improve the species or to make life more pleasant.

2　Replication of those adults proven to be healthy, bypassing the risk of genetic disease inherent in the chance mechanism of sexual recombination.

3　Acquisition of large numbers of genetically identical humans for scientific studies, e.g., the relative importance of nature and nurture for various aspects of human behavior as in the determination of intelligence.

4　Provision of a child to an infertile couple.

5　Acquisition of a child with a genotype of one's own choosing—someone famous, a departed loved one, one's spouse, or oneself.

6　Control of the sex of future children (the sex of a cloned offspring must be the same as that of the adult from whom the donor nucleus was taken).

7 Production of sets of identical persons to perform special occupations in peace and war.

8 Production of replicas of each person who would be the equivalent to identical twins. These could be frozen away at some stage in development until needed as a source for personal organ transplants.

9 Prevention of a "cloning gap," that is, to beat the Russians and Chinese.

Do any of these have appeal?

Embryos can be maintained in culture for relatively short periods of time while they are growing, but they cannot be stored for a prolonged time as is frequently desired for some kinds of research. For example, if the scientist wants to keep a desirable strain of experimental animal for later research, the animal must be maintained in breeding colonies, a process which is both time-consuming and expensive. It would be far better if the organisms—or their embryos—could be stored until they were needed. Recently, researchers at the Oak Ridge National Laboratory in Tennessee found that they could freeze mouse embryos, thaw them out, and reimplant them in foster mothers where they completed development into normal mice. Using this method, frozen embryos can be stored, thawed, and grown to full term in foster mothers. Embryos have been freeze-stored for as long as one year with 80 percent survival of the thawed embryos. Rabbit embryos, too, have been frozen and successfully revived to develop into normal healthy rabbits. (See Fig. 3.7.) The particular significance of this later work with the larger, more sensitive, and complex rabbit embryos raises the real possibility that these or similar procedures may be applicable to the primates. For such freeze-thawed individuals, time has stopped during the period when they are frozen.

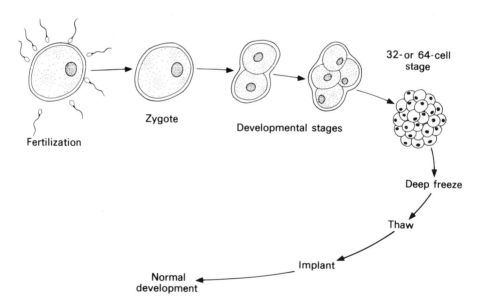

Fig. 3.7 *Freeze-storing of embryos.*

The potentials for this technology are great. For instance, this method has already been used to ship embryos long distances. Frozen embryos are cheaper and easier to transport since they do not require special handling during shipment and they are much smaller than an adult animal; they also are less likely to carry diseases, such as hoof and mouth disease, across boundaries. Application of this technique to humans should be obvious. Couples may be able someday to store their own conceptuses produced at a time in their lives when they themselves are most healthy and bring them to term later when they decide to live a more settled life. It is generally agreed that persons in their early twenties are at their reproductive optimum. On the other hand, if they decide not to personally bring the stored embryo to term they could contribute them to other couples in whom there is mutual sterility or uncorrectable genetic hazards. Further, banking ova will eliminate the need of repeated surgical extraction of eggs for egg transfer from wife or donor. Genetic twinning may also be possible. An embryo could be grown using an adult nucleus, transplanted to a human egg, and stored away frozen until such time as a spare organ is required. At that time it could be thawed and grown to the proper stage in a foster parent.

In the matter of organ transplants, it might prove safer or more efficient to transplant ovaries or tubes rather than eggs to females suffering from defects in these organs. Much progress of late is being made in understanding the immune reaction with the very real possibility that it will someday be controlled. Testes could also be transplanted, obviating the need to go to sperm banks. But whose genes are being transferred in reproduction?

Another line of research using mild enzyme treatment has succeeded in dissociating embryos at early stages. In these experiments, two sets of parents are involved. Each parental set produces an embryo in the normal way. Enzyme treatment breaks up the resulting embryos into single cells. The cells of two or more such dissociated embryos are then combined. Upon removal of the enzyme, the mixture of cells will reaggregate to form one whole embryo. The reaggregated embryo continues the developmental process as if nothing happened. Reimplantation in a female completes fetal development. (See Fig. 3.8.) Such individuals would be normal except that they would have more than two parents! Offspring of more than two parents are called allophenes, or more properly, chimeras. These kinds of experiments reveal that mammalian embryos are much more malleable than was formerly thought. This approach for producing offspring in humans has not been done, although some of the techniques coming from chimera research suggest ways for propagating segments of foreign mammalian DNA in recipient mammalian organisms—a topic we will return to shortly.

The human placenta, that vital link between the fetus and the mother, is perhaps one of the most remarkable of all structures associated with the creation of a new human being. The placenta acts as a lung, liver, and kidney for the growing fetus. As a lung, it takes oxygen from the mother's bloodstream and passes it through its own blood vessel in the umbilical cord to the fetus inside the uterus; as a liver, it nourishes and protects the fetus; and as a kidney, it removes wastes from the growing embryo. These several functions are accomplished by millions of tiny finger-like projections called villi that root the placenta into the endometrium of the

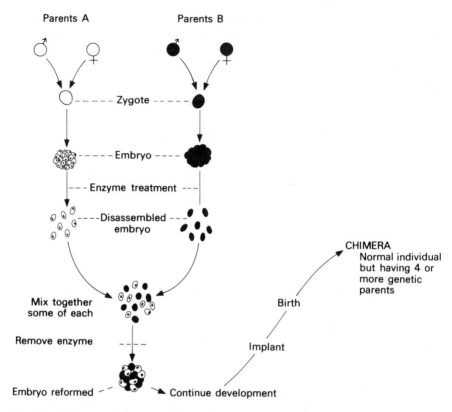

Fig. 3.8 *Chimera production—the product of four or more parents.*

mother. One means of visualizing the complexity of this unique organ is to imagine that if the number of villi were laid end to end, they would form a carpet extending 30 miles. Through the placenta and umbilical cord to the fetus pass as much as 75 gallons of blood a day toward the end of pregnancy. (See Fig. 3.9.)

Despite its complexities, scientists hope to duplicate the placenta in the laboratory. If they can, it will provide a marvelous tool with which to study the fetus. At Stanford University, one such artificial womb has been developed. The artificial womb, or fetal incubator, is an extremely complex apparatus. (Some have called its product a test-tube baby, but it is much more than a test tube.) It is built of stainless steel, about twice the size of a pressure cooker. Feeding in and out of the chamber are numerous tubes to carry nutrients and oxygen, along with gauges and valves controlling what goes in and out. The fluid inside the chamber is under intense pressure equal to 540 feet beneath the surface of the sea. Eight-, nine-, or ten-week fetuses, the products of spontaneous abortion, have been placed in the artificial womb. The womb has kept them alive for up to 48 hours. The problem lies in the incompleteness of the system; the artificial womb cannot dispose of wastes, such as CO_2 and urea. It is important to note that these experiments using aborted human fetuses have been discontinued as a result of a recent government ruling barring this

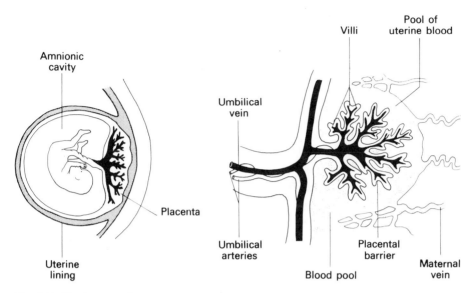

Fig. 3.9 *The human placenta.*

form of fetal research (see Chapter 5e, Experimentation using the human fetus). However, work with nonhuman organisms is continuing. Experiments using fetal lambs have kept some of these alive for 55 hours. Here, too, we can expect improvement in the technology, if that be our wish.

Considerable progress has been made in growing other mammalian embryos in the laboratory and research is proceeding with them. Mouse and rat embryos have been grown for about one-third of the total gestation period, up to and including the beating heart stage.

It should be emphasized that although no scientist at present appears to be interested in going from fertilization to birth entirely in the laboratory, the technology to do so is gradually being worked out piece by piece. It should be stressed that these techniques are being studied to better understand human embryonic and fetal development, with the objective being to improve the quality of babies born, *not* to bring about the baby hatcheries of the kind described in Aldous Huxley's *Brave New World*.

For example, perhaps the most dramatic practical advances have been made in the treatment of premature babies. Less than two decades ago, hope was slim for most of 233,000 babies born prematurely each year. Many died soon after birth. Now thousands are being saved, and many others who might have been permanently incapacitated or retarded are growing up to be normal, healthy children. Among the methods commonly used to save premature infants with breathing difficulties is a technique known as CPAP—continuous positive airway pressure. By inserting a tube in the baby's windpipe or placing a pressurized hood around the head, doctors can direct a continuous supply of low-pressure air to the sacs of the immature lung, preventing them from collapsing. Newborn intensive-care units, also, use skin sensors that continuously monitor oxygen and other blood gases, and use infusion pumps that deliver intravenous fluids to the infant's bloodstream at a preset rate through a tiny tube inserted in the umbilical cord. But, putting these techniques aside since the preemies are already born, one could quite rightly ask—why do these researches? Would there be any value in ectogenesis (birth outside the womb)? Some affirmative answers can be given:

1 Improvement of fetal medicine, including fetal surgery (as one doctor in the area says, "We don't even know what a sick fetus looks like; how can we effectively treat it?" Fetal medicine has been compared to a doctor administering to a patient who is contained inside a barrel on the dock).

2 Immunization of the fetus against childhood diseases.

3 Reduction in birth defects (fetal incubators do not smoke, drink alcohol, contract measles, or fall down stairs).

4 Fuller realization of one's genetic potential (oxygen deprivation, especially during the late stages of development, frequently results in lowered physical and mental abilities in the newborn).

5 More efficient sexing.

6 Convenience.

7 Population control.

8 Others?

Do these seem to present valid justification for the continuation of research on fetal incubators? At this point in time, society shows much hesitation in pursuing this work further, although some scientists disagree with this point of view.

If much of the present research in genetics and development has as its objective the alleviation of human suffering, especially at the beginning stages of life, how significant are congenital defects in the total field of medicine? The answer is that they are enormously significant. Birth defects still loom as one of humankind's serious problems even in affluent societies. Defects at birth dooming the individual to an early death or to a lifetime of illness take an enormous toll of human life and human potential. For example, a deformed child is delivered into the world once every 30 seconds. Hospital records in widely scattered parts of the world reveal that approximately one percent of all infants born alive suffer serious disorders ranging from harelip to anencephaly (a condition in which the bony braincase of the brain itself is absent). In other words, one baby in 100 who survives fetal growth is born with a defect so serious that the infant either dies early or is severely handicapped. In the United States alone, 250,000 infants are delivered each year with significant birth defects with 20 percent due to known genetic causes.

Then there are defects that are not noticeable at birth. Some manifest themselves during the first year after birth (e.g., Tay-Sachs disease); others appear only after many years (e.g., Huntington's Chorea or Chronic Brain Syndrome). When we group together the figures reported for fetal mortality—the stillbirths and spontaneous abortions, the malformations present in infants at birth and abnormalities that do not show up until later in life—the total percentage of major problems in humans is about 5 percent, or one in 20!

Part of body with defect	Frequency of defect per total number of births
Brain and spinal cord	1 per 326
Eye, ear, and nose	1 per 994
Face	1 per 326
Respiratory system	1 per 2000
Heart and circulation	1 per 252
Digestive system	1 per 435
Genitalia	1 per 1151
Urinary system	1 per 1140
General skeletal defects	1 per 994
Congenital hip dislocation	1 per 917
Clubfoot	1 per 524
Limbs reduced or absent	1 per 917
Skin, blood, or endocrine glands	1 per 524
Metabolic defects	1 per 917
Trisomy 21 (Down's syndrome)	1 per 1839
Whole body malformations	1 per 3000

More than 2000 genetically distinct defects are known, as opposed to those imperfections caused by flawed development (e.g., thalidomide babies). One percent of all children born have an abnormal chromosome number; 25 percent of all conceptions are lost through spontaneous abortion, usually because of genetic abnormalities; one of every five sperm or eggs produces one mutation that didn't exist before; there is a 3–6 percent risk with every pregnancy for some major defect. Of all deaths in children's hospitals (not including accidents of one sort or another), 40 percent can be attributed to diseases that are wholly or partly genetic in nature. Today, at least 25 percent of all hospital and institutional beds are occupied by persons suffering from some degree of genetic malfunction. (A more complete treatment of this topic is contained in *Biosocial Genetics* or *Human Heredity and Birth Defects*.[5])

What can be done? The unborn fetus of course has no control over the genes it will inherit; neither does the mother, at least within certain limits. The unborn fetus has no control over the environment it must inhabit, but the mother has some. Increasingly, control can be exerted, and here three levels can be identified—at the preconceptive, at the prenatal, and at the postnatal levels. On all three fronts, breathtaking progress is being made.

At the preconceptive level, the most direct method is to prevent conception from occurring if negative genetic factors are suspected. A number of conception-preventers are available, with the pill and the IUD among the more widely used, although both of these are under suspicion as causing undesirable side effects.

Most of the promise in birth control, both in the recent past and in the foreseeable future, is on the female side. Although in principle, an oral contraceptive for men is entirely feasible, there are a number of practical reasons why such advances are not being made. One is that most research on reproduction has concentrated on the female, probably because (1) the woman's reproductive cycle is more easily manipulated (the male reproductive system, while seemingly simple, is tremendously complex); and (2) the woman's reproductive role is more apparent—she bears the higher cost of reproduction both physiologically and socially.

Alternatives to the daily pill are being tested or marketed. In early 1976, Alza Corporation began marketing Progestasert, a membrane-enclosed, controlled-release drug reservoir. Inserted directly into the uterus, it releases a continuous low dose of the female hormone progesterone. The drug presumably prevents conception by acting directly upon the uterus, rather than suppressing ovulation, as oral contraceptives do. A pregnancy rate of 1.5 percent per year was obtained in experimental testing, as compared to 4 percent for IUD and 6 percent for pill users. Because the drug dosage is low, systemic effects are undetectable and the user has a normal menstrual cycle. Progestasert normally remains effective for about a year, but the device can be removed at any time if the user wants to become pregnant. Clinical tests reveal no signs of the blood clotting disorder that can cause strokes and other vascular problems of the kind arising from the use of oral contraceptives.*

A birth-control pellet that can be implanted directly under the skin by needle and may prevent conception for up to three years is being tested on human volunteers. The pellet, completely absorbable and implanted under the skin of the forearm, may prove effective in men as well as women. The pellet is different from other types of experimental, under-the-skin contraceptives in that it dissolves completely during its one- to three-year life span so the casing does not have to be removed surgically after the drug has been exhausted. The pellet is made of pure progestin, an artificially synthesized birth-control drug and blood-fat concentrate, a type of cholesterol. The progestin is identical to the birth-control drug contained in oral contraceptives. However, because absorption is better than it is when a pill is taken by mouth, the implantation device can use less progestin. It seems likely that the side effects of oral contraceptives would be minimized. If the present tests prove successful, the pellet should be available by the early to mid-80's at a cost that would be only about 1 percent of that using oral birth-control methods.

Another experimental development is an antipregnancy vaccine that would protect a woman against conception for six months to three years. The vaccination could be repeated as often as desired to prevent conception.

A new class of chemicals, the prostaglandins, have proved effective as "morning after" pills. The chemicals, which in effect are chemical abortifacients, have been cryptically named menstrual stimulators, since to some, abortion is a morally repugnant procedure. Prostaglandins are smooth muscle stimulators found widely distributed in the body. By inserting them directly into the uterus which itself is a smooth muscle organ, contractions are initiated and the uterine contents are expelled; hence the name menstrual stimulators. We can expect that continued

---

* Depo-Provera, an injectable contraceptive, has been shown to be one of the most effective contraceptives known. A single injection provides up to three months' protection against pregnancy. It has not yet been approved for sale in the United States, however, since it is associated with an increased possibility of cancer later in life both for users and for their children.

pharmacological research will result in still safer and more effective contraceptives in the future, including chemical control in males.

No method of chemical contraception is as simple and as safe as sterilization. Sterilization is now the most popular method of fertility control throughout the world. The estimated number of users of the main contraceptive methods worldwide in 1977 were approximately as follows:

Sterilization	80 million
Oral contraceptives	55 million
Condoms	35 million
IUD's	15 million
Other assorted techniques	65 million

Voluntary sterilization is much in demand because of the simplified methods for achieving it and the almost zero care required afterwards; it is simple and it is safe!

Male ligation, or vasectomy, is now a routine office procedure requiring only a few minutes. Millions of these procedures have been performed. Female sterilization by laparoscope, a lens and electrocoagulating instrument inserted through the abdomen, takes only a little longer. The now familiar "band-aid" or "belly-button" surgery are examples. Both operations are legal in all 50 states. Efforts at perfecting reversible surgical sterilization are proceeding and reports of success are publicized by the news media quite regularly. Such devices as a removable metal or plastic plug in the duct or a microvalve which can be turned off and on will make surgical sterilization still more attractive to many in the future.

Contraception and sterilization only control quantity; quality control can also be achieved and a variety of new procedures are now making this possible or are under development:

1   *In vivo* diagnosis of the fetus in combination with fetal medicine and selective abortion.

2   Genetic counseling.

3   Artificial insemination.

4   Eugenics, both positive and negative.

5   Euphenics.

6   Direct genetic manipulation.

Contrary to what was formerly thought, the womb is quite a dangerous place. A growing fetus is vulnerable to many kinds of ills. Congenital defects may be of two kinds: those resulting from environmental factors, such as Rh incompatability, thalidomide, rubella, or ionizing radiation, and those that may be of genetic origin. The three-prong combination of genetics counseling, prenatal monitoring, and selective abortion of seriously defective fetuses has become an effective system of control today. We will postpone a discussion of genetic counseling and abortion until a later time. A more comprehensive study will be devoted to the many psychological and ethical problems involved in their practice (see Chapter 5b and d). Directing our attention to *in utero* diagnosis and prenatal medicine, we see that many dramatic

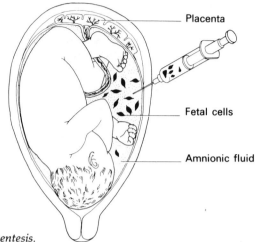

Fig. 3.10 *The technique of amniocentesis.*

advances are being made. In fact, fetal medicine is one of the fastest growing areas of medical specialization today.

The technique called *amniocentesis* is used to detect some genetic defects of fetuses still in the womb. This was one of the first of the genre of methods for *in utero* monitoring. The principle involved is this: The fluid surrounding the fetus contains, among other things, a great many cells derived largely from the skin and respiratory tract of the fetus. In amniocentesis, a small amount of this fluid is withdrawn by needle puncture of the pregnant uterus or extraction through the cervical opening, usually 12 to 16 weeks after conception (Fig. 3.10). The living cells are then removed from this fluid and either directly examined or grown in nutrient broth. After a number of cells have been grown, examination for defects can be carried out. All chromosomal irregularities in which the number or the structure of chromosomes may be abnormal can be identified, as well as about 60 biochemical or metabolic disorders. Rapid progress is being made in the use of this method for diagnosis of metabolic genetic defects. It is predicted by some that by 1980, over 500 biochemical deficiencies may be determined using this method. The latter number interestingly enough represents only about one percent of all metabolic diseases suspected. Therapeutic abortion or treatment of the defect if the technology exists may then follow.

A recent finding (1977) reported that it may soon be possible to use microchemical techniques to detect the presence of genetic disease in fetuses very early. At present, for all practical purposes, tests to detect genetic defects are not possible before the sixteenth or seventeenth week of pregnancy. This poses a serious dilemma. By that time in development, elective abortion becomes more and more fraught with risk to the female. The preferred solution is to carry out the screening at an early stage so that abortion, if it is used, is done at a relatively safe stage. New research may soon make possible the detection of a number of genetic diseases by measuring chemical reactions in single cells extracted from the amniotic fluid or by detecting the presence of abnormalities in the amniotic fluid itself. Prenatal or even preconceptual screening on a large scale will soon probably be possible, reducing the incidence of many genetic disorders.[6]

It has been claimed that fetal medicine is the only branch of medicine in which the patient must be treated without being seen, but direct visualization of the fetus, using fiber optics and magnifying lenses, brings the developing fetus into viewing range of the physician. A large number of abnormalities will become amenable to treatment when this procedure, known as fetoscopy, becomes routine. In Culdescopy, pictures—even motion pictures of the intrauterine environment and its contents—can be made for subsequent study. The instrument used is an endoscope, a tubular, light-bearing device that is inserted into the vagina and placed against the cervix to afford a good view of the uterine contents. For example, in the late stages of pregnancy, if the amniotic fluid appears to be a greenish-yellow rather than amber, the fetus has secreted a substance called meconium. This is a warning sign that the fetus is suffering from oxygen deprivation and must be delivered as soon as possible.

Ultrasonic, high-frequency sound waves are being used to obtain pictures of the placenta and the position of the fetus. A quartz crystal is placed on the woman's abdomen and high-frequency sound waves (2 million cycles per second) are beamed toward the fetus. When the waves reach the fetus, they bounce back and are transformed on an oscilloscope screen into a highly detailed picture of the fetus, the placenta, and other features of the womb. Unlike x-rays, ultrasound does not carry the risks, yet provides more information, since soft tissue can also be depicted. With ultrasound, the physician can determine the exact placement of the fetus, the size of the head, and the location of the placenta, all vital information for predicting complications in labor and delivery. Ultrasound can also be used to guide the physician's needle during amniocentesis, preventing any possibility of harm to the fetus. It can detect fetal life or death, measure growth, and identify a host of possible disorders, including hydrocephalus (water on the brain), uterine tumors, and ectopic pregnancies (pregnancy outside the uterus).

Today, many major hospitals regularly use electronic fetal monitors to keep a careful, moment-to-moment survey over the progress of a mother's labor. The fetal heartbeat may be checked by introducing a thin wire, with an electrode attached, into the uterus and attaching it to the fetus scalp. A slender plastic tube is also placed in the uterus to measure the mother's contractions. Both instruments are connected to a portable recorder that collects data from mother and fetus on a moving graph.

Infrared thermography, radio-opaque dyes, microphones, and other devices are making it possible to monitor, diagnose, and treat problem fetuses. Many fetuses that formerly were lost will be saved, and many others who might have been permanently damaged are growing up to be normal, healthy children. We can expect continued progress here.

Among the therapies available to treat detected problems, complete fetal blood transfusions have enjoyed some success. Rh disease, which less than a decade ago killed 10,000 American infants and caused many thousands more to be born deaf, retarded, or palsied because of the condition, is now virtually a thing of the past. Earlier approaches elected complete intrauterine blood transfusion to remove the destructive antibodies made by the mother. More recently, techniques (since 1968) using a vaccine prevents the formation of destructive antibodies by the mother in the first place. The vaccine must be administered within 72 hours of the mother's first birth, abortion, or miscarriage.

As we learn to more fully diagnose fetal infections, we may be able to inject requisite drugs to fight parasites, bacteria, and viruses like infectious hepatitis, polio, and rubella. Even fetal surgery, still in its experimental stages, may soon deal directly with lung hernias, hydrocephaly, tumors, and cardiovascular defects. A promise of things to come is revealed by a recently reported procedure which involves operating on just-born infants by first draining their bodies of blood followed by dropping their temperatures to about 60°F. Infants can be kept in this condition for up to one hour before being revived. They are, for all intents and purposes, dead. This procedure permits surgeons to perform complex repairs of such defects as malformed arteries or leaky heart chambers, repairs that would not be possible otherwise.

The techniques discussed can be used to detect a variety of defects on fetuses while they are still in the womb, where they can be treated, or, if no treatment is available, they may be aborted. What, however, can be done once the defect is found in a newborn infant? As already mentioned, complex surgery can be performed almost immediately after birth, if need be. In other cases, the missing or defective gene *product* can be supplied to the newborn deficient in that substance. This method is named replacement therapy. Insulin for diabetics or blood clotting factor for hemophiliacs are two examples of this therapy. However, in some genetic defects this method is not effective. Absence of enzymes may result in the build-up of harmful substances in the bloodstream to dangerous levels. Here the attending doctor may take one of several approaches. He may reduce the patient's exposure to the offending material through dietary restriction, if that is the route of entry. For example, PKU can be controlled by placing the child on a low phenylalanine diet. Another approach now being studied is to supply the missing enzyme to the patient in microscopic chemical "cages" implanted under the skin. These allow small amounts of the missing enzyme to leak out into the bloodstream, facilitating cellular uptake of the absent molecule. Direct injection of the missing enzyme is also being tried and shows some positive signs of success, especially in lipid-metabolism defects. Still another experimental approach has attempted organ transplantation to replace the defective organ unable to produce the enzyme(s) lacking. For example, a bone marrow transplant from a normal donor to a patient suffering from some forms of anemia (e.g., thalassemia) may reinstate the vital blood-forming function. Also through bone marrow transplants, immune function has been successfully instituted in infants born without an immune system. Genetically abnormal kidneys can be replaced by normal ones. Although the rejection phenomenon still remains a major obstacle to any of these later procedures, the conquest and control of immune function could make transplantation the major therapy of the future. Collectively, all of these techniques fit under that category of therapies loosely called phenogenesis or euphenics—the control of the development of phenotype or physical expression of the organism.

The best and ultimate treatment would be to correct the actual genetic defect, and recent experiments have shown that this may be theoretically possible in some cases. Man's knowledge in the field of genetics is increasing so rapidly that the ability to manipulate genes inside the living cell in a planned manner is rapidly approaching.

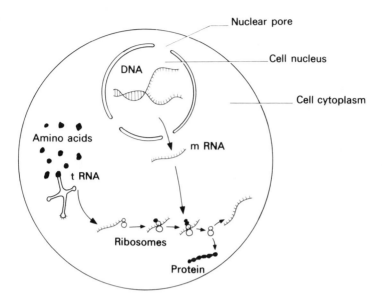

Fig. 3.11 *From DNA to RNA to protein.*

GENETIC ENGINEERING

DNA, the genetic unit of heredity (deoxyribose nucleic acid), is the material equivalent of the gene. It is located in the nucleus of the cell where it acts as a template to produce RNA (ribose nucleic acid). The smaller RNA then passes out from the nucleus into the cytoplasm where it acts as the working blueprint to link together some twenty different amino acids in various combinations to form a vast variety of proteins (Fig. 3.11). The proteins are the "work-a-day" molecules that actually regulate life and, in fact, determine whether or not life will exist at all. The thousands of enzymes that regulate the daily activities of the organisms are proteins, as are many of the structural molecules that provide for the organization of the body.

As a real and identifiable entity, DNA can be artificially changed by direct experimental manipulation. Molecular geneticists estimate that within five to ten years, the following accomplishments will be a reality as a result of genetic and cellular manipulations: production of designed organisms for industrial and environmental processes such as the extraction of gold from low grade ore or the cleanup of oil spills; production of plant cells with transplanted nitrogen-fixing capability; modification of the protein composition of food strains for cereal and cattle feed; the artificial production and cloning of desirable crop strains; the use of artificially synthesized cell systems to produce genes, hormones, phamaceutical products, and food stuffs in volume; and the transplantation of genes for pathogen resistance into crop strains. Within ten to twenty years it is predicted that large-scale tissue and organ culture may be directed for the synthesis of transplantable human tissue such as bone and pancreas. Synthetic "new animals" and "new plants," mutant insect viruses functioning as pesticides, and chimeric animals may also be possible. The treatment of monogenic human diseases may occur in the latter part of this century or the early twenty-first century. Monogenic diseases are the result of single gene mutations. Treatment of polygenic human diseases is not considered likely within the predictable future.[7]

Research related to the above areas is proceeding at a rapid rate with little public attention. Much of the funding to support the research is from private industry, hence not in public view. Thus, breakthroughs in these areas may occur much sooner than predicted, since there are economic considerations at stake. Let's examine some of this work.

The first fully functional gene was chemically synthesized at Massachusetts Institute of Technology in 1976. A research team, headed by Nobel Laureate Har Gorbind Khorana, used a lot of chemistry to synthesize the first human-made gene that worked when it was placed back into a living organism. The gene, a bacterial gene, required nine years to complete. It consisted of 126-nucleotide units composing the structural portion of the gene, plus a 56-nucleotide start signal, and a 25-unit stop signal. The double-stranded synthetic gene also contains overlap of single strands at the ends for joining it to recipient DNA.

The next phase of this team's work will deal with how the structure of the gene influences its function. Since the gene is chemically put together, it is possible to manipulate its structure in a controlled manner to study the influence of structure on function. It is anticipated that much fundamental understanding of gene action will come out of this. The specificity which comes from the chemical synthesis of the gene has the advantage of minimizing the unintended inclusion of other genes which can happen if a gene is taken directly from a living organism. At present, efforts are being made to chemically manufacture the gene for insulin.

Molecular biologists have developed a relatively simple method for introducing specific genes from vertebrates and other organisms into the genome of a host organism. "Alien genes" grafted into species where they were not previously present may be fully functional in the host. The mechanism for doing this is based on an earlier discovery, the discovery of the M-R enzyme system in many cells, including bacterial cells. (The letters M-R stand for modification and restriction enzymes.)

Many cells in their natural environment routinely encounter a variety of foreign DNA's. Foreign DNA is usually present as the breakdown residues of other cells, as, for example, part of the general intestinal milieu resulting from digestion of food stuffs. Organisms can incorporate small amounts of environmental DNA into their own genome usually during reproduction of the cell when internal molecular reorganization and reproduction is taking place. Fragments of incorporated extraneous DNA could genetically alter the host cell but this is undesirable from the cell's point-of-view since its genetic message would become permanently altered if foreign DNA uptake and incorporation occurred. To reduce the chance that this will happen, nature has invented the M-R system. The objective here is to maintain the original cellular DNA while at the same time eliminating extraneous DNA that accidentally enters the cell.

In M-R function, if modification enzymes chemically react with a DNA chunk, that fragment or unit is protected from destructive enzymic action. The protection of this DNA is done by methylating it at certain recognition sites. In this process, a chemical molecule called a methyl group is chemically bonded to the DNA. This stamps the DNA as being "self," hence, safe from destruction. If, on the other hand, methylation does not occur, then the DNA is not recognized as self; restriction enzymes then degrade the DNA into smaller units at the recognition sites since they are not protected by methyl groups. Further enzymic activity ultimately results in the complete molecular fragmentation of the alien molecule, and the integrity of the host cell is maintained intact.

Seizing upon one part of the M-R sequence, scientists recognized that restriction enzymes (there are several of them) in isolation could cleave large DNA macromolecules into fragments, some of which are whole genes. A second fortuitous outcome of this cleavage is that these double-stranded fragments have single-stranded "sticky ends," called that because under appropriate conditions these sticky or single-stranded ends can chemically recombine with other DNA molecules that too have been exposed to restriction enzymes. The result is the formation of a hybrid DNA molecule (Fig. 3.12).

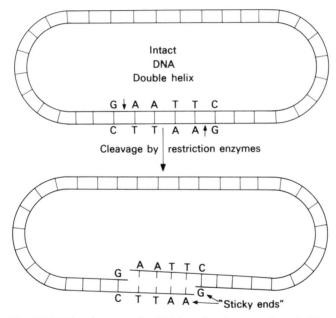

Fig. 3.12 *The cleavage of a DNA molecule to produce "sticky ends."*

The technique using restriction enzymes to form new and sometimes exotic combinations of DNA has become known as *in vitro* recombinant DNA formation or, more commonly, gene-splicing. This process involves taking donor DNA from various sources, including animal and plant cells, and fusing it to a bacterial plasmid. Following successful incorporation into the host bacterial cell, the hybrid DNA synthesizes the product of the introduced gene. Gene-splicing is presently being carried out in bacterial cells because they are simpler to manipulate than those of higher plants or animals.

The typical bacterial cell contains two kinds of DNA: a thread-like chromosome made of DNA and the plasmid (Fig. 3.13). The chromosome has basically all of the genetic information for making the cellular proteins required for overall func-

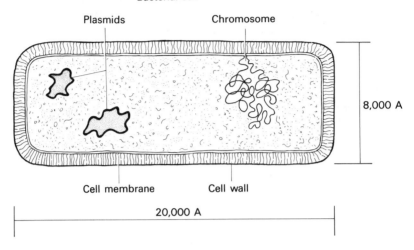

Fig. 3.13 *A bacterial cell.*

tion. Anywhere from 2000 to 3000 genes code for these essential proteins, many of which are the enzymes used by the bacterial cell to perform normal metabolic activity. Plasmids are much smaller than the chromosome; they specify enzymes that perform special functions, for example, the genes coding for antibody resistance. The bacterial cell needs these genes only when there are antibiotics in its environment. The plasmids are also double-stranded DNA but are only about 1 percent of the size of the chromosome. An average plasmid has, therefore, anywhere from twenty to thirty genes. A bacterial cell may have one or many plasmids but only one chromosome. Plasmids then are basically small units of DNA occurring in bacterial cells that carry specific information for secondary characteristics. Secondary responses are usually needed by the cells only in extreme environments.

Since they are discrete units, the plasmids can be isolated from fragmented bacterial cells. The isolated plasmids are fractured using restriction enzymes. Linear fragments of donor DNA similarly treated are then joined with the cleaved circular plasmid by another enzyme called ligase, resulting in the ligation or joining together of a portion of donor cell genes to the bacterial plasmid (Fig. 3.14).

By using a technique called transformation, this hybrid plasmid can be reintroduced into a bacterial cell where the recombined DNA will be replicated as part of the natural bacterial plasmid. Plasmid uptake is facilitated by treating the bacterial cells with calcium chloride. The treatment with calcium chloride presumably makes holes on the cell surface of the bacterium so that plasmids can penetrate the cell. The potential applications of this technique are very great; and, in fact, the promise by enthusiasts that recombinant DNA technology would someday bring handsome dividends seems to be coming true ahead of schedule. A research team at the University of California in San Francisco, headed by Dr. Herbert Boyer, successfully moved the insulin gene from a rat to a bacterial cell by attaching the gene to the bacterial plasmid.[8] However, there was no gene expression. More recently (June, 1978), it was reported by a Harvard research group that a functioning rat insulin gene has been obtained in experiments with the bacterium, *Escherichia coli*. This procedure

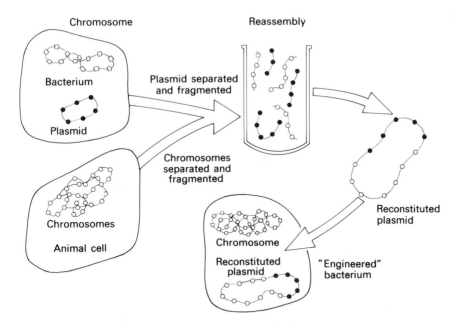

Fig. 3.14 *The formation of an "engineered" bacterium. (From "Biologists draft genetic research guidelines," BioScience 24 (December 1974: 692. Used with permission.)*

whereby enzymes or biological molecules are synthesized under artificial experimental conditions is called enzyme xerography. Of course, for such research to benefit the estimated sixty million diabetics in the world, human, not rat, insulin production is needed. And in fact, the awaited event was announced in September, 1978. Using gene-splicing techniques, a team of California researchers produced human insulin using bacteria into which the human gene for this hormone had been introduced.

The first successful use of recombinant DNA techniques to get a bacterium to produce a substance from a gene of a higher organism was reported in late 1977. Again, it was Dr. Herbert Boyer and his associates at the University of California Medical Center at San Francisco who fused the gene sequence for the human hormone somatostatin to the *E. coli* genome. The combination multiplied and began manufacturing somatostatin. Somatostatin is a hormone in the brain of mammals that inhibits the secretion of pituitary growth hormone. The achievement was hailed as "a scientific triumph of the first order" by Philip Handler, president of the National Academy of Sciences. And indeed it is, for the researchers who first isolated somatostatin from natural sources needed nearly half a million sheep brains to produce a mere 5 milligrams (0.00018 ounce) of the substance. Using recombinant DNA techniques, the California group required only 2 gallons of bacterial culture to obtain the same amount.

Ultimately, such manipulations may make it possible to introduce into human patients genes which will free them from the debilitating effects of a variety of crippling, monogenic, recessive genes. In 1975, researchers synthesized a mammalian gene for the first time. A Harvard research group successfully employed a multistep procedure to construct a rabbit hemoglobin gene. Another recently discovered enzyme, reverse transcriptase, was essential to this synthesis. Reverse transcriptase has the property of reversing the more general flow of gene information: DNA — RNA — protein is reversed to read RNA — DNA. A Nobel prize was awarded to David Baltimore and Howard Temins for the discovery of reverse transcriptase in 1975.

The Harvard scientists began their synthesis of the hemoglobin gene by isolating a purified strand of rabbit messenger RNA that carries the genetic instructions for building rabbit hemoglobin. Using reverse transcriptase enzyme, they were able to make a DNA single-strand coding for the hemoglobin. By using another enzyme, DNA polymerase, a second complementary strand of DNA was attached to the first. Transferring this gene to the plasmid of a bacterial cell, relatively large quantities of genetic material can be synthesized quite easily. This process of manufacturing copies of a single gene is called gene cloning. (See Fig. 3.15.)

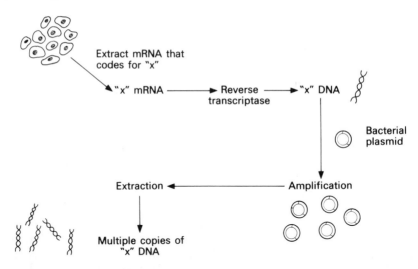

Fig. 3.15 *The method of gene cloning.*

Using these procedures, it is theoretically possible to take any purified messenger RNA and make from that the double-stranded DNA. Incorporating these genes into genetically deficient adult individuals or into embryonic or fetal tissue identified to be genetically defective using the techniques earlier described, the defects could be corrected and normal functions restored. Indeed, this is the latest theory for combining a variety of techniques discussed in this chapter to correct genetic defects or, alternatively, to incorporate new (i.e., superior) genetic information into a recipient organism.

A source of preferred donor DNA is either the method using reverse transcriptase or the restriction enzyme procedures. This purified DNA is cloned in procaryotic organisms (bacteria) by plasmid incorporation. The numerous copies of the preferred DNA are then introduced into a cell culture of mammalian cells where uptake into the mammalian genome will occur, albeit at this time at a rather low level of incorporation. The transformed mammalian cells are injected into an early embryo (at the blastocyst stage) to form a chimera. Implantation and subsequent development in a mammalian uterus could result in an organism fully possessing the introduced genetic features.[9] In principle, every one of these steps is feasible; experimentally, all have been researched. Their coming to fruition awaits only technological refinements. And that doesn't seem too far away!

Some scientists are optimistic that genetic engineering can be used to increase plant productivity and thus help ease the world food problem. Using the new gene-splicing techniques, genetic material may be moved from one organism to another entirely different life form, not only to bacterial cells. In the case of food production, biologists are working on the problem of increasing the efficiency of nitrogen fixation or nitrogen capture systems. These systems are controlled genetically. To accomplish this objective, the genes for nitrogen fixation, called *Nif* genes, may theoretically be spliced into the genome of common food plants that do not fix nitrogen. Nitrogen is an important plant nutrient and is usually supplied as a chemical fertilizer in modern technological agriculture. A significant advance in that direction came in a report from Dr. Fred Ausubel of Harvard University, whose laboratory has succeeded in establishing the sequence of gene coding for nitrogen capture in a bacterium called *Klebsiella*. This kind of information is basic to controlling the nitrogen fixation process. Enhancement of the capacity to fix nitrogen may be only a few years off for the legumes—soybeans, alfalfa, clover, and peanuts; some time after that, cereal plants such as wheat and corn may have the nitrogen fixing genes as part of their genetic makeup.

The range of applications of the new recombinant DNA techniques is limited only by the imagination of the scientists. Other benefits, present and potential, suggested by researchers in this area, include the following:

Basic research

Cloning quantities of complex animal DNA for study material;

Transferral of animal or plant genes from their normal environment into bacteria to study mechanisms of gene action;

Additional tool for study of cancer viruses;

Advancement of understanding of bacterial virulence and drug resistance.

Practical applications

Construction of bacterial cells as "factories" for synthesizing medically valuable biological substances such as insulin, pituitary growth hormone, human antibodies, human interferon, or viral proteins for vaccine production;

Gene transplantation to help cure human hereditary diseases;

Use of engineered organisms to clean up environmental pollution such as oil spills;

Genetically construct new organisms for weapons in biological warfare;

The extraction and purification of minerals from low grade ore.

It would seem that recombinant DNA techniques have brought us to the threshold of direct genetic intervention into areas as far apart as industry, agriculture, medicine, and war. Sidney Brenner, a British molecular biologist, captured the essence of this capability in the following words:

> I would expect this technique to be comparable in impact to the use of radioactive isotopes as tracers in biology . . . It's going to be very widespread. Simply, it's going to allow us to tackle for the first time problems of the molecular genetics of higher organisms—*of anything:* elephants, sea urchins. It'll make a lot of things obsolete, the possible easier, the impossible possible. It is fully as important as radioactive isotopes— probably no more profound in the questions it can reach. Why? Because these things self-replicate. You have a way of enhancing yield. You can detect things. You can put together combinations . . . even biological systems since the dawn of time have not had an opportunity to explore the complete range of combinations now suddenly possible. And, in principle, for any new combination we can make the probability (of success) one. One is a very large number (in matters such as these). We can put duck DNA and orange DNA together—with a probability of one.[10]

To some people, the possible applications of recombinant DNA molecule research are a cause for concern. Like many scientific discoveries, this one, too, carries the potential for evil as well as good. A discussion of this matter follows in Chapter 4.

The widely publicized experiments with hybrid DNA represent only a small part of the studies in what might be called molecular genetic engineering. The literature describes an enormous number of experiments in which genes have been manipulated either as donor genetic material or as host genetic targets. One area that particularly attracted attention is the insertion of alien genes into recipient organisms.

A number of approaches to inserting genes into a host organism have been tried. One experiment used the so-called "piggyback" technique. This is done by hitchhiking a gene to an infectious but non-disease-producing virus particle in piggyback fashion. The virus infects a cell in normal viral fashion and in the process deposits the new gene in that cell. The host cell accepts the alien gene as one of its own and manufactures the product of that gene (Fig. 3.16). A genetically diseased cell can theoretically be restored to normal if the correct gene can be inserted. In fact, this experiment has been successfully carried out in bacteria. Galactosemia is a genetic defect in which the gene for the manufacture of the enzyme galactosidase is missing. Bacterial cells defective in this function can be given the specific gene, using virus carriers, permitting the cell to manufacture the missing enzyme. Laboratory-cultured human cells deficient for a specific enzyme have had the missing function restored by inserting the gene, using a bacterial carrier as well.

Two German children suffering from a genetic disease argininemia were treated with a virus carrying the gene for the enzyme arginase. The disease results in a disruption of the urea cycle because the enzyme arginase is missing. In the case of the children, they were also epileptic, spastic, grossly retarded, and becoming progressively worse. Injection of the virus particles did provide momentary remission. Thereafter, the children generally improved. However, it was not certain whether this improvement was related to the virus-carried gene or was an effect of the low protein diet on which they were also placed.

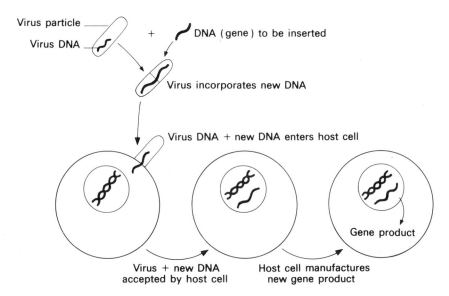

Fig. 3.16 *The piggyback technique of inserting foreign DNA into a host cell using a virus particle as carrier.*

Purified DNA has been introduced directly into mammalian cells. Hypertonic shock or calcium phosphate gel can increase the uptake of foreign DNA manyfold over that which might normally enter via virus infection. Cultured mammalian cells are capable of taking in whole mitotic chromosomes added to the medium. These extranumerary chromosomes, or chromosome fragments, occasionally become established in the cells and replicate. Cell fusion techniques previously discussed have been used to introduce whole chromosomes or parts of chromosomes into cells. In all of these experiments, the yields were not high—the rate of successful and subsequent functional uptake is generally in the neighborhood of one percent or less. There may be mechanisms within cells which prevent massive incorporation of foreign DNA. If these mechanisms can be found, cells could be manipulated to enhance the success rate.

Transplantation of tissue to transfer genes has been referred to earlier. In certain genetic diseases the deficient protein is intracellular and cannot be successfully introduced from the outside. Transplantation of normal cells or organs is a way around this. An example is bone marrow transplantation in sickle cell disease or thalassemia. However, this is not a satisfactory general solution now. The problem of transplant rejection is a limitation; furthermore, the involved organs are not always those that can be transplanted readily (e.g., liver).

One way around some of these problems of DNA incorporation uses whole sperm. Sperm are haploid cells; that is, they contain but half of the genetic information of the future organism. Under experimental conditions, sperm taken from subjects normal for some trait can be induced to enter cultured cells. The host cells may be deficient in that trait. In a fraction of these cultures, sperm spontaneously fuse with the cultured cells, contributing a part of their genetic material to these deficient cells. According to this scheme, inborn errors of metabolism might be corrected by growing deficient cells in tissue culture along with sperm from a normal individual. After a period of time, the transformed cells could be reinjected into the patient. As the cells begin to multiply, the person suffering from the deficiency would be able to produce enough enzyme to restore metabolism to some normal level. This procedure may circumvent the immune rejection mechanism, the problem encountered when whole tissue transplants are used.

SOME RESERVATIONS CONCERNING GENETIC ENGINEERING

In this chapter, we have glimpsed a few of the many developments arising from the rapidly growing field of genetics and development. Many more could be described. Enough has been said, though, to communicate the idea that genetic and developmental engineering is not science fiction. Rather, the research presently going on and the speed at which new knowledge is being gained in these areas suggest that at least this phase of the biological revolution is real. Of Fletcher's eight ways of baby-making, modern medical and biological science has something to contribute to each. While there are still great gaps in our knowledge of how many of these mechanisms will find application in humans, it is highly probable that within the next few decades we shall be able to duplicate many of them in human subjects. Great benefits for humankind can be realized; alternatively, a veritable Pandora's box of evil may be opened.

To conclude this section, some reservations about genetic manipulation need to be expressed. According to some expert opinion, much more is being promised than can possibly be delivered, at least within the foreseeable future. A number of reasons can be advanced to support this claim.

First, most traits in humans are not controlled by single genes; rather, they are polygenic—many genes contribute to a single trait. For example, according to some estimates as many as 250 genes may be involved in the expression of the single trait of human intelligence. Moreover, each gene itself is polymorphic; that is, it is capable of existing in a variety of forms called alleles. Although protein products of alleles are similar, they are not identical; they differ markedly in activity. The genes that control eye color are one example. The pupil of the eye can take a variety of shades, including none at all. It is thought that the vast majority of human traits—literally hundreds of thousands—and especially those most important in determining humanness—intelligence, temperament, personality, physical structure—are polygenic. This compares to probably a few hundred that are monogenic. With polygenic traits geneticists are not talking about a single gene as the determiner of phenotype for a given trait but about a large number of genes; each contributes something and each may take one of a great variety of forms. Add to this that our understanding of polygenic inheritance is still extremely primitive compared to what is known about single-gene inheritance and it becomes highly problematical, if not impossible, that the simple insertion of single genes can significantly alter human behavior. At least for now it is but the far-out stuff of which science fiction is made. Understanding of the distinction between monogenic and polygenic inheritance is clearly important if the public is to distinguish between realistic and wild projections for future developments in genetic intervention in humans. Gene insertion for a few monogenic genetic defects which behave according to classical Mendelian theory and where the mechanisms and biochemistry of that particular gene are understood may soon be possible. But scientists have a very long way to go before they can actively select for highly polygenic *behavioral* traits.

Another hesitation has been expressed in the matter of gene action. Assuming that one has succeeded in incorporating the alien gene into the host's genome, the mechanism whereby that gene is turned on or turned off on schedule must also be functional. In the eucaryote cells of animals and plants, we know next to nothing about the mechanisms of genetic control. Although some understanding has been gained on control mechanisms in procaryote cells, that is, bacterial cells, there is still a giant gap between those cells and mammalian cells. So not only must one isolate and purify a specific gene or gene system out of thousands within the cell, but also the donor DNA must be functional as well. There is no guarantee that insertion will result in expression. (Incidentally, we still do not even know with any certainty the number of genes which comprise the human genome. The number 50,000 structural genes is one frequently referred to "ball-park" number.) What we do know about regulatory function is that it is an extremely complex phenomenon probably involving a variety of factors, genetic as well as environmental. Further, and more serious, when tampering with genetic control mechanisms, the danger of untoward side effects is especially grave since one theory of cancer relates the disease to a genetic control system that has gone awry. The insertion of foreign DNA may significantly increase the risk that the cell or tissue will inadvertently become oncogenic. For these reasons, this single problem of gene control could well prove to be unsolvable and may serve as the ultimate barrier to successful infusion of alien DNA into higher organisms.

But still another problem exists. Even a full set of relevant genes does not fixedly determine a corresponding trait. Rather, most genes contribute to determining a *range of potential* for a given trait in an individual while the past and present environments determine the actual phenotype within the range. Although the study of behavioral genetics in human population is still at an early stage, one can conceptualize the problem with this simple equation: $P_v = G_v + E_v$, where P_v is phenotypic variation, G_v is genotypic variation, and E_v is environmental variation. Heritability, that fraction of phenotype that is due to genes, is not easily determined, at least in humans. The infamous and recent IQ/Race controversy, for example, highlights this difficulty; according to some, IQ has a low heritability of 0.2, while others contend a value of 0.8. No amount of argumentation has yet settled the question. The mechanisms of interplay between genes and environment are certainly complex ones, where predictability, if possible at all, is statistical only. The lesson here is quite clear: Even though one may have within his or her genome the genes of an Einstein, there is no reason at all to predict that an Einstein, in fact, will be the product. It has been shown that one cannot produce identical personalities even when identical genes are present, as, for instance, with identical twins. A genotype does not predict in anywhere near linear fashion a specific phenotype.

What these few examples illustrate is that genetic engineering—at least in humans—is still largely one of theory rather than practice. "Humans are less likely to improve by newer genetic technologies than by manipulation of the environment or enhancement of educational techniques," says Sir Francis Crick, Nobel Laureate of "double helix" fame.

REFERENCES

1 Joseph Fletcher, *The Ethics of Genetic Control* (Garden City, N.Y.: Doubleday/Anchor Press, 1974), p. 40.
2 H. J. Muller, "What genetic course will man steer?" *Bulletin of Atomic Scientists* (March, 1968): 6–12.
3 Mark S. Frankel, "Human-semen banking: social and public policy issues," *Man and Medicine* 1, 4 (1976): 289–309.
4 Duane C. Kraemer, Gary T. Moore, and Martin A. Karmer, "Baboon infant produced by embryo transfer," *Science* **192** (1976): 1246–1247.
5 Gerald James Stine, *Biosocial Genetics* (New York: Macmillan, 1977); E. Peter Volpe, *Human Heredity and Birth Defects* (Indianapolis & New York: Bobbs-Merrill, 1971).
6 "Single cell analysis aids clinical chemists," *Chemical and Engineering News* (April 11, 1977), pp. 39–40.
7 B. B. Hoskins, J. T. O'Connor, T. A. Shannon, R. Widdus, and J. F. Danielli, "Applications of genetic and cellular manipulations to agricultural and industrial problems," *Bioscience* **27**, 3 (1977): 188–191.
8 "Insulin gene transferred to bacterium," *Chemical and Engineering News* (May 30, 1977), p. 4.
9 Robert Pollock, in a book review *(Teratomas and Differentiation), Science* **194** (1976): 1272.
10 Sidney Brenner in "Fearful of science" by Horace Freeland Judson, *Harpers Magazine* (June 1975): 70–76.

BIBLIOGRAPHY

Etzioni, Amitai, *The Genetic Fix* (New York: Macmillan, 1973).
Halacy, D. S., Jr., *Genetic Revolution* (New York: New American Library/Mentor, 1974).
Lappe, Marc, and Robert S. Morrison (eds.), *Ethical and Scientific Issues Posed by Human Uses of Molecular Genetics* (New York: New York Academy of Sciences, 1976).
Leach, Gerald, *The Biocrats* (New York: McGraw-Hill, 1970).
Ramsey, Paul, *Fabricated Man* (New Haven: Yale University Press, 1970).
Rorvak, David, *Brave New Baby* (New York: Doubleday, 1971).
Rosenfeld, Albert, *The Second Genesis: The Coming Control of Life* (New York: Arena, 1972).

4

SHOULD GENES BE TAMPERED WITH?— THE RECOMBINANT DNA CONTROVERSY

THE PROBLEM

Gene-changing experimentation and the related reproductive technologies are now burning social issues. The fantasy that was science fiction but a few years ago has turned into near-reality. The fact that it is happening is not at all surprising, for the tremendous successes of science over the past few decades have made the understanding of the processes related to life's beginnings inevitable; what is amazing is the astonishing rapidity with which it is happening. It has been only a little over ten years that the first cloned vertebrate, a toad, was reported by John Gurdon in England; five years ago, through the chemical manipulation of the genetic machinery of bacteria, it became possible to use the bacterium *Escherichia coli* as a factory for the preparation of segments of DNA from any organism.

The popular media call public attention to one interesting development after another: Scientists successfully synthesize a gene; clonal reproduction from cells of a single frog; offspring produced by embryo transplants; the genetic nature of a cell changed by injecting a deficient cell with healthy genetic material drawn from another totally different species; plant and animal chimeras; and gene-splicing. The list seems almost endless. These and other related developments call our attention to the fact that we are on the brink of a "genetic revolution." The formulation of this new technology could change society at least as profoundly as has atomic energy. This is what Robert Sinsheimer, molecular biologist from the University of California, observed at a recent conference on recombinant DNA as he exclaimed, "Science has not taken so large a step into the unknown since Rutherford began to split atoms."[1] And, indeed, one reporter likens the discovery of gene-splicing to the development of the first atomic devices. Robert Oppenheimer, one of the prime scientists in the World War II Manhattan Project, is reputed to have said following detonation of the first bomb, "Physicists have now known sin." Biologists, too, may be moving out of the age of innocence with the discovery of the new method for genetic manipulation using recombinant DNA techniques.[2]

One of the most controversial issues in recent years to agitate the scientific community, government officials and lawmakers at federal, state, and local levels, and the general public is the question of how we should deal with research on recombinant DNA. Should it be done at all? And if so, under what limits and safeguards? And who should set the limits and enforce safeguards? Concern for these questions has aroused concern at the highest levels. Former President Ford in September of 1976 sent a memorandum to the heads of all major federal departments and agencies. The memo related the formation of a new Interagency Committee of the federal government whose mission was "to review federal policy on the conduct of research involving the creation of new forms of life."

The main ground of the recombinant DNA debate is by now well trodden, but the arguments go on. The literature is literally overwhelming, and the relative positions continue to arouse an unusual degree of antagonism and vituperation between conflicting scientific camps. This conflict has generated a push calling for federal legislation and regulation. This is a first-time event in the history of science in the United States. Needless to say, some scientists warn that legislation could endanger free scientific inquiry in general and the future of a whole field of highly valuable research in particular. Determining the course of basic laboratory research by legislative fiat constitutes a dangerous precedent for future government intervention into the whole scientific enterprise. On the other side is the public anxiety that, while the research could increase our understanding of genetics and result in benefits to humankind, it may also be responsible for the creation of new diseases or ecological disruptions or of doing irreparable genetic damage to future generations.

It early became recognized that there are real ethical implications associated with this state of the art. And these ethical dilemmas transcend the domain of the molecular biologist. The consequences may have heavy impact on the public so that the issue of regulation can no longer be considered solely an internal problem to be settled by the biologists. Social, political, and philosophical factors have become part of this volatile matter. The wisdom over proceeding with this research, as well as the controversy over the adequacy and enforcement of present safeguards regulating it, continues to vex scientists, lawmakers, and the concerned public.

To examine the nature of this issue, we will consider the following questions as they were raised by various groups during the gene-splicing controversy:

1   What are the real biological and environmental hazards of this research? What are the benefits of continuing with this work?

2   Should we proceed in an area of potential danger when experts agree that both the risks and benefits of the research are unknown?

3   What safeguards will adequately protect citizens from the dangers of recombinant organisms—assuming the research will continue?

4   What assurances are there that any safeguards will actually be followed and who is to enforce them?

Admittedly, the recombinant DNA question is but a tip of the iceberg in the broader issue of genetic technology. As an earlier discussion demonstrated, far more than gene-splicing research is being conducted in laboratories worldwide. A few of these areas will be taken up in Chapter 5. The furor raised over recombinant DNA research, however, offers an excellent case study to assess effects and guide development of a new technology from a very early stage. No doubt the experience gained here will have application to the other parts of the "genetic revolution." First we will question the benefits as against the risks.

BENEFITS VERSUS RISKS

It is impossible to foresee all the possible uses of so versatile a tool. Here we can note briefly a few of the potential uses. Stanley Cohen, a molecular geneticist at Stanford University, divides these benefits into two principal categories: (1) advancement of fundamental scientific and medical knowledge; and (2) practical applications.[3]

It is with first group benefits—insights into fundamental knowledge—that research biologists are excited; it is this area that the most reliable predictions can be made concerning the uses of these new techniques. Two research problems, especially, lend themselves to these methods: (1) mapping and sequencing of genes in cells including those of humans, and (2) analyzing the mechanisms of gene action including regulation.

Gene regulation is one of the greatest challenges in biology today. The knowledge whereby genes are turned on and off to control differentiation from fertilized egg to mature organism, or the regulation of everyday activities in the cell by gene-switching, is still exceedingly primitive. Further, the loss of normal gene regulation is thought to be a key failing in cell growth, resulting in cancer. What is lacking is a fundamental understanding of the structure and function of genes, and the new methodology provides a strategy for approaching these difficult problems. For example, scientists can begin to learn how defects in the structure and function of genes results in genetic disease and can begin to work out corrective therapies by altering gene function or structure by inserting a missing gene or correcting its malformed parts.

Gene sequencing is also very crucial to a full understanding of regulation. It is now becoming clear that spatial relationships of genes on chromosomes largely determine their function. The presence of a gene or gene complex is not the only requirement that must be met if a certain gene product is to result. Other genes within a complex frequently play "off-on" roles. This, too, will be valuable information for understanding fundamental processes and will also be essential knowledge if gene transplants are to be successful.

On a more practical level, recombinant DNA techniques may permit the construction of bacterial strains that can produce biologically important substances such as antibodies and hormones (see Chapter 3). These approaches could revolutionize the production of antibiotics, vitamins, and medically and industrially useful chemicals by eliminating the costly and exotic procedures presently followed. In the area of vaccine production, we can expect the construction of specific bacterial strains able to produce desired antigenic products so that killed or attenuated disease-causing viruses need not be used. Specific cancer antigens may also be produced in this way.

Other benefits from recombinant DNA research may be realized in the area of food and energy production. The incorporation of genes for nitrogen fixation has already been mentioned. Certain algae are known to produce hydrogen from water by using sunlight and energy. This process, if it could be harnessed, would yield a virtually limitless supply of pollution-free energy; recombinant DNA methodology offers a way in which this problem may be solved. Oil-spill cleanup can be facilitated by manufactured bacteria that have super appetites for the numerous hydrocarbon components of raw petroleum; General Electric has received a patent to manufacture such a bug.

Concerning these later benefits, it is perhaps ironic that some of the most vocal opposition to recombinant DNA research has come from those concerned with issues of the environment. The ability to manipulate the genes of microorganisms offers the potential of more food, more effective utilization of energy resources, and approaches to cleaning up the environment; yet some environmentalists and environmental groups—for example, the Friends of the Earth and the Sierra Club—have taken strong antirecombinant DNA positions.

With regard to the possible risks of these researches, a number of fears about potential hazards have been voiced both from within and outside the scientific community. The capacity to revise and move around genetic materials with relative ease increases the number of potential biohazards. The molecular biologists who developed and first began to use these techniques became anxious about the chances of engineered organisms carrying health-challenging genes being released into the environment. Two classes of hypothetical risks can be conceived: (1) voluntary insertion of a bacterial or viral gene known to be important in disease; and (2) inadvertent change in the biology of a bacterial cell resulting in a severe epidemic. It is the second concern especially that has attracted the general public and is the one most discussed in the current debate. Cause for alarm stems from two sources, namely, the use of E. coli as the experimental organism of choice and the so-called shotgun experiment.

Escherichia coli is a human gut bacterium. It also lives in fish, insects such as beetles, grasshoppers, and flies, and the soils of both densely and sparsely populated regions. It is one of the several hundred different varieties of microorganisms found in the lower bowel of the intestinal tract where it makes up about one to two percent of the total population. It is generally quite harmless and indeed, probably plays an important role in the further breakdown of food particles not digested by our own digestive enzymes. Genetic information in E. coli is carried by both plasmid and chromosomal DNA.

Why would scientists choose a microbe which has cohabited, more or less happily, with us for eons of time to carry out their potentially dangerous research? The answer is that we know so much more about E. coli than about any other organism, including humans. The enormous quantity of accumulated information about this critter dictates that, despite the hazards of genetically changing it into a "new" organism, it remains the experimental organism of first choice. Already, about 20 percent of its genes have been accurately mapped, and its major metabolic pathways have been studied. According to some reports, banning the use of this microorganism would set back genetic research a number of years, since to obtain the same information for another, more acceptable organism would require some time to search out.

E. coli, like all other bacteria, is not a true species. Species boundaries in bacteria are not as sharp as they are in eucaryotes (i.e., cells with nuclei). Genes may transfer from one organism to another, usually mediated by plasmids or viruses. In a process called transformation, an entirely new genetic characteristic or characteristics may be moved from one group to another. Many bacteria, especially evolutionarily related strains, freely exchange genetic information. *E. coli*, then, is a name given to a range of strains with certain features held in common and also with a variety of differences—surface molecules, nutritional requirements, growth rate, and sensitivity to various factors in the environment. There is an almost astronomical number of distinct strains of *E. coli* varying by as much as 25 percent in their genetic compositions. The strain most often used in biological research is designated K12 or a genetically disabled derivative of it. Strain K12 is not a predominant species in the large bowel and, in fact, the available evidence indicates that *E. coli* strain K12 rarely establishes itself as a viable resident in the human gut.[4] Darwinian fitness of an organism is a very important consideration here. Let's examine what this means.

In the gut there is intense competition between bacterial strains and other inhabitants; variables in growth rate, nutritional requirements, adherence to the gut wall, and antimicrobial factors in the host determine survival. Hence, most novel strains are quickly extinguished in the competition with other intestinal residents for available niches in true Darwinian fashion. With bacteria, the battle between strains is over very quickly since generation time, i.e., the life cycle, is as short as twenty minutes and the selection pressures in the intestine are very intense. Strain K12, therefore, is generally incapable of surviving for long outside the laboratory environment. It has been living in laboratories for so long that it has probably lost its power to infect humans. The disarmed bug would then seem to make gene-shuffling experiments relatively safe, for even though a microbe carrying a new genetic combination which contained a pathogenic gene did enter a human host, it would not live long enough to cause an infection whether in the exposed person or in the general public.

What has been said is generally correct, but there is a catch here. As described earlier, DNA can be exchanged between strains in the process called transformation. The donor bacterium need *not* be alive to effect a transfer; a dead cell will do. Now a real risk is encountered since innocuous strains that normally are quite benign in the bowel can be transformed into virulent live strains. For example, if an *E. coli*, K12, carrying the gene for a potent bacterial toxin was taken up in large doses by a human host, the disease-producing gene could be transferred via the plasmid to an actively reproducing and related strain to cause the disease. A strain carrying a tumor virus might also be hazardous. An added difficulty may be encountered here since humans are immunologically unprotected against those bacterial hosts that are indigenous. If a natural inhabitant of the bowel is converted into a pathogen via transformation, it could conceivably initiate a worldwide pandemic since the human immunologic system would not be triggered to destroy the recombinant organism. This is the fear of many who are opposed to recombinant DNA research. Some, like Erwin Chargaff, a biochemist at Columbia University, insist that a complete prohibition against the use of strains found in humans is the only way to prevent this from happening.[5]

Another unpredictable biohazard is made possible by the technique referred to as the shotgun experiment. In this procedure, the whole DNA genome of an organism is chopped enzymatically, using restriction enzymes. Segments of a few genes are then inserted into bacteria for cloning. This kind of experiment is especially advantageous for advancing our understanding of mammalian genes. There is a great deal of uncertainty with these kinds of nonspecific experiments for no one knows what genes or gene fragments are likely to be implanted into the DNA of the bacterial plasmids. If they are incorporated, the host bacillus will continue multiplying them indefinitely. When one clones a gene, he may not only clone one desirable genetic feature but also a strip of DNA with unknown characteristics. The most dangerous of all possible shotgun experiments, some people believe, are those involving the genome of organisms closest to humans, such as other primates, or the human genome itself. In a genotype as large as that found in humans, there probably are some genes of definite potential hazard. For example, the probability exists, though admittedly low, for forming a bacterial strain with a toxic product or for a tumor virus, either one of these picked up from normal donor tissue. Even a gene specifying a human or primate hormone or enzyme could be hazardous to a human host if it were expressed in *E. coli* while in residence in the lower bowel. In 1000 cases maybe nothing would happen and then in one case something very unpleasant might occur. Nobody can predict what form the experiment will take or what the effect of these scenarios might be on a human host—*E. coli* producing estrogen in abundance in the male lower intestine or testosterone in excess in the female gut; or cellulase, an enzyme for breaking down cellulose, a plant structural molecule, becoming widespread in the bowel of either sex. Cellulose, being indigestible by humans, gives bulk to the feces. Should such an *E. coli* gain a selective advantage and spread throughout the population, the result might be a large number of people suffering from chronic, maybe fatal, diarrhea. Or what would be the effect of a bacterial population in the gut actively synthesizing insulin? (*Hint*: Have you ever heard of insulin shock? It can be fatal!) Some of these projections are not as far-fetched as they may sound. A cellulose-containing *E. coli* was put together by scientists at General Electric. The plan was to use the organism to break down plant cellulose and use the products of the digestion—a universal sugar molecule called glucose—in various commercial processes. The human hazards of this research, however, moved the researchers to destroy the organism before any of the scary effects could be realized.

Add one more to these serious reservations: the almost irreversible nature of the mishap, should it occur. If the manufactured organisms escape, and there are some critics who contend that this is inevitable, there is no way to recapture them. The hazard is not like DDT or PCB's or aerosols which can be stopped simply by not using or manufacturing them. These chemicals are ultimately degraded by the environment. Not so with exotic bacteria. They are alive and they may be reproducing out there in you, your children, and your children's children. To some, this is one of the greatest potential threats.

The fears discussed earlier about potential hazards of recombinant DNA research are seen largely as health and safety questions. But these issues are secondary to what Sinsheimer sees as the far broader implication of this research, namely, producing adverse effects on the human gene pool, and closely related to it, the very old worry of human genetic engineering. Sinsheimer, in testimony before the Senate health subcommittee summarized these concerns succinctly:[6]

Senator Kennedy: Do you agree that in terms of magnitude this is of as great significance as the splitting of the atom?

Sinsheimer: What this technology does is to make available to us the complete gene pool of evolution. We can take the genes of one organism and recombine them with those of others in any manner we wish. To my mind this is an accomplishment as significant as the splitting of the atom.

Senator Schweiker: Are you saying that all that has gone before, we now have the power to change in some way—the evolutionary process?

Sinsheimer: Yes.

On the first issue of adversely affecting the human pool, we are dealing with an ethical problem perhaps more than with one in public health. In the words of Erwin Chargaff, "the principal question to be answered is whether we have the *right* to put an additional fearful load on generations that are not yet born." By additional, he means the genetic problem on top of the existing and unresolved fearful problem of the disposal of nuclear wastes. "Our time," he frets, "is cursed with the necessity for feeble men, masquerading as experts, to make enormously far-reaching decisions." Is there anything more far-reaching than the creation of new life forms? Once released, one cannot recall a new form of life. This would constitute an irreversible attack on the biosphere, something Chargaff asserts is "so unheard-of and so unthinkable to previous generations that I could only wish that mine had not been guilty of it."[7] The potentially grievous risks to which he refers might be the spread of slow viruses, a newly discovered class of viruses thought by some to be a cause of cancer, or other new and exotic diseases some of them not yet "made." In plain words, he is saying that we are simply not equipped, intellectually or morally, to deal with dilemmas of such far-reaching import. Truly imposing safeguards bordering on police-state powers must be implemented if this problem is to be dealt with at all warns biologist Chargaff.

In Sinsheimer's view, the question is whether, in the light of what we know of the processes of evolution, it is at all prudent to continue with recombinant DNA research. Interestingly, Sinsheimer, a molecular biologist of some renown himself, was an early advocate of genetic engineering. As late as 1970, he expressed the view that human genetic engineering was the way to escape the bad aspects of our heredity and to improve human intellect and other crucial capacities. Now he believes just the opposite; he warns of the dangers that may accompany the new knowledge, especially the so-called evolutionary question. Why did he change?

In his earlier days, he envisioned genetic engineering as a carefully conceived and controlled process with little or no chance of error. It never occurred to him, for instance, that anyone would do a shotgun experiment. But we can be deceived by our own technology. Biologist Richard Novick poses the problem this way: Suppose a well-intentioned scientist wants to do a potentially dangerous experiment. How should he evaluate whether or not to proceed? Novick claims that the scientist may, in fact, be unable to distinguish between the two alternatives. He is caught up in a conflict of interests as revealed by these positions:

1. I am convinced that the procedures really are not dangerous, and therefore it is okay to do them; or

2. I have convinced myself they are safe precisely because I want to do them![8]

Since one's self-interest is involved, it is terribly difficult, if not impossible, to determine whether or not the experiment should be done. Wide-scale use of these powerful techniques without adequate controls has turned Sinsheimer from an advocate to a critic.

Turning to the evolutionary question, Sinsheimer means by this that some of the genetic manipulations made possible by the new technique may be of a kind which evolution has strongly tried to prohibit. Technically this has been given the name the procaryote/eucaryote barrier. What this means is that in nature the cells of simpler organisms do not routinely exchange genetic material with cells of higher organisms. According to Sinsheimer, this apparent barrier between procaryotes (e.g., bacteria) and eucaryotes (e.g., mammals) has evolved for good evolutionary reasons. For example, the barrier might be there to protect the genetic machinery of higher cells from procaryote take-over. Many recombinant DNA experiments require the insertion of genes of higher organisms (i.e., eucaryotes) into procaryote cells. Transgressing the barrier by artificially creating procaryote/eucaryote hybrids in hundreds of laboratories throughout the world is to risk causing unpredictable and irreversible damage to the evolutionary process brought about by massive mixing of unrelated genomes.

Another belief held by a number of critics (e.g., George Wald, Nobel Laureate in Biology at Harvard University), is that one step leads to another. The recombinant DNA technique is the beginning of the genetic engineering of bacteria, then of plants and domestic animals, and ultimately of humans. This requires that we take on the enormous responsibility for life on this planet and in doing so, we will take future evolution into our very hands. Sinsheimer again provides the clincher to this argument: He insists that we aren't anywhere near clever enough to know what the long-range consequences will be, so we shouldn't even try!

Dr. Harry Hollis, Director of the Committee on Family and Special Moral Concerns of the Christian Life Commission of the Southern Baptist Convention, mirrors this view in these words:

> I feel very strongly that Huxley's warnings have a bearing for us today. After Dachau and Watergate, we shouldn't take lightly what human beings are capable of inflicting on each other. This is not just science fiction. Genetic engineering for the worst of reasons is a possibility in this world in which we live.[9]

The issue of who has the authority to develop and produce new life forms is perhaps the single most important question any society has ever had to grapple with.

The potential for misuse has been seized by a number of other critics. Dr. Ethan R. Signer of the Massachusetts Institute of Technology sees the technique being used by the military for the development of weapons. Drug companies will use it in secret for competitive profiteering. Jonathan Beckwith, also of MIT, refers to advances in genetics along with amniocentesis and postnatal screening for genetic defects, as but another ruse for carrying out social engineering. He raises the specter of a creeping eugenics movement buttressed by "scientific fact." Dr. Beckwith is alarmed over a possible genetic fix for solutions to social problems. He expresses it this way:

> What can be seen is an attempt to transfer social and political problems out of the realm where analysis of the *political system* comes into question, into an era where medical and genetic solutions can be proposed. Political issues are wrapped up in the antiseptic white coat of medicine and the scientific experiment.[10] (Emphasis added.)

This recitation of risks and benefits could continue—for example, on the one hand, the genetic control of human behavior; on the other hand, insertion of a normal hemoglobin gene to correct sickle-cell anemia so prevalent in black populations. However, the major points of contention have been introduced. Let us turn our attention now to the second question posed at the beginning of this chapter: Should we proceed in an area of potential danger when experts agree that both the risks and benefits of the research are unknown?

THE WISDOM OF RESEARCHING THE UNKNOWN

Stanley N. Cohen, who was one of the first scientists to use these new techniques, contends that all objections based on potential risks derive whatever validity they may have from hypothetical, speculative possibilities, not from known, demonstrated phenomena or even from generally predictable events. In an article appearing in the highly respected professional journal *Science*, titled "Recombinant DNA: Fact and Fiction", he says:

> Much has been made of the fact that, even if a particular recombinant DNA molecule shows no evidence of being hazardous at the present time, we are unable to say for certain that it will not devastate our planet some years hence. Of course this view is correct; similarly we are unable to say for certain that the vaccines we are administering to millions of children do not contain agents that will produce contagious cancer some years hence. We are unable to say for certain that a virulent virus will not be brought to the United States next winter by a traveler from abroad, causing a nationwide epidemic of a hitherto unknown disease—and we are unable to say for certain that novel hybrid plants bred around the world will not suddenly become weeds that will overcome our major food crops and cause worldwide famine.[11]

In fact, he goes on to point out that there is no zero-risk in anything that we do using already existing technologies—from influencing the earth's weather, to exploring space, to breeding hybrid plants and animals. Improperly, he states, much of the speculation about potential hazards has been interpreted as being actual fact. Intuition, emotion, and individual value systems are the decisional factors used by many of these critics, rather than data or theories generally accepted within the scientific community. Scare scenarios can be framed on any activity or process and these may be based on much, little, or no fact. It is the latter two categories, he claims, on which much of the opposition to recombinant DNA research bases its stand. "But we must distinguish fear of the unknown from fear that has some basis in fact; this appears to be the crux of the controversy surrounding recombinant DNA."[12] Answering critics became almost a full-time preoccupation for a number of scientists, judging by the number of times their names appeared in print or they were called upon to testify before local, state, and federal agencies and boards.

Moving on to address the specific objections raised by the critics, these responses were given—first, regarding the use of *E. coli* as the experimental organism. Contrary to implications of a number of opponents, the probability of an *E. coli* strain K12 or a disabled derivative of it surviving in the large bowel is almost zero. A very large safety factor is provided by using methods wherein strains of *E. coli* K12 are drastically impaired in their ability to multiply or transfer their plasmid

except under very special conditions provided in the laboratory. One strain designated EK2, for example, has several stable mutational defects (i.e., gene deletions)
that prevent it from multiplying under the nutritional conditions of the human gut.
One of the genetic deficiencies in one strain of EK2 even codes for its own self-de-
struction. These lethal mutant cells require diaminopimelate to form cell walls.
Under laboratory conditions, this chemical (an exotic amino acid) is included in the
culture medium on which the bacteria are grown. Without diaminopimelate, the
cells can continue to grow but they cannot form cell walls, hence, they will lyse or
burst. In the gut, diaminopimelate is always absent; consequently EK2 cannot multiply. It has been found that fewer than 1 cell in 100 million survives after 24 hours.
To ingest 100 million cells at all, a person would have to literally feast on cultures of
the bacterium—and that would be no accident!

Any experimental organism to be used in this research must first pass strict tests
to establish that it is, indeed, unable to live in natural environments. Only then
can it be certified for use by the National Institutes of Health (NIH) for use in experiments that carry a high risk of environmental contamination or are a threat to
personal safety. The tests, furthermore, must prove that the chance of spread in the
event of an accident must be less than 10^{-8} (1 chance in 100 million) before certain
kinds of more exotic experiments are permitted. Probabilities as low as that afford a
high level of confidence, considering the small numbers of organisms that could escape as a result of human error or flaws in the experimental procedure. The defenders of existing techniques insist that thirty years of study with *E. coli* provide reasonable assurance to any rational person that enough is known about them to prevent a contagious epidemic. While some have suggested that an alternative to *E. coli*
K12 be investigated—that is, engineer an organism that is completely and totally
helpless outside of the laboratory environment—it is not at all certain that useful
and safer organisms can be found.

The risk of *E. coli* recombinants—the transformation of benign to virulent
strains—is a real problem, but the risk here, too, as claimed by proponents, is very
small. Despite widespread apprehension over the presumed production of genetic
chimeras, the recombinants envisaged will still be 99.9 percent genetically *E. coli*
with less than 0.1 percent foreign DNA added. This, to be sure, could change the
toxicity of the organism but it would not be enough of a genetic change to radically
expand the habitat of the bug outside the gut. It would certainly be no worse than
the present communicable enteric pathogens such as those that cause typhoid or
dysentery. The Andromeda strain scenario could never be realized by this method.
The problem of minimizing this small risk could be dealt with by following strict
laboratory procedures of the kind presently in use for handling dangerous pathogens. There is, therefore, no realistic basis for public anxiety over this issue, any
more than over the way laboratory work on known pathogens is being conducted
routinely.[13] This was the judgment of those in favor of carrying on experimentation.

A further safeguard against recombination is provided by using the genetically
weakened cells previously mentioned. EK2 cells, for instance, are severely impaired
in their ability not only to multiply in the environment but also to transfer plasmids
to other cells. Certain genes that code for this transmission from donor to acceptor
cell are absent from EK2 plasmids. It has been estimated that the probability of plasmid transfer in the human gut is far below 10^{-16} per recombinant cell per day.

The dangers attendant with shotgun experiments were also enormously exaggerated, insisted the advocates of continued research. Mammalian donor cells have literally tens of thousands of genes, while each bacterial recombinant can contain at most a very few genes (recall the size of a plasmid from the previous chapter). The probability of isolating a strain with genes for a toxic product or for a tumor virus, picked up from tissue presumed to be normal (no experimenter would voluntarily select diseased mammalian cells), is exceedingly low. The laws of probability simply militate against this uptake of extraneous and dangerous alien DNA by a bacterial cell.

In addition, assuming uptake, there is absolutely no guarantee that a gene or gene combination will ever produce anything at all in the new host cell. In fact, there is a good deal of data to suggest that the mechanisms of control here are probably absent and must be actively inserted before the transplanted genes can be made active. For example, researchers succeeded in inserting the insulin gene into a bacterial plasmid but it was still nonfunctional.

Still another rejoinder to the opposition could be best stated in the form of a question: Do the products of shot gun experiments represent a truly novel class of organisms? Newer data suggests that the so-called procaryote/eucaryote barrier is, in fact, breached over and over again in nature. It has been shown that bacteria can take up naked DNA from solution under experimental conditions. In the gut, intestinal bacteria are constantly exposed to fragments of host DNA released by the death of cells lining the intestinal wall (epithelial gut tissue is exceptionally short-lived with a maximum life span of about 38 hours). One can expect, then, that there is a considerable amount of the DNA from these cells present in the contents of the gut. To be sure, the survival of free DNA in the gut is very brief since digestive nucleases readily degrade it; further, the efficiency of DNA uptake by bacteria is very low. But the sheer magnitude of this event in the collective human intestines in the world—around 10^{20} bacteria are excreted daily by the human species—makes it virtually certain that eucaryote/procaryote recombinants have been formed innumerable times over the millions of years of evolution. And, judging by the observation that we are still here, life has managed quite nicely in spite of this event.

Moreover, Cohen suggests that there is no evidence that the evolutionary process is under delicate control in nature at all. Even if true, humans have for thousands of years modified the process of evolution. From the early domestication of plants and animals to the more recent use of antimicrobial agents to treat infections has the delicate control of evolution been irreversibly changed to an advantage, without encountering the conjectured disasters. We certainly do have "the right," Cohen insists, to counteract the evolutionary wisdom of millions of years which gave us the gene combinations for bubonic plague, smallpox, yellow fever, polio, diabetes, cancer, and other diseases. Warfare against these delicate balances in the form of modern medicine must be part of any humanistic concern for fellowpersons.[14]

James D. Watson, a molecular biologist and corecipient of the 1962 Nobel prize in biology, became an early vocal advocate of continued recombinant DNA research. In testimony at a public hearing to determine whether or not the state of New York should enact legislation controlling gene-splicing research, he caricatured the opposition's arguments as "an imaginery monster." In his testimony he insisted that recombinant DNA technology can provide the wherewithal to do experiments that would be impossible without it. And, one might ask, how highly do we value this information? Watson is of the firm opinion that the knowledge gained outweighs the risks by many magnitudes of difference. To claim that any of this research poses a threat to humankind "is total nonsense." It is Watson's position that the whole matter has become hopelessly overblown, mostly because it was scientists themselves who initially expressed publicly some reservations about their work. But by being "responsible," the controversy took on the features of a "black comedy." A parallel used by Watson on a number of occasions likens the whole affair to the fallout shelter debacle of the early 1960s. There was, as subsequent events pointed out, no substance to the fear that these shelters were needed or in fact whether they would even have worked; it was much ado about nothing, probably designed by our political leaders to foment patriotic enthusiasm. So with recombinant DNA research; it too is much ado about nothing:

> I'm afraid that by crying wolf about dangers which we have no reason at all to worry about, we are becoming indistinguishable from my two small boys. They love to talk about monsters because they know they will never meet one.[15]

This position coincided closely with the European view where opposition to recombinant DNA research is not nearly as widespread nor is it publicly expressed. Sir John Kendrew, Director General of the European Molecular Biology Laboratory, encapsulates their position in these words:

> Ignorance is the ultimate enemy. We have a new and powerful weapon in this technique. I hope it will be fully exploited in the USA, Europe and throughout the world.[16]

Perhaps the most significant long-term fear uttered by antagonists was the ultimate extension of genetic engineering to humans. Defenders of continued research claimed that molecular DNA recombination was no more radical a step toward engineering that were the many other developments in genetics (see Chapter 3). For the most part, other developments in genetics have aroused little public terror. And besides, as far into the future as can be reasonably projected, the medical aim of gene manipulation in humans is the alleviation of human suffering through gene therapy. To accomplish this, a large number of technically complex problems must first be overcome. By some estimates, we are a long way from achieving the goal. But even if the guess is wrong, the step to manipulating polygenic, behavioral traits is still so far into the future that it is impossible at this time to even hazard a guess when, if ever, it will be achieved. Moreover, in already developed organisms like adult humans, no conceivable amount of manipulation of DNA could reorganize the behavior—most assuredly not the complex wiring of the brain. Experience with the environment plays the commanding role here. The possibility of tyrants manipulating their subjects by genetic engineering is too remote to even justify concern.

Lastly, there was the practical question about doing science. There is a maxim that says, "that which has been learned, cannot be unlearned." For better or for worse, if certain research is restricted in one country, there is no guarantee it will not continue in another. We may indeed be entering dangerous territory in exploring recombinant DNA, but we are surely in dangerous territory if we start to limit this exploration simply because we lack the long-range vision to assess its consequences!

Needless to say, the opponents did not take these rejoinders seriously. A general meeting was convened by the National Academy of Sciences in March of 1977 called the Forum on Research with Recombinant DNA. Once more the major players were called back onto the stage and both sides repeated their positions and counterpositions. On the pro side, David Baltimore, Nobel Laureate in Biology from the Center for Cancer Research, MIT, admonished the audience: "Don't (let's) allow ourselves to be frozen by the fear of the unknown." The contrary view was summarized by Stephen E. Toulmin, Professor of Philosophy, University of Chicago: "The recombinant DNA case is a historic first . . . I can think of no prior case in which the actual conduct of experiments in a basic natural science itself directly posed a threat of general public harm." Mistrust at the meeting was evident from the start. A few hours before the Conference began, a newly organized group calling itself the Coalition for Responsible Genetic Research, demanded "an immediate, international moratorium on all research that would produce novel genetic combinations between distinct organisms which have not been demonstrated to exchange genes in nature." The provisions of the ban would cover all research—academic, industrial, or military—and would remain in effect until there has been broad public debate and a full assessment of all dangers.[17] (The Coalition numbers among its hundreds of sponsors, Nobel Laureates George Wald of Harvard and Sir MacFarlane Burnet of Australia; Aurelio Peccei, founder of the Club of Rome; Lewis Mumford, author and philosopher; environmentalist groups, Friends of the Earth and the Phi Beta Kappa Environmental Study Group of New York; and the activist groups, Science for the People and the Boston Area Recombinant DNA Group, of which Jonathan Beckwith and Ethan Signer—earlier mentioned critics—are members.) Another group carried placards about the hall proclaiming, "We will not be cloned." By and large, the position of the supporters of recombinant DNA research was exemplified by the remarks of Anthony Mazzocchi, a director of the Oil, Chemical, and Atomic Workers International Union: "It's not a case of 'if' but 'when'."[18]

The phraseology uttered was much the same as that voiced on numerous other occasions and such discourse will probably continue for some time to come, for if the debate truly broadens, as both sides urge, the pros and cons of gene-splicing research should be on the program of PTA's, civic organizations, professional clubs, and high school classes. It is apparent then at this writing, that no definitive answer can be given to Question 2: Should the research be done in the face of so many uncertainties? So, adopting the advice of George Wald given at the NAS forum described above: "The broad questions have not really been addressed. We turn with relief to problems of safety because they are easier," we, too, here turn to the problems of safety.

SAFEGUARDS AND GUIDELINES

Question 3 asked, what safeguards will adequately protect citizens from the dangers of recombinant organisms? The whole concern over recombinant DNA research was initiated by a group of scientists at a Gordon Research Conference, a scientific meeting on nucleic acids held in New England, in the summer of 1973. As a result of concerns expressed by participants at that meeting, an open letter was sent to the editor of *Science*, requesting the National Academy of Sciences to study the problem of recombinant DNA research and after study to set some guidelines for using these techniques. This was beyond doubt an historic event, evidencing a new moral concern by scientists.

A committee was called into being by the National Institutes of Health (NIH) under the chairmanship of Paul Berg, a Stanford molecular biologist and one of the original signers of the 1973 letter to *Science*. This group, officially known as the Recombinant DNA Molecular Program Advisory Committee to NIH, more often simply as the Berg Committee, recommended that a general moratorium on all recombinant research be voluntarily honored by scientists until the hazards could be thoroughly investigated. In February of 1975 an international conference, attended primarily by molecular biologists from around the world, was convened at the Asilomar Conference Center in Pacific Grove, California. Five days of almost day and night sessions concluded with the passage of two resolutions: (1) a moratorium on recombinant DNA research voluntarily accepted by scientists should be lifted (the intent of the moratorium which went into effect in 1974 was to allow time for studying the issue before proceeding further with research), and (2) that future research should be conducted under a set of guidelines. The NIH Advisory Committee then went to work on refining the suggestions offered by scientists at Asilomar to develop the guidelines.

Thus, the very first thrust of the recombinant DNA debate was within the scientific community itself. The Berg Committee raised the moral issue that some of the proposed research could be dangerous to the general public. It was largely this proposition, put on the table of the conference not without opposition from scientific colleagues, that drew public notice to the whole matter. It is interesting to conjecture what would have happened had the scientific community not attracted attention to itself. In the eyes of the public, the Berg group performed a responsible and self-cleansing action which reflected to the credit of science. From within that community, the accolades were not as congratulatory. Norton Zinder, one of the signers of the 1973 *Science* letter, laments in this way: "There are people who say, 'If you guys hadn't opened your mouths, nothing would have happened; it would all have blown away'."[19] Whatever may have been must remain pure speculation for the moral issue has been joined—science (the "is") can no longer be isolated from its applications (the "ought").

During 1975, the NIH Advisory Committee developed guidelines and in December of that year submitted a draft to the NIH Director. After nearly a year and a half of study, NIH formally issued on June 23, 1976, its official guidelines based on that draft. The strategy behind the guidelines was how to take the step of control in a way that would bring the most benefits to science and society while keeping the public risks at a minimum. Thus, the emphasis was on *containment* rather than cessation of this kind of research. The guidelines were written expressly for technical people by technical people, most of whom were doing this research. Critics of the guidelines insisted that public input was not commensurate with the magnitude of the risk to which the public would be exposed nor to the interest they had demonstrated. This continued to be a point of irritation to some.

In arriving at the guidelines, the NIH panel followed these recommendations laid down at the Asilomar conference:

1 There are certain kinds of experiments involving recombinant DNA molecules that are so hazardous that they should not be attempted at all now.

2 There are experiments where the risks and scientific benefits weighed are justifiable at this time, providing "appropriate safeguards" are taken.

3 The level of containment should match the degree of hazard of the experiment.

4 The guidelines will be updated at least annually to take in new knowledge about biohazards of recombinant DNA.

The guidelines in brief are these:[20]

Physical Containment

P1 (minimal): strict adherence to standard microbiological practices;

P2 (low): limited access to laboratory during experiments; precautions against the release of aerosols and the prohibition of mouth pipetting;

P3 (moderate): laboratories equipped to ensure inward flow of air (negative air pressure); biological safety cabinets; wearing of gloves; decontamination of recirculated air;

P4 (high): special facilities of the kind used in biological warfare research—installations such as isolation by airlocks, clothing changes and showers, decontamination of all air, liquid, and solid wastes.

Biological Containment (applicable when using *E. coli* K12)

EK1: use of *E. coli* in its usual form;

EK2: use of modified *E. coli* K12 so that *E. coli* hosts or modified plasmids have a survival rate of less than 10^{-8} (1 in 100,000,000 million) in the natural environment, if the host organism should escape from the laboratory;

EK3: use of EK2 systems for which the increased containment has been independently confirmed by animal tests.

Experiments prohibited:

1. Experiments taking their DNA from highly pathogenic organisms.

2. Experiments in which the DNA to be joined contains gene for production of highly toxic agents.

3. Experiments in which the DNA is derived from a plant pathogen if the host may acquire increased virulence or range.

4. Experiments involving uncontrolled release of organisms containing any recombinant molecule.

5. Transfer of genes conferring drug resistance to microorganisms not known to acquire such resistance naturally, when the resistance may compromise clinical use of the drug in medicine or agriculture.

6. Large scale experiments with recombinant DNA's known to result in the formation of harmful products; exceptions may be approved by the NIH Recombinant DNA Advisory Committee.

These guidelines relativize the risk for a range of experiments and provide a taxonomy (a way of naming) for permissible genetic recombinations. Each potential *donor* of DNA (e.g., primate, bacteria, plant, etc.) is assigned a containment requirement consisting of both physical and biological parameters. This two-dimensional containment space can be represented by a matrix as shown below.[21] Included are a few examples for each containment coordinate into which the alien DNA will be inserted. (See Fig. 4.1.) Note that some donors are double listed. For example, primate DNA can be implanted into *E. coli* under EK3 conditions or under EK2 + P4 conditions.

Physical containment levels _____ Safer ⟶

	P1	P2	P3	P4	Banned
EK1	Bacteria naturally exchanging DNA with *E. coli*	Plants (no known pathogen)	Plant viruses		Venoms from insects and snakes, genes for botulinum toxin
EK2		Cold-blooded vertebrates (frogs), plant viruses	Nonprimate mammals (cats), birds	Primates (monkeys), animal viruses	
EK3			Primates (monkeys), animal viruses		

Biological hosts (E. coli strains)

Figure 4.1 *(Reference 21. Reprinted with permission of the copyright owner, The American Chemical Society, from the May 30, 1977 issue of* Chemical and Engineering News.*)*

As might be expected, the publication of the NIH brought immediate and vocal remonstrations from the scientific community. To some, the guidelines were much too strict and would have the effect of seriously curtailing scientific research. To others, they did not go nearly far enough. This latter opinion raised the crucial question: Ought the burden of proof to go ahead with recombinant DNA research fall on those who support it, or on those who oppose it or at least want much tighter controls?[22] The implied answer is that the burden of proof lay with the opponents of continued research.

There are obvious errors in the guideline's approach to assignment of risk. For instance, a great deal of responsibility is placed on the investigators. Individual human beings usually do not consider low-probability risks serious enough to take precautions to protect against the risks. The guidelines depend upon the conscientiousness of the worker. Workers frequently become habituated to danger. Furthermore, laboratory workers are motivated by temperament, training, and employment to do their work and to undertake associated risks or get out. To make the guidelines effective, almost constant alertness to the dangers of the research is required. It can be questioned whether this is within the range of human capabilities.

It is generally conceded that the guidelines represent a compromise between two fears: (1) that of conceivably creating dangerous new organisms, and (2) that of not bridging in, by excessive regulation, the search for new knowledge. These were the same fears that prompted the Asilomar conference; they are still with us today. As with most compromises, neither side felt that it had been treated fairly. But we must live in a world of compromise; compromise determined the guidelines, too. Had a long-term moratorium been declared, charges of unnecessary governmental intrusion both within and without the scientific community would have echoed across the land. If no action had been taken at all, it is almost certain that research would be going on at a much faster pace than it is now and the public would know much less about these matters.

A host of other objections to the guidelines were raised, many related to the earlier discussed positions: the fear of environmental contamination, the possibility of large-scale epidemics, and the like. But one which attracted much attention was voiced by Senator Edward Kennedy in a speech at Harvard in May of 1975:

> It was commendable that scientists attempted to think through the social consequences of their work. It was commendable, but it was inadequate. It was inadequate because scientists *alone* decided to lift it. Yet the factors under consideration extend far beyond their technical competence. In fact they were making public policy. And they were making it in private.[23]

Before the publication of the guidelines, there was very little public input either in discussions leading up to them or in their formulation. But that all changed with their publication. Although the guidelines still stand, the manner in which they were developed kindled public resentment that science was thrusting an unprepared and reluctant humanity into a world which it neither knew nor even wholly wanted. Community after community jumped on the recombinant DNA bandwagon calling for their own investigations and the possible spelling out of the terms under which the research might proceed in their locales.

Cambridge, the home town of MIT and Harvard, was the first. Though the mayor wanted to ban all P3 and P4 research, the city council endorsed the NIH guidelines but with added restrictions: for example, a city biohazards committee should be created to oversee all recombinant DNA research in the city. San Diego, the site of the University of California, San Diego campus, accepted the NIH guidelines with the reservation that no P4 experiments be done in the city and that the city be notified if any P3 experiments using EK3 containment were undertaken. Madison, and the University of Wisconsin, set up a citizens' committee to publicly debate the issue. Ann Arbor, Bloomington, Urbana-Champaign—the list was added to almost daily—also have had public debates.

At the state level, New York State, after lengthy public hearings, prepared a bill to control the research. A most significant inclusion in the bill was the requirement that everyone engaged in gene-splicing research must obtain a certificate from the state health commissioner who would also specify training and health-monitoring programs. California contemplated legislation. New Jersey and Michigan did the same. A common feature of all these efforts is that they all accepted the NIH guidelines but usually with specified extra restrictions of their own. Whatever further restrictions are placed on the research, it will at least be proceeding on the basis of informed public consent. Certainly this is an innovation in the matter of scientific research.

There is still one very large area which has eluded the sort of regulation contained in the NIH guidelines. The guidelines as they were designed cover only government-funded research. This includes both NIH and NSF funding which together makes up about 95 percent of all federally financed research. But a great many worries have been expressed about the lack of supervision in the private sector, most especially the drug industry. Pharmaceutical firms and chemical and agricultural companies are understandably interested in recombinant work since the technique provides an almost unparalleled opportunity to easily and cheaply mass produce a variety of drugs, chemicals, fertilizers, and food. General Electric is already out in front with the announcement that it has received a patent on a microorganism that can eat up oil spills.

In what is considered a landmark decision, the U.S. Court of Customs and Patent Appeals ruled in October 1977 that an inventor can patent new forms of microorganisms. The case was brought by Upjohn Company which sought to patent the microorganism it manufactured to produce the antibiotic lincomycin. In a second case, the same court in March 1978 decided that General Electric could patent a manufactured strain of bacteria that eats up oil more efficiently than do naturally occurring organisms. The new strain was developed by experimentally altering the plasmids so that a variety of hydrocarbon-degrading enzymes could be synthesized by the bacterium. Both decisions were based on the judgment that the transformed microorganisms were "not found in, and are not a product of, nature." The altered microorganisms were interpreted to be "a kind of tool used by chemists and chemical manufacturers in much the same way as the chemical elements and compounds which are not alive. . . . (are used) to produce new compounds."[24] These Court decisions affirmed the position that manufactured microorganisms are in the same category as chemical compounds, not living organisms. The way is opened for inventors to patent all sorts of novel organisms.

While the commercial prospects for the new technology promise benefits to both citizen and mercantile interests, the potential dangers connected with its further development and application for commercial purpose pose perhaps the most serious challenge to the use of these new techniques. The problem was spotlighted by a *Washington Post* story (September 26, 1976), which reported: "U.S. health officials acknowledged that the government does not know what companies are trying to create revolutionary new forms of life or the whereabouts of their laboratories."[25] In other words, up to now there has been no federal agency supervising research being done by private industry using recombinant DNA.

Companies are in general agreement with the NIH guidelines but with these significant reservations. The guidelines call for disclosure of research plans; companies cannot accept this for competitive reasons. They are concerned about protection of proprietary rights; obtaining a patent for publicly disclosed procedures may be difficult. The guidelines specify *E. coli* mutants as vectors; companies might want to use other hosts. Knowing the detailed biology of the microorganism is not nearly as crucial when the motive is profit. And then there is the matter of commercial production; the guidelines place a 10-liter limit on each experiment. Pharmaceutical manufacturers require batches produced in many-liter quantities. Lastly, companies see a need to harmonize with what is occurring internationally. By restricting research and development here, overseas firms, notably in Europe, will be able to move ahead of the United States in certain areas of pharmaceutical production.

THE FEDERAL GOVERNMENT AND DNA RESEARCH

The original hope that motivated the scientific community to regulate this potentially hazardous research itself was thus dashed. The discussion leading up to the formulation of the guidelines and their publication could not be contained. The debate gathered its own momentum and moved into the political sphere. Both House and Senate subcommittees held public hearings on legislation that would regulate this research and that would apply to both academic and commercial research. At least three bills were introduced into the House and one in the Senate during the 1977 Congressional session. None of these reached either floor of Congress. Another effort was made in the 1978 Congressional session. Under the leadership of Representative Paul Rogers (D–Fla.), a new draft bill was devised. Its salient features were an extension of the NIH Guidelines for two years and makes them applicable to both private and industrial research; inspection and enforcement authority would be placed in the hands of the Secretary of Health, Education, and Welfare; and provision was made for a study commission having a majority of nonbiologists as members to assess the long-term applications of gene splicing. A controversial issue was the inclusion of a preemption clause which precludes from enacting local authorities of regulations more severe than those stipulated in the federal legislation.[26]

A number of research scientists continued to insist that no federal legislation was needed. The scientific community, it was argued, is fully capable of policing itself and besides, insists Dr. Paul Berg, one of the early leaders in the push for a voluntary moratorium in 1973, "the possibility that experimental organisms will be hazardous or released is extremely small." Continued Berg, "legislation of the type that so far has been proposed would inhibit basic research on important biological and medical problems."[27] The future of recombinant DNA legislation is still undecided but whether scientists like it or not, politicians will continue to call for some kind of regulation of its activities (see Chapter 13).

An unfortunate spin-off of this whole affair is that it may be a long time before scientists raise another issue for public debate. The bitterness engendered within the scientific community and the negative responses generated from so many quarters both within and without the sciences suggest that scientists in the future will conscientiously avoid drawing public attention to themselves and their work. This can be quite disconcerting, for society must depend upon its scientists to be informed on matters which concern both. A withdrawal from the public arena by scientists can only lead to greater polarization and suspicion.

And so, in answering the question, What safeguards will adequately protect citizens from the dangers of recombinant organisms?, we have responded to the next question, too: What assurances are there that any safeguards will actually be followed and who is to enforce them? Quite clearly, the scientific debate here is over. Biologists will no longer dominate the discussions. California Institute of Technology economist Roger G. Noll declared at the earlier mentioned NAS forum: "In the future biologists will not be the movers of policy, but the suppliers of technical data."[28] It only remains to be determined whether the subsequent actions that are taken stand to harm or benefit either or both the scientific community and the society which it serves.

There is still the matter of the international scene. England has already developed a set of guidelines very similar to those of the NIH. A central feature of their code requires that all genetic manipulation first be screened by a centralized advisory group—the Genetic Manipulation Advisory Group—whose main function would be to take account of the specific aspects of the proposed experiment and advise on the application of the code. The Soviet Union is considering a version patterned after both the American and the British guidelines. A new committee on genetic manipulation has been set up by the International Council of Scientific Unions. The ICSU coordinates scientific activity on a worldwide basis. For example, it has committees on space, solar and terrestrial physics, oceanic, antarctic, and water research, the environment, and the teaching of science. The genetic manipulation committee will not conduct research itself but will attempt to monitor experiments in progress throughout the world and serve as a channel of communication among the scientific communities engaged in such research. According to Sir John Kendrew, ICSU general secretary, committees to prepare guidelines similar to those adopted by NIH have been organized in all countries known to be carrying genetic research. These include nations throughout Western Europe, the USSR, Hungary, Australia, and Japan.

ETHICAL ASPECTS OF GENETIC RESEARCH

To borrow a phrase, the nuclear genie (of another kind) has been let out of its bottle. This nuclear genie, like its predecessor, brought to birth a technology so potent that misuse may cause grievous perturbations in society at large. For good or ill, the time of grace is passed and now decisions must be made regarding the present and future use of this new technology. What should be the decision, since the consequences represent unknown risks? How do we even go about deciding? Do ethical and moral considerations provide any direction here? In partial answer to at least the last question, the response must be in the affirmative, for if one of our earlier assumptions is reasonably correct, then ethical reasoning should provide some assistance in working through this problem.

Essentially, the value object reduces to this question: Can we justify the goals and the methods of molecular genetic research? The "we" in this proposition is used in the broadest context to include the scientists who carry out the research; the general public who may derive great benefits from this technology as well as bear the brunt of the hazards; the government who is morally and legally obligated to protect its citizens and further, will provide a large share of the funding for these researches; the physicians who are charged with alleviating human suffering; and commercial enterprises which undoubtedly stand to gain extensive profits utilizing this technology. Any ethical analysis that can do justice to the question while at the same time appeal to these many and varied interests is indeed an enormous undertaking. Here we can but make a beginning.

As a start, we turn to the two major ethical theories introduced in Chapter 2: consequentialism and deontology. Consequentialism derives validity based on the consequences of a certain action. A consequentialist reasons from the data at hand pertinent to an actual case or problem and then chooses the course of action that offers an optimum or maximum of desirable effects. Central to this position is the question of means and ends, or of acts and consequences. Does a morally desirable end ever justify a questionable means? Alternately, could a good means ever justify an evil end or justify the consequences if the evil end was not foreseen or the result was not intended? The consequentialist would answer yes to both questions for as the previously noted Jeremy Bentham (see p. 53) would have it, "no act, strictly speaking, can be evil in itself." For the consequentialist, results are what counts and results are good when they contribute to human well-being. On the basis of this, then, the real issue ethically is whether genetic manipulation will, in its foreseeable or predictable results, add to or take away from human welfare.

There is a second factor to be included in a consequentialist analysis, namely, that each situation is to be apprised separately. Since categorical rules or dogmatic positions are nonapplicable, the making of decisions empirically requires that every problem be approached open-ended, that is, not settled in advance. Here the question becomes, When would it be right, and when would it be wrong? The obvious implication framed by this question is that sometimes it may be right, at another time it may be wrong; an act may be right in one circumstance, but the same act could be incorrect in another instance.

When might a situation of using genetic manipulation be justified because of the good to be gained? Using Joseph Fletcher's term, when would the "proportionate good" be great enough to justify the use of these techniques? The step to solution is the familiar cost/benefit analysis. For example, if by inserting a gene to correct a genetic defect the person is freed from the disease or deformity, or the process ameliorates the effect of the deficiency, then all other considerations must be set aside. If research requires human embryos or fetal tissue to provide the means to treat or prevent the disease, even though they must be sacrificed, then the assigned priorities are in favor of the research. Consequentialists would advance the same logic in support of other applications of genetic manipulations, or on a larger scale, to the many other reproductive technologies mentioned earlier such as cloning, chimeras, and ectogenesis. If our actions are tailored by a loving concern for human beings to achieve the greatest good for the greatest number, then as Fletcher admonishes, "we need not be afraid."[29] But the task is made enormously difficult because we cannot see the promises and the dangers that are in front of us. It is fear of the unknown that holds us back, for people in this situation generally choose the safe side, the let's-go-slow, or what's-the-rush side. Fear, as Fletcher would have it, is at the base of the present debate on genetic manipulation: fear of consequences, fear of science, fear of the power this new technology will give to those with evil intent, fear that some of our most highly prized beliefs—the rightness of heterosexual coitus, the natural way for reproducing offspring, the wisdom of nature in directing life processes—will be denied fruition if we let down our guard against human intrusion into these very vital processes. Most of all, there is the fear of the playing of God in making decisions reserved only for Him. But fear can be overcome; any action guided by a compelling love for our fellowperson is the right action, no matter what means are employed or if unforeseen bad consequences result. "To be (human)," Fletcher concludes, "we must be in control. That is the first and last ethical word. For when there is no choice there is no possibility of ethical action."[30]

Turning now to a deontological approach, ethical judgments derive from general propositions and/or universal axioms. Here, rightness or wrongness is determined according to whether an action complies with broad moral principles or derives from prefabricated rules. The Kantian admonition, "never treat people as means," would be an example of a decision based on moral rules. The rules of morality exist in advance of any specific problem; thus, certain acts are always wrong—lying or stealing, for instance.

Deontologists, therefore, might say that therapeutic or corrective goals are not enough to justify genetic manipulation no matter how desirable they may be. Good consequences, in and by themselves, can never justify any act or procedure. Dr. Leon Kass, molecular biologist now at the University of Chicago, put this position with these words:

> Morally it is insufficient that your motives are good, that your ends are unobjectionable, that you do the procedure "lovingly" and even that you may be lucky in the results; you will be engaging in an unethical experiment upon a human subject.[31]

This also is clearly recognized to be the position of Paul Ramsey who, among others, believes that these procedures are wrong because they violate the natural order; they are wrong because they are antihuman (see p. 57).

Sumner B. Twiss, philosopher from Brown University, strikes for a more reasoned approach in effecting a solution to the genetic manipulation issue. He states his position in a paper delivered at the Conference on Ethical and Scientific Issues Posed by Human Uses of Molecular Genetics, sponsored by the New York Academy of Sciences in May of 1975.[32]

Challenging the usefulness of the cost/benefit approach, Twiss sets out to identify criteria which may be helpful in morally justifying the use of gene manipulation techniques. Cost/benefit analysis is of limited usefulness, since the issue (or almost any other issue for that matter) cannot be settled by it. He reasons that even if it were possible to align all of the costs against all of the benefits—and there is no guarantee that all of either will be on the list—a decision for or against still involves the moral values of those doing the deciding, and if these have not been clarified in advance, the moral ideal as imbedded in choice may or may not be realized. (See the earlier discussion on metaphysics, p. 60.) Twiss uses the following case as an example: Suppose a choice had to be made between developing an effective gene therapy for a disease and a prenatal diagnosis/selective abortion program for the same disease (see Chapter 5c). The cost/benefit analysis would not settle the matter, since all of the moral and social issues relating to abortion and the definition of personhood would dominate the discussion. Choosing to await the success of a speculative technology would be totally unsatisfactory in this case.[33] No amount of cost-benefiting would set priorities here. (It might be added parenthetically that cost-benefit is used more often than not to justify a previously determined position on a value question—environmental impact statements are classical examples. This is probably one of the major problems in the gene-splicing controversy— neither side cares one bit about the other's arguments, each using a preferred cost/benefit set to support its previously established position.)

A variation on this theme poses the problem in risk/benefit terms rather than cost/benefit. The objection to cost/benefit comparisons as applied to recombinant DNA research (or any other activity with an uncertain future) submits that these two terms are not symmetrical—they are not comparing the same thing. Risk, as used here, implies uncertainty; unforeseen consequences may arise but they also may not occur. Benefit, on the other hand, carries with it certainty. Certain gains are to be expected if some activity or policy is engaged in. A better way of posing the bargain might be—harm versus benefit, or risk versus possible gain. In these comparisons, the two potential outcomes are equally paired.

Twiss suggests a method for dealing with ethical problems of this kind. Setting *value priorities* and then measuring the projected action against these may be more useful. This is the methodology outlined in Chapter 2 with the addition that the reference values are evaluated on a more universal scale—on the order of those in deontological theory. Twiss proposes five ethical questions applicable to genetic technology:

1. What moral values are relevant to justifying proposed genetic goals and guiding the legitimate use of genetic technology?

2. What are the limits of moral responsibility for the unintended consequences of developing and implementing genetic technologies?

3. Given the economic constraints implied by scarce resources, what norms should govern the allocation of these resources in applied genetics?

4. Assuming that many of the benefits and risks associated with genetic technologies have a potentially profound impact on future generations, what obligations do present generations have to future generations for the development and implementation of genetic technologies?

5. Assuming that moral appraisal is a significant element in projecting priorities in the use of genetic technology, what implications do the answers to the first four questions have for setting up a priority schedule in applied human genetics?[34]

A full presentation of his discussion of these ethical questions cannot be carried out here and the interested reader is referred to his excellent paper. Even a summary of his analysis cannot do justice to his well thought-out ideas, but the following presentation makes an effort.

Confining his concern to medical genetic applications (i.e., gene therapy), he submits these responses to the ethical questions previously introduced:[35]

Moral values

1. The protection of individual rights is the baseline for moral reasoning.

2. The obligation of medicine is to administer to the health needs of people, both as individuals and as a community (i.e., public health).

3. The treatment of genetic ills is included in value 2, hence, health-oriented genetic technology is justifiable.

Conclusion: Genetic technology is morally desirable and ethically mandatory—research from this perspective has high priority.

Long-range responsibility

1. It is morally imperative to acquire relevant predictive knowledge before implementing a new technology with uncertain consequences, some of which could be harmful.

2. Ignorance about indirect, delayed harmful consequences, particularly if they are irreversible, constitutes a moral reason for being cautious in developing and implementing a technology.

3. "Do not undertake an important experiment whose results cannot be evaluated."

4. Researchers are morally accountable to coworkers and the larger community if their work carries the potential for harmful consequences.

5. Public policy-makers share some of the responsibility for preventing social abuses.

6. Long-term prospects to improve the condition of future generations, especially if benefits accrue to the least advantaged, assigns high priority to research (see Rawls, p. 58).

Conclusion: The moral imperative of acquiring predictive knowledge before acting and the possibility of indirect consequences balanced against the potential benefits to future generations assign this medium priority; the priority could go up or down as new knowledge concerning consequences is gained.

Allocation of resources

1. Genetic research will become progressively more expensive as the problems become more and more refined.

2. Medical care ranks high among the needs of society.

3. Accessibility to medical care should not be based solely on costs but on the principle of equity.

4. In a society having limited resources, not all claims can be honored simultaneously.

5. The principle of efficiency—the highest return for the resource allocated—is to be balanced by the Rawlsian principle of equity.

Conclusion: The principles of equity and efficiency favor the allocation of scarce resources to research in molecular genetics, hence a claim of high priority.

(This matter dealing with long-range responsibility in scientific research will be taken up in Chapter 13 under the heading, An Ethos of Science.)

A study of this summary probably leaves the reader still quite uneasy. The answers, if there are any here, do not seem any more satisfying than the two positions of consequentialism and deontology. But to advance a completely defensible ethical case in the matter of recombinant DNA research would require a completed technology, including an assessment for each projected application as well as a perfected public policy whose position is ethically and/or morally acceptable to all. Neither of these requirements can be met at the present time. The best an analysis like this can do is to identify certain ethical issues which are relevant to the problem at hand. If this has been achieved, then this study has been successful.

As this entire discussion has shown, decision-making on the use of genetic technologies is a complex matter involving points of moral contention at every step. The world, fifty or so years from now, no doubt will study with interest the quality of our arguments on the matter of genetic manipulation. How favorably they will be impressed will be determined by what is being said today.

Postscript: The problem of how to regulate recombinant DNA research is still far from resolved although legislative ardor has been significantly reduced. Many scientists, too, who originally raised concerns about the safety of such research have since modified their position in the light of more complete information, concluding that there is little, if any, hazard resulting from recombinant DNA research especially when performed under the NIH guidelines. Controversy continues, however, particularly concerning two points. The first point still considers some form of federal legislation which extends the updated guidelines (see below) to non-federally funded agencies, while the second concerns some sort of preemption stipulation (see p. 119).

The Senate has urged that HEW control rDNA research while HEW has asked for specific legislation to regulate DNA experiments (September, 1978). In either case, it has been suggested that the standards for rDNA research should be similar, if not identical, to those required by the NIH guidelines. The matter of preemption has not been resolved, either.

Three changes appearing in the revised guidelines also reflect the position that rDNA research is not as hazardous as formerly thought. Specifically, experiments utilizing *E. coli* no longer require high-level containment procedures since it is now believed that the enfeebled *E. coli* laboratory version K12 is unlikely to be converted to a pathogen (P4 physical containment and EK3 biological containment are abolished—see p. 115). A second change allows experiments using whole virus DNA to be conducted at the P1 and P2 levels rather than the previous P3 and P4 levels. And lastly, shotgun experiments are permissible under P2 conditions rather than P3 and P4 as formerly stipulated. (See Nicholas Wade, "New Rulebook for Gene Splicers," *Science,* August 18, 1978, pp. 600–601, Vol. 201.)

VALUES PERTAINING TO THE RECOMBINANT DNA RESEARCH ISSUE

1   To settle for what we know now is to condemn future generations to all the existing ailments plus all those new ones that keep turning up.

2   If we have the means of preventing, curing, or significantly alleviating human disease, or improving upon the human condition, then a choice not to proceed would be a choice against humanity and is contrary to ethics.

3   No one can ever guarantee total freedom from risk in any significant human activity; therefore research promising great benefits is to be preferred over not proceeding at all.

4   Much of the controversy concerning recombinant DNA research is based on persons who are poorly informed, some who are well-meaning but misguided, and some who are self-serving; their opinions do not represent the real world of research, hence they should not be taken seriously.

5   Freedom to do scientific research is not absolute but must be constrained by ethical and social considerations of the society in which it operates.

6   Biological scientists cannot be the sole judges of what is good or bad for society.

7   The acquisition of new knowledge is the sole and ultimate criterion for carrying on research—knowledge is always good.

8 The NIH Guidelines drawn up by scientists for scientists are only a form of "self-serving tokenism" and do not adequately reflect public interests.

9 We do not have a right to put additional genetic burdens on generations yet unborn.

10 The acquisition of genetic knowledge and its implementation in technology requires that unethical experiments be performed on human persons, be they embryos, fetuses, or fully mature individuals.

11 In every instance of conflicting claims involving humans, human needs should always determine the course of right action.

(The values included in the preceding study could be added to this list.)

REFERENCES

1 Robert L. Sinsheimer, in "Stellar cast; gripping plot; but no new message," by E. M. Leeper, *Bioscience* **27**, 5 (1977): 319.

2 Nicholas Wade, "Recombinant DNA: guidelines debated at public hearing," *Science* **191** (1976): 834.

3 Stanley N. Cohen, "Recombinant DNA: fact and fiction," *Science* **195** (1977): 655.

4 Maxine F. Singer, and Paul Berg, letters "Recombinant DNA: NIH guidelines," *Science* **193** (1976): 186.

5 Erwin Chargaff, letter "On the dangers of genetic meddling," *Science* **192** (1976): 938.

6 Robert L. Sinsheimer, in "Recombinant DNA: a critic questions the right to free inquiry," by Nicholas Wade, *Science* **194** (1976): 303.

7 Erwin Chargaff (in Reference 5), p. 938.

8 Richard P. Novick, "Present controls are just a start," *Bulletin of Atomic Scientists* **33**, 5 (1977): 16.

9 Jeremy Rifkin, "DNA: have the corporations already grabbed control of new life forms?" *Mother Jones* (Feb/Mar, 1977): 39.

10 Jon Beckwith, "Social and political uses of genetics in the United States: past and present," in *Ethical and Scientific Issues Posed by Human Uses of Molecular Genetics*, Marc Lappé and Robert S. Morrison (eds.), (New York: New York Academy of Sciences, 1976), p. 52.

11 Stanley N. Cohen (in Reference 3), p. 654.

12 Stanley N. Cohen (in Reference 3), p. 655.

13 Bernard D. Davis, "Potential benefits are large, protective methods make risks small," *Chemical and Engineering News* (May 30, 1977), p. 30.

14 Stanley N. Cohen (in Reference 3), p. 655.

15 James D. Watson, "An imaginary monster," *Bulletin of Atomic Scientists* **33**, 5 (1977): 13.

16 Sir John Kendrew (in Reference 1), p. 319.

17 E. M. Leeper (in Reference 1), p. 318.

18 Anthony Mazzocchi (in Reference 1), p. 319.

19 Norton Zinder, in "Gene-splicing: critics of research get more brickbats than banquets," by Nicholas Wade, *Science* **195** (1977): 466.

20 "The guidelines in brief," *F.A.S. Public Interest Report* (Recombinant DNA Issue) **29** (1976): 8.

21 Sheldon Krimsky, "Public must regulate recombinant research," *Chemical and Engineering News* (May 30, 1977), p. 21.

22 Daniel Callahan, "Recombinant DNA: science and the public," *Hastings Center Report* **7** (1977): 21.

23 Edward Kennedy, in "Kennedy: pushing for more public input in research," by Barbara J. Culliton, *Science* **188** (1975): 1188.

24 "Court permits patent of new microorganisms," *Chemical and Engineering News* (October 17, 1977), pp. 5–6.

25 Washington Post (in Reference 1), p. 25.

26 Nicholas Wade, "Congress set to grapple again with gene splicing," *Science* **199** (1978): 1319–1322.

27 "DNA research: no federal regulation now," *Chemical and Engineering News* (Nov. 21, 1977): p. 22.

28 Roger G. Noll (in Reference 1), p. 317.

29 Joseph Fletcher, "Ethical aspects of genetic controls," *New England Journal of Medicine* **285** (1971): 776–783.

30 Joseph Fletcher (in Reference 29), p. 782.

31 Leon Kass, "New beginnings in life," in *The New Genetics and the Future of Man*, Michael Hamilton (ed.) (Grand Rapids: Eerdmans, 1972), p. 30.

32 Sumner B. Twiss, Jr., "Ethical issues in priority-setting for the utilization of genetic technologies," in *Ethical and Scientific Issues Posed by Human Uses of Molecular Genetics*, Marc Lappé and Robert S. Morrison (eds.) (New York: New York Academy of Sciences, 1976), pp. 22–45.

33 Sumner B. Twiss (in Reference 32), p. 37.

34 Sumner B. Twiss (in Reference 32), p. 24.

35 Sumner B. Twiss (in Reference 32).

BIBLIOGRAPHY

Etzioni, Amitai. *Genetic Fix* (New York: Macmillan, 1973).

Fletcher, Joseph. *The Ethics of Genetic Control* (Garden City: Anchor/Doubleday, 1974).

Hamilton, Michael (ed.), *The New Genetics and the Future of Man* (Grand Rapids: Eerdmans, 1972).

Hilton, Bruce; Daniel Callahan; Maureen Harris; Peter Condliffe; Burton Berkley. *Ethical Issues in Human Genetics* (New York & London: Plenum, 1973).

Lappé, Marc, and Robert S. Morrison (eds.), *Ethical and Scientific Issues Posed by Human Uses of Molecular Genetics* (New York: New York Academy of Sciences, 1976).

Ramsey, Paul. *Fabricated Man* (New Haven: Yale University Press, 1970).

Rogers, Michael. *Biohazard* (New York: Alfred A. Knopf, 1977).

Wade, Nicholas. *The Ultimate Experiment* (New York: Walker and Company, 1977).

5

REPRODUCTIVE TECHNOLOGIES: A SAMPLER OF ISSUES

A. THE ETHICS OF GENETIC RESPONSIBILITY

Major ethical issues arise directly or indirectly from the new genetic knowledge and the correlated technologies that are concerned with human reproduction. With the coming of a better understanding of genetics and development, the means exist for control over the process of child-bearing. It is now practicable in a number of cases to predict characteristics of a developing fetus far in advance of its birth. A growing number of elegant therapeutic procedures administer to the ailments of the growing fetus. Safe abortion techniques allow the easy removal of fetuses determined to be grossly defective. Even before procreation, the new insights permit a degree of counseling to prospective parents that can predict the probabilities of occurrence of certain traits among offspring not yet conceived. The desire of every parent not to have defective or abnormal children is being made possible by the dramatic advances in reproductive technology. The conscious guiding of human procreation from start to finish is becoming more and more solely dependent on the parent's desire to have normal children. But availability does not imply use. Some of the major obstacles to implementing reproductive improvements are psychological and ethical, based on traditions which are sometimes hard to break. The classical sanctity-of-life ethic, for instance, is still preferred by some over a quality-of-life one.

Society, too, has a fundamental interest in the wise use of this new knowledge. Not only do parents and families gain by healthy children but the community prospers as well. The promotion of the common good is dependent upon the active participation of all its citizens; the caring for people is best facilitated when they are robust. A reasonable number of inhabitants who are physically and mentally sound is much preferred by any society over unmanageable masses or excessive numbers of sickly and deformed bodies supported by public welfare. This reciprocal relationship benefiting both parents and society can be served by the wise use of the new genetic technologies. Hopefully, humankind will learn that new knowledge can be brought to bear on fostering the common good in matters of reproducing the next generation. And so it is in order that a discussion of the major ethical issues arising from the uses of the new genetic knowledge should begin with the larger question: What responsibilities do parents and society have over insuring the genetic good health of offspring?

The proposition contained here is not simply a philosophical one nor is it empty of practical implications. Rapid progress in the whole area of human procreation has made it possible to implement whatever choice individuals and/or society will make. Furthermore, and in a more general way, the position taken on the matter will largely determine one's response to other issues as well. For example, if it is decided that society has an important stake in the quality of the children born into it, then precise measures—coercive or whatever—must be enacted to guard against transgressors who would ignore the common good. Thus, genetic responsibility and eugenic responsibility are seen as part of the same cloth. Persons who have a genuine sense of their own responsibility will take seriously the genetic health of the next and subsequent generations.

Sumner Twiss approached the issue of genetic responsibility by posing several questions, graded in order of insistence upon compliance.[1] The first gives unobstructed freedom of choice exclusively to parents:

> Do parents have the right to determine the genetic quality of their offspring according to any criteria acceptable to them alone?

The second question raises the urgency of the issue to a higher level of insistence by designating the responsibility a *duty* borne by parents.

> Do parents have the duty to avoid bearing children with serious genetic defects when it is possible to do so?

The third question is the most demanding of the three for it removes the matter of genetic responsibility from the parents and places it on society.

> Does society have the right to intervene in parenthood?

Before proceeding further, it will be expedient to arrive at some semantic clarification, at least tentatively, if not satisfactorily. Two value terms were introduced by the questions above: right and duty. Much philosophical debate has gone into analyzing the meaning of these. On the one hand are those, like Joseph Fletcher, who insist that the designation of rights is purely arbitrary. Society deals out rights in accord with certain human needs and as needs change, so do rights. On the other side are the moral intuitionists who talk about such things as rights being inalienable. Certain behaviors are permissible simply because membership in the human species is held. In this view, rights are self-evident, primitive, and fundamental; they need no further justification than their mere utterance. Between these two is the contention that to designate a claim to be a right it must be derived from moral principles, much as a metaphysics grounds an ethics. To cut through these abstractions—and many more could be cited—let us use the following criteria so that discussion can proceed.

Two kinds of rights can be delineated, *legal* rights and *moral* rights. A legal right bestows to individuals certain privileges and freedoms and the exercise of these is guaranteed by law. Legal rights provide persons with a sphere of autonomy in which they are free to act as they choose and others are obligated to respect behavior properly exercised within that domain. While acting within it, anything not expressly forbidden is permissible. This, of course, is recognized as the rule of law as established by the United States Constitution. A moral right has a higher level of persuasion on its side. Moral right is, therefore, *a prima facie* right to something. No legal constraint can block the performance of it. If the free exercise of moral rights is somehow hindered, persons may justly demand that they be honored and society is obligated to provide the wherewithal for their attainment. In the assigning of rights the principle of equity must be honored; all persons have equal claims to rights.

A *duty* is an obligation to perform certain acts and one is justly subject to moral criticism or legal punishment if he/she fails to perform the designated action. The privilege of choice is not included here.

In the questions above, we will construe right to be a moral right in the first question and a legal right in the third. Duty will be used in the sense that moral criticism and/or legal punishment can be leveled at those who fail to perform according to prescribed standards.

A consideration of the issue of genetic responsibility will most certainly implicate a variety of values since persons may view the matter in a number of ways. Some relevant values are listed below along with a discussion of each. These can provide a starting point in working through the alternatives posed above. As will be noted, they vary considerably relative to these questions—some are supportive of one opinion while others stand opposed to it. They are not given in any preferential order nor is the list all-inclusive. You are encouraged to add to them.

1 *The broad category of personal inviolability includes freedom of choice in matters of reproductive behavior.* Personal inviolability is guaranteed in the Constitution under the Ninth- and Fourteenth-Amendment rights; the Ninth Amendment speaks to the reservation of rights to the people and the Fourteenth Amendment, the right to privacy and personal liberty. Personal liberty permits persons to act in ways judged by themselves to be in their own best interests. There is considerable judicial and legal precedent that supports this principle with court rulings declaring that there are certain activities which are beyond the power of the government to regulate (e.g., Roe vs. Wade (1973), the right of the woman to the use of her own body; Griswold vs. Connecticut (1966), in which a marital right to privacy in reproductive matters was judged to be protected as a constitutional right). The newer reproductive technologies have widened the exercise of this freedom by allowing more choices (e.g., contraception, legal abortion, etc.). In any of these matters, the freedom to choose carries with it at the same time the freedom not to choose. Compelling any reproductive behavior, whether it be coerced abortion of defective fetuses or the legal requirement that a genetic screening test be a prerequisite for a marriage license, can never be tolerated.

2 *Setting criteria for child-bearing is a dangerous threat to the fundamental right of individual self-determination.* To ensure that only "good babies" will be born, a list of qualifications would necessarily be drawn up by someone or some group. These criteria may be applied to prospective parents or they may be used to measure the fitness of a fetus/infant. This application would make a sham of personal liberty and rights to privacy and would carry with it the potential for erosion of individual freedom in many other areas. Once the government inserts itself into this matter by

setting standards, the way is open to set arbitrary criteria in any other area of political, social, or economic life. The very roots of our democratic society would be undermined by insisting that only those certified could bear children and only qualified fetuses/babies would be allowed life.

3 *It is the right of every child to be born with a sound mind and body insofar as is possible.* This is the ethical dictum of human geneticist Bentley Glass. The new reproductive technologies make this increasingly possible. It is right and good to use these devices to insure that children will be sound, since it is they who must live in the world after they are born. Genetic health is taken as a given. If this right cannot be fulfilled, then it is better not to be born at all. The maxim of love for their children will compel parents to do all in their power to insure that their offspring will have an opportunity for the "pursuit of happiness" guaranteed them under the Constitution. Further, all persons are morally obligated not to knowingly bring pain and suffering into the world as would be the case if defective children were born when the genetic risks were understood in advance.

4 *It is part of the parental role for parents to determine what is best for their children.* Parents exercise this responsibility throughout that period of the child's life when they are under parental care. Judgments about what is right and good for children, frequently without their consent, is an important part of parental duty. Again, judicial opinion strongly supports this aspect of responsible parenthood. Parents who abuse their children or are in other ways negligent in discharging their parental responsibilities may lose custody of their children to the state. If parents can make these judgments after children are born and must live with the consequences of these decisions, then by extension, they should be allowed to make responsible choices prenatally for they are in the best position to weigh the factors and their consequences.

5 *As good citizens, parents are obligated to act in ways that promote the common good.* Promotion of the common good requires both those actions that actively contribute to the betterment of society—that is, those obligations that generally designate good citizenship—and actions that would contravene in the common good. Since in many cases, physically and mentally handicapped persons must rely heavily, frequently totally, on public resources, bearing defective children is an act of poor citizenship. Increasingly, public resources become more and more limiting with the consequence that the common good begins to suffer. Some programs are cut back, others must be cancelled. Placing extra demands on societal resources by knowingly bearing defective children must necessarily dictate a shift in allocation away from programs where the common good is promoted to those few individuals who many times are incapable of making any significant contribution to society. They are doomed to a life of institutional living. This constitutes an unconscionable act of poor citizenship.

6 *It is a case of discrimination to prohibit persons who carry "bad" genes to reproduce.* Persons have no control over the genes they inherit. Nor do they voluntarily place themselves in the position of being a carrier of genetic disease (e.g., sickle-cell). Since possession of genes judged to be undesirable did not result from an act of commission, individuals cannot be deprived of other but related rights. To do so is to single out certain persons and afford them different treatment. This is clearly

a violation of the principle of equity. Further, the persons identified to be undesirable are frequently members of the already disadvantaged social classes—the poor and unwanted ethnic groups. This compounds the dangers of discrimination by adding the charge of group or race genocide. Still another factor: Recessive carriers represent a statistical, not an actual, risk. It is quite within statistical possibilities that even carriers can bear normal children, or alternatively, normal individuals can conceive genetically defective offspring.

7 *Determining what is genetically normal or acceptable is fraught with hazards.* The whole problem of what constitutes normal, whether it be genetic, behavioral, educational, or whatever, is a question over which there is little consensus. Here we are caught up in the classical line-drawing problem. Where is the line that constitutes sufficient "quality" to enable couples to reproduce or fetuses to live? Any cutoff point will be arbitrary for all but a few cases where gross abnormalities occur (e.g., anencephaly). Furthermore, almost every genetic defect runs a continuum of seriousness and the degree of seriousness many times cannot be determined in advance. For example, mental retardation in Downs syndrome persons can be very mild on the upper end (i.e., lower average) to very severe on the lower end (i.e., imbecile). And besides, it is biologically unrealistic to insist that children be born with a sound mind and body; this condition can never be guaranteed even if genetically healthy parents are crossed. All of us harbor some deficient genes; new genetic defects may appear for the first time in the conceptus as the result of spontaneous mutations in the parental germ plasm. Spontaneous mutation occurs at a continuous and measurable rate. Still more, there is no technology available that can detect all genetic defects; only certain well-studied ones. Because of these factors, there is no point in trying to establish what is genetically normative.

8 *It is morally irresponsible to knowingly bear defective children.* To conceive children in the full knowledge that there is a substantial risk of their being defective—that is, higher risk than what is known to occur in the general population because of the randomness of sexual recombination or spontaneous mutation—constitutes a prima facie reckless, inhumane, and morally irresponsible course of action. This judgment arises from value 3, the child's right to an acceptable quality of human life. Moral recrimination is justified in this situation since the act is an intentional one done with full knowledge. A person is morally responsible for his actions if he freely performs them and with full knowledge of what the consequences may be.

9 *Caring for the handicapped, including the genetically handicapped, is part of society's larger role.* One of the major reasons persons organize themselves into societies is for mutual assistance; this includes caring for those unable to care for themselves. And here there is much precedent: state mental hospitals, alcohol rehabilitation programs, free neighborhood clinics, planned parenthood programs, and the like. Also, society frequently assumes the paternalistic position as, for example, when it protects people against themselves even when the coerced protection is against personal wishes (e.g., suicide). It is a humane, democratic society that helps bear the costs of exercising individual freedom.

10 *Society has a stake in individual reproductive behavior.* Not infrequently, defective children become the wards of the state. According to some estimates, the

public treasury spends about $1.7 billion annually to institutionalize persons suffering from Down's syndrome. The cost to treat one case of Tay-Sachs each year is about $25,000; hemophilia, about $15,000. Most certainly, these costs, if borne by the public, represent a drain on social resources which deprives other social programs of opportunities to improve the common good. It is a principle of moral philosophy that a society can take steps to protect itself if there are basic threats to such values as security and survival, or freedom and justice. It can be argued that large numbers of long-term institutionalized patients and those requiring special attention do pose such a threat. Euphenic solutions, that is, environmental manipulations to optimize gene expression (e.g., administering insulin to diabetics, providing a special diet to PKU children, physical therapy for the palsied, etc.), are much more expensive and resource demanding than eugenic solutions (i.e., improving the genotype through selective breeding). It is well to remember that the day is long past when parents were the sole providers for their children. Therefore, since society must bear some of the cost, it must also exercise some control. Parenthood, then, is not a right but a privilege and as a privilege, obligations and duties are inferred. Also, a well-functioning society clearly needs the fullest participation of all its members. The genetically "unfit" simply are not in a position—physically or mentally—to participate fully; hence their numbers should be minimized by selective procreation.

11 *Under conditions of conflict, fetal rights take precedence over parents' rights.* If the circumstance should arise where an abortion of a defective fetus is considered, than the fetal life must take priority over parental wishes. This is argued on the weakest party principle (see p. 58). The fetus, in this instance, cannot argue its own case—whether it should or should not live; consequently, it is to be accorded the privileged position.

12 *Defective children are a public health hazard.* Although this argument may sound trivial, there may be a ring of truth in it that has application to the issue of genetic responsibility. Society designates certain diseases as public health hazards if they are debilitating, are contagious, and/or can be spread to other people through contact (e.g., TB). Genetic disease, by this definition, is a public health hazard since it too is debilitating and is communicable. Further, as with the massive debilitating effects of epidemic disease, genetic disease can do irreparable harm to the gene pool of a population through the introduction and multiplication of bad genes—in every respect an epidemic although its expression may be more long-term. Just as society quarantines to check contagious disease, so enforcement of genetic criteria to control genetic pollution is warranted. Genetic disease is an immediate public health hazard, too, since it can deprive society of valuable resources required in the present (e.g., hospitals, health personnel, tax monies, etc.).

13 *Rather than considering the genetically handicapped as public health hazards, it is preferable to consider them a positive sign of genetic diversity.* The previous argument, labeling the genetically handicapped as public health hazards, is specious. Much study has gone into the question of whether or not the human gene pool is, in fact, deteriorating and at least some expert opinion does not agree that it is. The immensity of the pool makes it unlikely that deleterious genes will take over in the foreseeable future. Furthermore, the natural conditions required for increasing the number of defective genes in the population are not present; continued outbreeding between unrelated couples, a feature of modern society, coupled with the fact that more genes are lost in any one mating than are ever passed on, makes the whole argument for genetic deterioration speculative at best. Theoretical studies, furthermore, suggest that the spread of deleterious genes through a population is a phenomenon that requires many generations and is not likely to occur within at least several generations even if it could be demonstrated that genetic pollution is a real event. If the evidence is not convincing, then should society base a genetic policy on such flimsy data and argumentation? It is better to consider the genetically different as a sign of good health, indicative of genetic diversity. And here, there are a number of valid models to support the view that genetic diversity rather than homogeneity is to be valued for long-term survival. George Gaylord Simpson, the evolutionary biologist, clinches this position with the assertion "that there is no one best genotype or even a few best genotypes, and that a gene that might in itself seem defective may nevertheless be desirable in the gene pool of the population as a whole"[2] (also see pp. 137, 138).

14 *Using cost-benefit judgments to determine social worth is dangerous.* Social worth can never be evaluated in dollar-and-cents terms. Socially it is wrong because future worth can never be predicted with certainty. History has shown repeatedly that persons with physical deficiencies in one part of the body compensate for that loss by emphasizing or developing another part to a point of excellence (e.g., Charles Steinmetz, a brilliant electrical engineer, mathematician, and inventor was born a cripple and a dwarf). Intellectual or artistic achievement and physical weakness is not an uncommon combination. Thus to judge social worth early, as in the fetal or infant stage, would be at best a very questionable social practice. But it would be morally wrong as well, for it stands in direct contradiction to the moral principle that submits the infinite worth of every individual. Every life has some worth; there is no such thing as a life not worth living. Lastly, there is no political guarantee that resources saved by reducing the frequency of births of severely affected persons will be spent on socially desirable programs. The money saved could just as well be used for developing more exotic military hardware designed to create infirmity.

15 *The rights of other family members must be considered when defective children may be born into the family.* Here, there are at least two categories of concern: economic factors and psychological factors. In the first group, the need for costly medical or institutional care associated with rearing defective offspring can be staggering. This could and often does deprive other living members of the family of opportunities which might be afforded without the extra economic burden. Psychologically, the impact on the family can be devastating, even to the point of breakdown in the family unit. Emotional anguish is a frequent experience brought on by the tensions and pressures within the family and the feelings of unwantedness of other children simply because of the time devoted to caring for the defective child and the emotional drain it imposes on the parents. Alternatively, some families have been strengthened by the experience of caring for a defective family member. Greater cohesion, manifestations of love, care, and mercy—the highest of human virtues—can be fostered and strengthened in the experience.

16 *Children are not property to be kept or discarded.* The United States Constitution some time ago established the legal principle that persons cannot be considered property, to be exchanged or abandoned at will. Here, too, responsible parents do not want children just for their own convenience or utility, so that if the child doesn't measure up, it is simply given away to the state and another effort is made. The purpose of having children is not what one can get out of them—as things—but as fellowpersons, sharing in love-relationships and experiencing mutual happiness. Responsible parenthood is a deep human relationship between people and should not be taken lightly as can happen with a piece of property which may or may not be kept.

17 *If concern for population size requires that families have fewer children, then the children who are born should be healthy rather than defective.* This is the quantity-quality argument where if numbers must be limited as under population control conditions, parents will not want to risk any departures from the norm. The children a couple have should be as perfect as possible since the number of chances one is entitled to is reduced. It would seem expedient to make the most of the opportunities. The new technologies are seen as a means of quality control in a quantity-limited system.

18 *The determination of who is acceptable based on genetic categories can be all too easily extended to other categories of social usefulness.* Once the principle that the genetically unequal may be treated unequally is accepted, then grounds other than genetic may very well be implemented. History teaches us that the probability of this occurring is very high (e.g., Nazi Aryanism, black subjugation, the forced sterilization of welfare mothers in the U.S., etc.) Social usefulness as a criterion opens the way for abusive and restrictive programs without limit. In any system based on social utility, "some are (always) more equal than others." Certainly this maxim must be rejected by a democratic, free society.

19 *In a system where genetic criteria determine reproductive worth, the true aims of medicine cannot be realized.* The moral obligation of the medical practitioner is to minister to the health needs of all without discrimination. In a genetically guided society, the medical profession will necessarily be called upon to make numerous quality judgments; some will pass, others will be rejected on "good medical" grounds. Physicians then become technicians, engineering the procreation of society. Of course this must be done under legal sanction for doctors will do just what they are told to do. Medicine then becomes a legal arm of the state. In either case, involving themselves in the genetic selection of patients or acting as law enforcement agency of the state, the medical profession abdicates its traditional ethical position of duty first to those in need of its services. "Above all, do no harm," the primary injunction of the Hippocratic Credo, still dominates Western medicine. The responsible physician may very well consider the broader needs of the community when he practices medicine, but the needs of the individual patient must still come first. Judging the social fitness of lives is not part of humane medical practice.

20 *Individuals have a responsibility to protect the human gene pool.* This value carries the matter to a higher abstract level, namely, concern for the species. In the light of what has been discussed previously (both in value 13 and in Chapter 1—kin selection and the nature of altruistic species behavior), the issue can be argued as to whether there is any innate motivation to preserve the species' genetic heritage. The selfish-gene concept has as its goal the perpetuation of self. If there is such a drive, then it is unlikely that a valid biological defense can be made favoring this proposition. Culturally, though, as human beings we possess the capability to override selfish compunctions and it can be argued, as some have, that we do have intergenerational responsibilities, including species responsibilities. But these are self-assumed, not being derived from any fundamental or first principles. For instance, the idea that the lives of future persons ought ideally to be better than our own and certainly no worse is a matter of opinion only. Moreover, there need be no great concern over this greater species responsibility for this objective could be easily attained by showing active concern for one's own children without looking any further ahead than that. The argument in favor of protecting the gene pool is more theoretical than real.

The problem remains

As in other issues encountered in this text, no effort will be made here to suggest a resolution to the initial question: What responsibilities do parents and society have over insuring the genetic good health of offspring? Fortified with the discussion of some of the relevant values, the student is encouraged to return to the three questions posed by Professor Twiss at the outset of this discussion. They are unanswered in this text; there is still no consensus concerning them in society. What do you think is a proper position to take on these matters?

REFERENCES

1   Sumner B. Twiss, Jr., "Parental responsibility for genetic health," *The Hastings Center Report* 4, 1 (1974): 9–11 (a more comprehensive presentation of this paper by the author can be found in *Ethical, Social and Legal Dimensions of Screening for Human Genetic Diseases*, Daniel Bergsma (ed.), under the title, "Ethical issues in genetic screening" (New York and London: Stratton International Medical Books, 1974). 225–261

2   George Gaylord Simpson, *The Meaning of Evolution* (New Haven: Yale University Press, 1967), p. 59.

BIBLIOGRAPHY

Häring, Bernard, "Genetics and responsible parenthood," *The Kennedy Institute Quarterly Report* 1, 2 (1975): 6–9.

Ingle, Dwight J., *Who Should Have Children?* (Indianapolis and New York: Bobbs-Merrill, 1973).

Lappé, Marc, "Allegiances of human geneticists: a preliminary typology," *Hastings Center Studies* 1, 2 (1973): 63–78.

B. GENETIC SCREENING

At least three types of programs are becoming increasingly prevalent in the practice of genetic medicine: (1) screening for carriers of deleterious genetic traits, (2) prenatal monitoring of pregnant women, and (3) selective or therapeutic abortion.

Together, these have worked marvelously well in effecting quality control in the newborn. However, each is not without its problems. Let's examine some of them—first, screening for carriers of deleterious genetic traits.

About 90 percent of all people who turn to genetic diagnosis and counseling do so only after a defective child has been born; the rest seek professional assistance because they are worried about something "in their family." Inherited disorders usually show up in children because the parents were unaware that one or the other of them, or both, carried in the recessive state the gene for a genetic disease. When it is considered that each of us carries from six to ten genetic faults that may match up with our sexual partner, it is apparent that the potential for individual disaster and societal concern is significant. At present, about 300,000 couples per year are being counseled. A recent article in the *New York Times* suggested that up to five million couples are in need of genetic counseling. At the New York American Association for the Advancement of Sciences, the human geneticist Bentley Glass asserted that the number in need of counseling is closer to 100,000,000. According to proponents of screening, much tragedy could be avoided if people had some sort of record of their genotype to forewarn them. This knowledge, which should be private, could be used for making personal decisions on whether to marry and reproduce. Genetic screening by one means or another is the obvious way to fulfill our obligation to potential children as well as to the community which has to suffer when defective children are born. A reservation, though, should be expressed: Of the over 1800 Mendelian disorders in humans known to exist, only a relatively small number are suitable for genetic screening programs.

Genetic screening has been defined as the search for those suffering from or carrying a disorder of simple inheritance.[1] Simple inheritance as here used means the trait behaves in typical Mendelian fashion, obeying more or less, the law of dominance and recessiveness. In the carrier condition, affected persons have a single recessive gene for the trait under question. Individuals may or may not manifest clinical symptoms of the genetic disease. The more general case is that they do not, although there is some suggestion that even recessive carriers do show reduced vigor.* Full demonstration of the defect occurs when the person carries a double dose of the recessive gene. The dominant gene allele is not present as in the carrier state to suppress the expression of the disease. Double recessive can only come about if both parents carry the defective gene and the gene is passed on by each of the parents in sexual recombination.

The double objective of genetic screening is (1) to safeguard the human gene pool, and (2) to improve phenotypic expression through the management of genetic disease. The concept of a gene pool as the reservoir of the genetic information for a species is a relatively recent one. In many respects the concept is more abstract than real. The gene pool is not an entity confined to any individual or group of individuals but represents the vast constellation of all human genomes. To say the least,

---

* In phenylketonuria—PKU—heterozygote carriers may show a below-normal breakdown of the amino acid, phenylalanine; those suffering from the disease are unable to convert phenylalanine at all and manifest varying degrees of serious mental retardation. It is not known whether the carrier state results in any mental impairment although the suggestion that there is has been made.

this contains a gigantic amount of human genetic diversity since it now is an accepted fact that no two genomes, barring monozygotic (identical) twins, are similar. Hence, to take individual responsibility for the integrity of something so large is a rather ambitious, maybe even presumptuous, endeavor; and in fact whether or not single persons can seriously perturb it has been questioned. However, a number of population geneticists (e.g., James Crow and Cavalli-Sforza) have spoken strongly in favor of maintaining the integrity of this enormous pool. The fears are of two kinds: the loss of a critical portion of the genome that might in some way jeopardize our future as a species and the contamination of the pool through excessive introduction of deleterious or useless genes. Genetic screening is especially effective in addressing the second of these concerns.

The second objective of genetic screening is to improve phenotypic expression by the management of genetic disease. Here, several strategies may be followed: (1) emphasis on maximizing the expression of the genes present by providing them the best possible environment for trait development; and (2) gathering and communicating all relevant factors related to a specific condition so as to allow individuals the freedom to choose the appropriate reproductive behavior. In the first, a maximizing environment may include euphenic measures such as the administration of insulin to diabetics or treatment for sickle-cell disease. In the second, management is loosely interpreted to include responsible procreative choices encouraged by information and education.

Retrospective genetic screening

In general, genetic screening can be subdivided into two categories by method: *retrospective genetic counseling* and *prospective genetic counseling*. In retrospective counseling the parents already have a genetically damaged child and are concerned about recurring risks or there is a fear that one or both prospective parents may harbor deleterious genes because of indications in the family pedigree (a relative, near or distant, has demonstrated a genetic disease). Robert Murray, a physician and genetic counselor, lists the following as the traditional duties of the counselor:[2]

1. establishing the risk of recurrence of disease;
2. interpreting the risk in meaningful terms;
3. aiding the counselee to weigh the risk;
4. reaccessing the risk and estimating its effects on the counselee through follow-up counseling.

He would add to these the communication of all the medical, social, and genetic factors related to the condition, including consequences of alternative courses of action. Provision for emotional support should also be part of the counselor's role.

Counseling is usually given in the form of probability statements with risks of less than ten percent being considered low by most human geneticists. The aim of retrospective counseling is to provide all the relevant information including the nature and prognosis of the disease and its medical, social, and emotional impact on the parties concerned. The information should be provided in such a way that couples can make an independent and autonomous decision. Thus, the first commandment of genetic counseling is "be nondirective." The counselees, in other words, are not to be given advice as in the more general case of doctor-patient interactions.

There are, however, special problems involved in communication between the counselor and the persons seeking counseling: The very concept of the gene may not be easily grasped; its mode of inheritance and how it operates to produce disease may not be clear; the idea of statistical risk may be baffling; and the kind of language used may subtly reveal the counselor's bias. Linguists have shown that language can unconsciously shape courses of action. This may be true even when one is skilled in counseling. At the heart of the nondirective principle is the question: Did the couple fully understand the information given so as to arrive at a free and informed decision?

It can be argued that a completely free decision is not even possible once persons voluntarily seek out the assistance of a counselor. They are no longer completely free to choose. Some factor or factors compelled them to question their plans for a child in the first place. They are no longer objective searchers for information; they are directly involved. This may influence their decision. A further complicating factor is the conflict between the desire, frequently strong, to have children and the anxiety over bringing a defective one into the world. Frequently, the parents earnestly request that the counselor, presumed to be an expert, tell them what to do.

With the advent of the new technologies, the traditional role of information giver is changing. Whereas in times past the counselor could speak only in terms of statistical risk, now it is possible to ascertain the state of things more directly by prenatal screening. In some cases the counselor knows for certain what will happen, as in the case following amniocentesis. The chance discovery of unexpected conditions (e.g., the XYY syndrome) changes the conditions and the problem shifts to one of intruding personal values into the counseling setting. Should the counselor communicate the information obtained or not? What are the ethical connotations then?

Several other aspects of retrospective counseling have created ethical difficulties. There are approximately 700 practicing genetic counselors in the United States (1975 data); about one-half are clinical investigators (PhD geneticists), while the others are practicing physicians (mostly pediatricians). At present, the shift is toward more MD counselors as medical genetics becomes recognized as a medical specialty. Each group sees its obligation in a different way. The PhD geneticist, as a scientist, may manifest an allegiance to maintaining the quality of the gene pool, while the physician's concern is with the individual patient he faces. Physician counselors tend (but not always) to be nondirective, maximizing individual patient choice, while those who view their obligation as a societal one may favor policies which subordinate the individual to the greater societal good; that is, they are directive.[3] The defense of this latter position is that people frequently will not voluntarily use the information they receive. It therefore behooves the counselor as expert to use the authority of his/her profession by emphasizing the consequences if the advice is ignored.

A more practical problem in genetic counseling is the feeling of guilt or shame about carrying "bad genes." The guilt and humiliation of having one's inadequacies exposed, even if they are only pieces of DNA we call genes, can create significant problems. Tests and procedures, even when *fully explained*, arouse fears in patients. Many individuals become frightened when they learn they are carriers; others have no concept of what this even means, frequently confusing the disease itself with the carrier condition (a common occurrence with sickle-cell anemia). Still others suffer the emotional trauma arising from the obsession that they may never have normal children. Self-image suffers when persons learn they may be "abnormal." A sense of powerlessness can take hold leading to a fatalistic adjustment with life.

Can the knowledge that one is the carrier of a serious disease be so personally disruptive the harm of knowing outweighs any possible benefit? Dr. Richard Restak, a practicing neurologist, warns us of the "dangers of knowing too much."[4] He contends that genetic counselors hand out "unmeasured doses of dangerous information" to those who can't even understand it. John Fletcher describes the psychic response as "cosmic guilt"—an unusual sense of shame and guilt associated with genetic disease. Genetic screening may hold significantly different social and psychologic meaning for a person depending on when in his/her procreative life the knowledge is acquired. If it is obtained before marriage it may bring about changes in (1) a person's desire to get married, (2) the choice of an acceptable mate, and (3) the desire for children. If his/her carrier status is disclosed within an established family unit, husband or wife may experience severe dissatisfaction with each other as reproductive partners and possibly seek other mates.[5] Also, internal emotional strain may induce them to take the irreversible step of sterilization to correct their disorder even though the risks of the defect in offspring may be statistical.

There is no question that having medical information about oneself which signals actual or potential difficulties raises anxieties in most persons. The fundamental question here is how does one determine what is best for the counselee? Do the possible consequences of having affected children outweigh the possible benefits of freedom from anxiety based upon ignorance? It is these powerful emotions of guilt, fear, anger, and anxiety that the counselor is called upon to deal with, but may be unable to handle them effectively. Most counselors agree that these emotions should also be part of the whole counseling process but few agree on how they should be accommodated. (For the record, the majority of counselors are males; most of those coming for counseling are females. Men's and women's emotional perspectives do not always coincide. Should men, then, counsel women? Should whites counsel blacks?)

Another area of concern for the counselee is to what extent the genetic counselor will invade his or her privacy or the privacy of others. The genotype of relatives is frequently needed for purposes of constructing a family pedigree. Will the genetic counselor cause more or fewer problems by becoming involved with those not specifically coming to him/her for assistance? Can counselees themselves expect confidentiality about their defects when they voluntarily seek out consultation? Traditional medical ethics legally guarantees confidentiality. Heterozygote carriers might not wish to have their carrier status known to anyone but themselves since it might significantly retard their social mobility or status. What about confidentiality if other individuals are involuntarily drawn in as part of a family screening program? Who is privileged to this information not voluntarily sought? Does the counselor have some obligation to inform other family members that they may be at risk as carriers once it is discovered that a member of the family has a particular deleterious gene? Then is the issue of confidentiality still a private matter of one person? Should genetic information about him/her be given to other family members or even to those outside the circle of relationship? The information could be extremely valuable to relatives or even to others not related (e.g., a person who intends marriage with one of the potential carriers). The knowledge can act explosively on marriages, personal identities, and future plans. Also, if relatives did not seek out the information voluntarily they may not care even to know it. Should they be told if they are at risk? It is for reasons like these that some, even within the medical community, are not supportive of genetic counseling programs.

Defenders of screening programs, though, contend that they enhance the value of knowing. The assumption here is that it is better to know than not to know, especially when the knowledge offers parents positive options that will permit them to be in a better position to make choices. To be sure, the assessment of benefits is full of uncertainties. But the avoidance of emotional trauma is a matter of education and the counseling that should accompany genetic screening; screening per se ought not to be judged wrong because the potential for misuse or error exists. Benefits outweigh negative factors.

Prospective genetic screening

The second subdivision of genetic screening is prospective counseling. This is usually carried out as mass screening programs. Here the objective is identification of carriers before marriage or mating takes place. After identification, carriers can be counseled regarding genetic hazards. It must be insisted though that any genetic screening program must be considered preliminary and not definitive in determining carrier status. Initial detection as in mass screening must always be followed up with more rigorous and controlled testing to definitely establish the presence of the defective gene.

At the outset, genetic screenings were administered to large populations as part of public health programs. They were well-intentioned, supported by state and national governments. A great deal of money was appropriated and legislation was enacted to establish large-scale genetic screening programs, especially for several diseases. Lately, however, public mass screening has come into much disfavor and a number of the former statutes have been withdrawn. Let's examine this further.

Francis Crick, Nobel Laureate in Biology and Medicine, once said that "if we can get across to people the idea that their children are not entirely their own business and that it is not a private matter, it would be an enormous step forward." The biophysicist Leroy Augenstein estimated that of the six percent of the babies born defective each year in the United States, 40,000–50,000 "are so defective that they don't know that they are human beings." Sir Peter Medawar, immunologist Nobel Laureate in Biology and Medicine, stated, "It is a profound truth that nature does not know best; that genetical evolution, if we choose to look at it liverishly instead of with fatuous good humor, is a story of waste, makeshift compromise, and blunder." Joseph Fletcher says, "We are now approaching a situation in which genetic causes account for as many or more deaths than disease in the popular sense." It is against a back-drop of observations like these that the move for mass or social screening for genetic defects was initiated. Furthermore, screening is the obvious way to address the problem of continuing genetic deterioration in those populations that have access to modern medicine. Since the culling effects of natural selection are being thwarted in part, so one of the arguments goes, humans must take more direct action to minimize this potentially dangerous increase in the genetic load. Others would take the position that since it promotes the social good it is our moral obligation to undergo voluntary screening; and if voluntary screening proves inadequate, then screening should be legally compelled. A socially conscientious system might take the form of a national registry where genetic information would be filed. The information would be used for various purposes, such as marriage license applications and cross-matching for organ transplantation or blood typing.

As genetic screening programs become more routine and are coupled with other medical predictive testing, it is foreseeable that an extensive profile, including one's genotype and one's propensities toward disease (e.g., heart attacks, diabetes, cancer, etc.), could be developed for many individuals. Does it not seem intuitively correct that if health information about oneself is highly valued in certain circumstances then an increase in that information in the form of genetic knowledge should be most welcome? The possibilities of making more rational choices will be realized. It sounds good, but could such a system work? To obtain a position on the magnitude of the social and ethical problems contained in the single proposition of obtaining genetic information, we do have several real-life models to refer to: mass screening for sickle-cell disease and Tay-Sachs screening.

Sickle-cell screening

Sickle-cell, as it is known, occurs at much higher frequency in blacks than in any other group. Sickle-cell disease is an autosomal recessive condition, so that one may carry the gene for the trait but not personally demonstrate it. It is estimated that there are about two million black carriers in the United States; about 8 percent of the U.S. black population. The frequency of homozygotes is about 1/625 at birth and probably 1/875 among U.S. blacks as a whole due to mortality from the disease. The estimated frequency of the sickling gene in the white population is only 0.08 percent. There is no known treatment for the disease, although some promising experiments are being carried out that lessen the severity of so-called sickling episodes.

A relatively simple test for the sickle-cell carrier is based on differential solubility between sickle and nonsickle hemoglobin. Nonsickle hemoglobin is more soluble. Preliminary identification is followed up with confirmatory laboratory testing, for example, using the technique of electrophoresis. One should emphasize, though, that laboratory screening tests commonly in use have not always been reliable, and there is not yet perfect agreement on the best methods for follow-up analysis.

Regardless, in the middle and late 1960s a number of states and municipalities enacted legislation requiring the sickle-cell test for blacks in certain circumstances—in Washington, D.C. testing was required before a marriage license would be issued; New York State required screening before school entry; in Massachusetts the innocuous carrier state was legally labeled a disease; Georgia passed unanimously a newborn screening law.[6] Most legislators, including the bill's black sponsors, thought they were going after a serious and debilitating disease, not the carrier persons. But many viewed these laws as an ominous sign that the government was attempting to set criteria for childbearing. Others saw them as genocidal since only blacks had to undergo the required testing. The specter of eugenic sterilization, an extremely sensitive issue with minority and welfare groups, was seen by some as the motivation underlying this program.

By all accounts, sickle-cell screening was a disastrous chapter in genetic screening's brief history, probably because it was written into law. Participation was coerced. In general, the testing was harmful, uninformative, coercive, misleading, and chaotic. As Tabitha Powledge reports, "it has become increasingly clear that the arguments in favor of sickle-cell screening have had more to do with politicians' desires to do something dramatic and comparatively inexpensive for neglected segments of our population as well as doctors' desires to encourage black interest in health in general, than with the medical wisdom of a current program of carrier screening *'per se'.*"[7]

Many objections have been raised against the sickle-cell screening program. A central concern is that carrier status is often confused with having the disease. Just as before, there is something foreboding about being told that you are a carrier of a disease when it is not clear what is meant. One can only wonder about the propriety of having access to information which only confuses and causes emotional upset. But the implications are more than psychologically harmful to the carrier. *Stigmatization*, a new form of denoting status, marked individuals judged to be socially inferior. Higher insurance premiums, reports of job discrimination, and social ostracism were not the infrequent corollaries of stigmatization. To say the least, all of these can affect one's sense of personal worth, altering the degree to which he/she feels sufficiently competent to acquire and execute certain social roles.

Still another reservation objects to singling out only one group for testing, in the case of sickle-cell screening an already stressed minority group was the target population. In our culture, deviation from the "normal" identifies one as being somehow different, and different is frequently tantamount to inferior. Different genetically frequently means that such individuals be treated differently. Social duress of blacks has already been significant; why add more barriers to the struggle for social equality? Mass screening confined to single groups can easily become another way of categorizing people whom we don't like or fear.

The accusation that mass screening programs confined to one ethnic group correlates with race genocide has some substantiation on its side. Since there is no widely available prenatal test to detect the disease *in utero*, reduction of births by parents who are both carriers is the only sure way to reduce the frequency. Where both parents are heterozygote carriers, there is a 25 percent probability (1 in 4) that they will bear an affected homozygote child. On a population basis, reducing the incidence of the disease requires the elimination of four births in order to prevent the birth of one affected child. This can well be interpreted by the black community as disguised genocide. Of course, a solution to many of these problems is a thorough program of public education and enlisting the voluntary participation of the community rather than coercing by force of legislation. Mobilizing community agencies and resources so far to do this has not been very effective. But as a rejoinder, one might well ask why initiate a mass screening program that identifies sufferers only to inform them that we can do little or nothing about their condition? (A recent observation reported that sickle-cell homozygotes have for the first time been detected *in utero*. If this proves to be routinely possible, this argument against mass screening programs of minorities may become moot.)

The charge of discrimination may also have some fact on its side. Most knowledgeable blacks concur in the opinion that sickle testing in every black citizen should be as routine as vision and hearing tests. It is the mass crash approach, sometimes legally coerced, as well as the "Johnny-come-lately" attitude, that is irritating. The disease should really have been under surveillance for years. It has been known and clinical tests for its detection have been available for some time, but effective treatment is still not available. If this had been a white person's disease, exhibiting the same high frequency of occurrence, an enormous concentration of public funds on research, prevention, and cure would have been directed to it long ago. Overdue attention is now focused on the disease because it is only within the past few years that blacks have had any political power.[8] This is a serious charge with far-reaching moral and ethical overtones besides the obvious political and economic ones.

Screening for Tay-Sachs carriers

The second genetic disease for which an extensive screening program has been carried out is Tay-Sachs disease. Tay-Sachs disease is not common, even among the population where it is most frequent—Jews of eastern-European ancestry. It, too, is an autosomal recessive, with a carrier frequency in Ashkenazi Jews of about 1/30. About 50 children with the disease are born each year in this country. The infant at first appears normal and healthy but in a few months begins to degenerate. Blindness, paralysis, and general unresponsiveness mark the symptoms and death is certain usually before age 5 years. The financial toll on a family with a Tay-Sachs child can be devastating with up to $40,000 annually being required for its care. The more that is spent, the longer the child will live but in no case will it live to adulthood. Prenatal diagnosis is possible from cells cultured from the amniotic fluid. Therapeutic abortion of the affected fetus can follow. Using these procedures, a couple can be sure they will have children without Tay-Sachs disease. A simple, inexpensive test can detect carrier status, alerting would-be parents in advance to potential complications. Since the disease is irrevocably fatal and screening can help detect the carrier state in parents planning a family, it is difficult to argue against screening for this defect.

Different from sickle-cell screening, Tay-Sachs screening programs are well-organized and participation is voluntary. The careful and planned approach of enlisting the support, enthusiasm, and sponsorship of Jewish organizations has created a groundswell of demand within that community for the testing. This kind of community support appears to be important for successful mass screening.

The difference in the technology for controlling Tay-Sachs has also contributed to the effectiveness of the screening program. *In utero* identification of an affected fetus followed by therapeutic abortion does not pose a genocidal threat to the Jewish community since parents may try again for a healthy child if they desire.

Social and ethical issues in genetic screening

Here, then, are contrasted two prototype screening programs, one an unquestioned success, the other a dismal failure. There are lessons to be learned from these short episodes in genetic screening history. In the first place, it is apparent that like so many other technologies, genetic screening has presented us with many unanticipated side effects. What kind of answers can society provide to questions like these:

Is the social good to take precedence over individual rights?

Can the unattractive matter of race and ethnic designations be handled effectively?

Is compulsory genetic screening constitutional?

Should it be voluntary?

Who should have access to one's genetic information?

Will genetic screening provide precedent for other kinds of social screening, for example, psychological screening?

Do we want genetic criteria for having children and should they be set by the government?

How can the problem of personal and social stigmatization be more effectively handled?

Is there any point in testing when nothing can be done?

Should one diagnose incurable genetic diseases—e.g., Huntington's chorea?

Is there a right not to know?

Should life insurance companies or businesses insist on genetic tests along with physical examinations?

Is the collection and dispersing of individual genetic information an invasion of privacy?

Should screening be done when translation of the information gained into actual practice is low?

The list seems endless. The questions raised remain largely unanswered. The human rights of personal inviolability, self-determination in marrying and founding a family, and voluntary procreation imply unbridled freedom of parental choice in reproductive behavior. But parental rights may not be absolute. There are circumstances where marriage partners have the duty to avoid bearing children with serious genetic defects if possible. How far does parental freedom extend and at what point must other measures be taken? Humans have always been aware that sometimes children are born with gross differences. In some societies, these were omens of the gods; in others, they represented a visitation of evil; in either case, deformed fetuses were an inevitable consequence of nature at work. In our society, the new reproductive technologies, including genetic screening, give us the power to control and eliminate defective offspring. Many, though, are not convinced that this is a worthwhile goal.

Returning to the matter of screening for genetic disease, it would be well to review criteria that can be used for effective programs. Robert Murray suggests the following guidelines:

1. The techniques must be reliable.
2. The data obtained must be used effectively, that is, for health reasons only.

3. There should be a screening authority; for example, an effective supervisory state commission to minimize abuse.

4. The public must be prepared before screening.

5. A pilot study must first be run to see that all goes well before mass screening is tried.

6. There should be no compulsory screening—with positive options, high compliance can be expected.

7. Disturbance of the lives of individuals should be minimized as far as possible.

8. Only after all of these conditions have been successfully met should mass screening be implemented, and even then only with constant monitoring.

The emphasis in this list is on protecting interests of individuals in the several domains in which he/she operates: the psychological, the social, the economic, and the political.

Lappé and Ehrman present a second list of prerequisites for screening:

1. The disorder to be screened must constitute an important health problem.

2. The disorder to be screened must be reasonably understood medically.

3. It must be recognized in the presymptomatic stage.

4. It must be treatable, preferably at an early stage.

5. The tests must be sensitive enough to distinguish the disorder from subclinical deviations below normal.

6. There must be a cut-off point between those found to need or not to need treatment.

7. It must be cost-effective to screen and the test should be directed at the target population.[9]

This list places greater emphasis on the search for the disease—its identification and the test itself. In this latter regard, several other criteria for testing have been submitted that may help resolve some parts of this thorny problem. The test (1) must be easy, (2) must be oversensitive; some false-positives* are permissible but false-negatives are not, and (3) must be followed by treatment or at least some kind of benefit for the patient. On this last point, the dictum, "if you can't treat it, don't test for it" is a prerequisite for testing suggested by some. However, not everyone agrees. For example, there may be benefits in knowing even though no therapy is presently known, as in the case of the terribly debilitating Huntington's chorea. You might want to consider the rightness of this position.

We end this section with the following bits of verse. Although each paraphrase is humorous in its own way, both contain thought-provoking ideas. Think on them.

---

* False-positives are instances where individuals tested are initially determined to be carriers of the genetic defect but subsequent tests do not corroborate the first test.

False-negatives are instances where the initial test did not detect the carrier status and individuals are presumed to be free of the defect when, in fact, they are heterozygote carriers.

Soliloquy on Screening
with apologies to William Shakespeare

To screen or not to screen
That is the question!
Whether it be nobler to proceed
With a test for mutant genes
Only after the minds of all have been
prepared by proper education
Or to begin to test, anon, because
It is the thing to do.
One should not ask to test
Without informed consent
Alas, in time
Ignorance and confusion
In the minds of parents and screenees
May cause pain, suffering, stigmati-
zation
To those innocents who ask not
For the genes they are heir to

And, may at some distant day
Defame those who screen.
For whether one should test a
pound of flesh
A single cell of a drop of blood
It is that person tested who must
Live with and adjust to—the label
"carrier"
And therein lies the rub!

(Copyright, Robert F. Murray, 1974.
Used with permission.) (Robert F.
Murray, Associate Professor
Pediatrics and Medicine, Howard
University College of Medicine,
Washington, D.C.)

A Patient's Psalm

The Lord is my Genetics Counselor,
I shall not want for risks.
He maketh me to lie down in geneologies,
He nondirects me beside karyotypes.
He restoreth my inborn errors; He
leads me in the paths of reproduction
for my name's sake.

Yea, though I walk through the valley
of amniocentesis or under the
shadow of fetoscopy, I will fear no
evil; for thou, the Greatest Good
for the Greatest Number, art with me;
thy chromosome counts and thy enzyme
assays they comfort me.

Thou preparest multiphasic screening
before me in the presence of my

illness; thou anointest my head
with check-ups; my profile runneth
over.

Surely mutations and heterozygosity
shall follow me all the days of my
life; and I shall dwell in the
house of computerized biomedical
information forever.

Paul Ramsey, *Journal of the American
Medical Association*: 219(11)
(Mar. 13, 1972): 1476.
Copyright 1972 by American Medical
Association. Used with permission.

VALUES PERTAINING TO GENETIC SCREENING

1   Genetic counseling poses greater risks to individual well-being than there are benefits to be gained.

2   Individual liberties are best protected if genetic screening programs operate on a voluntary basis.

3   Benefits to both society and individuals are best achieved through compulsory screening programs.

4   Genetic counseling ought to be nondirective so as to maximize the exercise of individual freedom.

5   Genetic counseling ought to be prescriptive since the expert opinion of the counselor is more likely to be translated into responsible action by the clients.

6   Education and persuasion are to be preferred over compulsion.

7   If there are no benefits to be gained, screening should never be done.

8   The primary purpose of genetic screening is to benefit the family.

9   The primary purpose of genetic screening is to protect the human gene pool.

10 It is beneficial to screen for a genetic disease if the potential suffering of carrier parents and/or affected children is ameliorated.

11 No single criterion is sufficient in itself to determine which diseases should be screened for.

12 The severity of a disease should be the important criterion for screening.

13 No disease should be screened for that does not have a treatment.

14 In some instances of genetic defects, it is better not to be born.

15 In cases where it is determined that risks of having a genetically diseased infant are high, parents ought not to risk procreation.

16 If the genetic disease in question is not severe, then parents may rightly choose to reproduce.

17 Parents should avail themselves of all available means to bear healthy children.

18 If a specific therapy exists for a diagnosed genetic disease, parents ought to carry the fetus to full term.

19 Genetic knowledge about oneself is liberating and ought to be encouraged.

20 Genetic knowledge about oneself may lead to anxiety and to personal and social trauma so persons should have the right to refuse it.

21 Genetic information about oneself ought to be incorporated into decisions determining social action (e.g., marriage plans, desire for family, job, etc.).

22 Only married people or those planning marriage ought to be screened for genetic diseases.

23 Genetic screening is the first of a series of steps which can reduce the economic burden to society for the care of the genetically defective and therefore should be required where there is a significant risk of bearing affected offspring. This applies to either individuals or ethnic groups.

24 Genetic screening should not be used for trivial purposes (e.g., determine the sex of a fetus).

25 Legal constraints controlling reproductive behavior ought to be placed on persons with identified genetic abnormalities.

26 Respect for the dignity of others requires complete honesty and openness on the part of the counselor.

27 The medical profession is bound by a code of honesty in its dealings with patients.

REFERENCES

1   Tabitha M. Powledge, "Genetic screening as a political and social development," in *Ethical, Social and Legal Dimensions of Screening for Human Genetic Disease*, Daniel Bergsma (ed.) (New York and London: Stratton Intercontinental Medical Books, 1974), p. 29.
2   Robert F. Murray, "The practitioner's view of the values involved in genetic screening and counseling" (in Reference 1, Bergsma, ed.), p. 189.
3   Marc Lappé, "Allegiancies of human geneticists: a preliminary typology," *Hastings Center Studies* 1, 2 (1973): 63–78.
4   Richard Restak, "The danger of knowing too much," *Psychology Today* (September 1975): 21–23; 88–93.
5   James R. Sorenson, "Some social and psychologic issues in genetic screening: public and professional adaptations to biomedical innovation" (in Reference 1, Bergsma, ed.), p. 175.
6   Tabitha M. Powledge, "The new ghetto hustle," *Saturday Review* (January 27, 1973), pp. 38–40; 45–47.
7   Tabitha M. Powledge (in Reference 1), p. 37.
8   Lowell Elzia Bellin, "Conning blacks through tokenistic public health programs," *Man and Medicine* 1, 1 (1975): 13–21.
9   Marc Lappé and Lee Ehrman, "Screening for polygenic disorders" (in Reference Bergsma, ed.), p. 117.

BIBLIOGRAPHY

Other articles in Daniel Bergsma (ed.), *Ethical, Social and Legal Dimensions of Screening for Human Genetic Diseases* (New York and London: Stratton Intercontinental Medical Books, 1974).

Erbe, Richard W., "Mass screening and genetic counseling in Mendelian disorders."

Fletcher, John, et al, "Informed consent in genetic screening programs."

Green, Harold P., and Alexander M. Capron, "Issues of law and public policy in genetic screening."

Gustafson, James M., "Genetic screening and human values: an analysis."

Kaback, Michael M., et al, "Sociologic studies in human genetics: I. Compliance factors in a voluntary heterozygote screening program."

Lappé, Marc, and Richard O. Roblin, "Newborn genetic screening as a concept in health care delivery: a critique."

Mellman, William J., "Chromosomal screening in human populations: a bioethical prospectus."

Twiss, Sumner B., "Ethical issues in genetic screening: models of genetic responsibility."

Other references

Culliton, Barbara, "XYY: Harvard researcher under fire stops newborn screening," *Science* 188 (1975): 1284–1285.

Fletcher, John, "The brink: the parent-child bond in the genetic revolution," *Theological Studies* 33 (1972): 457–485.

Hilton, Bruce, et al (eds.), *Ethical Issues in Human Genetics—Genetic Counseling and the Use of Genetic Knowledge* (New York: Plenum, 1972).

Kopelman, Loretta, "Ethical controversies in medical research: The case of XYY screening," *Perspectives in Biology and Medicine* **21**, 2 (1978): 196–204.

Roblin, Richard, "The Boston XYY Case," *Hastings Carter Report* **5**, 4 (1975): 5–12.

Rosenstock, Irwin M., and Artemis P. Simopoulos, *Genetic Screening: A Study of the Knowledge and Attitudes of Physicians* (Washington, D.C.: National Academy of Sciences, 1975).

Whittier, C. F. "Sickle-cell programming—an imperiled promise," *New England Journal of Medicine* **288** (1973): 392–398.

Genetic Screening: Programs, Principles and Research (Washington: National Academy of Sciences, 1975).

C. PRENATAL DIAGNOSIS

Screening programs are justified only when they provide specific benefits for specific individuals and/or families. Can the same standard of benefit be applied to the issue of prenatal care? What ethical and psychological problems are raised when the techniques of intrauterine diagnosis are used to improve the quality of our offspring?

Prenatal care includes several *in utero* monitoring systems and fetal therapy including fetal surgery (see Chapter 3). In general, the techniques employed parallels the stage of fetal development:

First trimester: Ultrasound and hormonal tests; heartbeat can be examined and determination of imminent spontaneous abortion can be made.

Second trimester: Amniocentesis, ultrasound, fetoscopy, hormonal tests; monitors development of major body organs, structural and biochemical systems.

Third trimester: All of the above plus a variety of methods to evaluate fetal status in the last stages of pregnancy (see Chapter 3); measures placental function, lung development, metabolism, ability to withstand stress, etc.

Vigorous research and development in the new specialty of fetal medicine will add many more exotic procedures to the physician's available techniques. However, the extent to which these techniques should be utilized is one decision on which biomedical experts are not agreed. Take the case of amniocentesis.

Some ethical difficulties with *in utero* diagnosis

A recent survey revealed that a sizeable number (15–20 percent) of genetic counselors would not voluntarily mention the procedure of amniocentesis to their patients usually because they (the counselors) did not believe in abortion. Amniocentesis is of little significance if parents are not willing to at least entertain the thought of terminating a pregnancy if the diagnosis reveals some serious fetal defect. Dr. Carlo Valenti, a practicing obstetrician, notes, "The hope for treatment of most genetic disease 'in utero' is unrealistic and untenable. Although I would welcome an alternative to the abortion of a defective fetus, I reluctantly conclude that abortion must remain the solution to inheritable diseases."[1]

At least two criteria are invoked to justify the abortion of defective fetuses: (1) meaningful and rewarding life, including the necessary longevity to develop physical and mental capacities, is not possible; (2) normal development in early months of life will give way to extended deterioration thereafter (as in Tay-Sachs disease). This is a completely different approach to classical medicine for the cure here is not aimed at eradicating the disease but eradicating the patient. Leon Kass has pointed this out to us:

> In the case of what other diseases does preventive medicine consist in the elimination of the patient-at-risk? Moreover, the very language used to discuss genetic disease leads us to the easy but wrong conclusion that the afflicted fetus or person *is* rather than *has* the disease. True, one is partly defined by his genotype, but only partly. A person is more than his disease. And yet we slide easily from the language of possession to the language of identity, from "he has hemophilia," to "he is a hemophiliac," from "she has diabetes" through "she is diabetic," from "the fetus has Down's syndrome" to "the fetus is a Down's."[2]

There is, of course, another interpretation possible here—rather than describing the abortion procedure as resulting in the death of the patient (i.e., the fetus), designate it instead as a case of disease-prevention. The fetus may not yet be a living human patient and the disease is being stopped at an early stage. It can hardly be over-stressed, though, that fetal monitoring coupled with early abortion of defective fetuses is a brand new step in medicine, one that might legitimately be called the "ultimate preventive medicine."

It is fortunate, then, that most women who undergo amniocentesis for prenatal diagnosis of suspected birth defects are relieved of their anxieties—the fetus is found to be healthy. In a study done in 1974, 2187 women at 37 institutions had diagnostic amniocentesis during the second trimester of pregnancy. In 2125 cases, the fetus did not have the suspected defect. Of the other 62, 60 women had abortions and the defect was confirmed in the fetus; the other two aborted spontaneously.[3]

Several defenses have been advanced in support of the prenatal diagnosis/early abortion approach. Selective abortion is justified in these cases because it procures benefits for individual families by protecting them from the financial and emotional strain of bearing and rearing defective children. Furthermore, the option of selective abortion expands the exercise of freedom of choice since it is a cardinal rule in the practice of prenatal diagnosis that the ultimate decision for both diagnosis and abortion is to be made by the parents. Also, genetic good health is a fundamental right of every newborn—the right "to be born with a sound mind and body."[4] Probably other advantages of this medical procedure could be listed for, clearly, the abortion option is only one of several possible options following prenatal diagnosis. The monitoring is only an information-gathering procedure and the information generated can be used in a number of ways—one of which is therapy. But defective fetuses aside, most practitioners stress that diagnosis most often reveals a normal fetus and thus serves to reassure anxious parents.

Karen Labacqz, a medical ethicist, challenges the practice of prenatal diagnosis and selective abortion on the grounds that it (1) violates fundamental principles of justice, and (2) threatens the traditional life-preserving orientation of medicine.[5] If one grants that the fetus is human, then the question of whether one human being may remove another human being from her body becomes a moral issue. Quality-of-life questions are difficult to settle since the problems of drawing the line in prescribing the quality of life for another are impossible to resolve. Lebacqz prefers to identify a conflict of interest as the issue at stake here—the interests of the fetus to-be-born with the parents who desire a "good" baby. In situations of conflict, priority ought to be given to the weaker party. In this case, the fetus is that party since it cannot present its case. To overrule the unequal position of the fetus is to ignore the principle of equality. The only ethically valid course of action is maintenance of the fetus even if it is defective. Lebacqz's second objective will be discussed more thoroughly later but her meaning is readily evidenced by the statement (number 2 above).

Sociologist Amitai Etzioni interviewed a number of physicians to determine their attitude relative to using amniocentesis.[6] He found that one group was not even familiar with the procedure while another acquainted with the technique would inform a pregnant female about its availability only under special circumstances (e.g., the female is over 40 years of age or a high risk case). The reasons given for their reservation were varied:

1 The risk is too high; the procedure itself is dangerous in that abortion may be induced, infection may occur, damage to the placenta may result in hemorrhage, the fetus itself may be punctured, etc. The contrary opinion submits that there is no hard evidence to suggest that any of these are real threats. And in fact, the federal government has endorsed amniocentesis as a diagnostic procedure basing its position on the results of a 4-year study of more than 2000 women where it was determined that the procedure is safe and it is accurate.[7]

2 The procedure may place undue anxiety on parents since the decision to abort or not to abort must be made by them. John Fletcher studied 24 couples undergoing this diagnosis and found that 6 of the couples separated, although 4 managed reconciliation later. The strong desire for a healthy child combined with the knowledge that destruction of a life could follow if their desire was not realized created moral suffering of the highest order. Shame and guilt associated with genetic disease led to the judgment that one's marital partner was no longer compatible or the self-inflicted feeling of "guilt" on one member of a couple led to self-reproach, marital break-up, and divorce. What may be indicated by this study is that tension and stress can result from this procedure. However, these figures may not tell us much for we do not have backgrounds on these persons. In fact, these marriages may have been in trouble before they came to the counseling setting.

3 Amniocentesis is but the first step down the "slippery slope" for by making abortion the preferred option to deformed children, the easy solution of killing may become routine for any other defect judged socially unworthy. This position suggests that it is best never to open the issue by even suggesting amniocentesis for abortion on demand is a principle without limit. Contrariwise it is a fact that the abortion of defective fetuses is motivated by the most humane of reasons. In actuality, the parents strongly desire children; it is only because they want "the best" for their children that they even expose themselves to medical diagnosis in the first place.

4 Genetic intervention may threaten the race. The argument here is that some traits presently judged to be undesirable may prove to be essential for survival

in the future; don't eliminate them as would be the case if therapeutic abortion was the elected option. A negative argument suggests that if amniocentesis followed by selective abortion is not used, the most seriously afflicted children who will be born will not survive to reproductive age. With the option of abortion, carrier parents may be encouraged to have more children, some of whom may be defective but not enough to warrant abortion. The net result will be an increase in defective genes in the population. A circuitous argument, but perhaps it makes sense. The question of safeguarding the human gene pool has been discussed several times already so this objection to the use of amniocentesis will not be responded to here.

Etzioni is critical of any view which limits choice for the reason that as value judgments they are based on the biases of the individual physician, but their effect is on others, including the general public. An ethical issue raised here is the age-old one: Who speaks for society? Should the public, after being appraised of the facts and the consequences, be allowed to make up its own mind? Is an informed adult the equivalent of an expert in matters of value judgment? Should prospective parents be allowed the decision? As to the procedure itself, are the risks worth the benefits? Can a physician and/or a health department be held responsible for the birth of a deformed child if such a birth could have been prevented by fetal monitoring? Is it legitimate to bring malpractice suit against a physician who failed to suggest or make the procedure available if a child is born defective? Should, then, public health departments advertise the availability of such procedures? But where will the tests be carried out? It has been claimed that adequate amniocentesis testing could not be delivered if the demand for it becomes widespread. Even the pregnant over-35 class could not be accommodated entirely; and then who is to pay for the testing? The average cost per procedure is between $300 and $500. Where will the money come from if public funds must be used as under National Health Insurance or to those on public aid?

Can the prenatal diagnosis be abused? Probably so. A letter appearing in the *Journal of the American Medical Association* pointed this out.[8] A 38-year-old mother of one boy and two girls received an amniocentesis diagnosis to check for Down's (trisomy 21). The test confirmed that the fetus was not affected and that it was female. The patient thereupon stated she did not wish to bear another female child and she sought a therapeutic abortion. This situation may well become a common occurrence as the prenatal diagnostic procedures become improved and more widely available. The moral issue involves the concept that a pregnancy is conceived specifically with the plan of destroying a fetus if it is an unwanted sex. This raises two other questions: Is abortion an ethical option in sex selection? and Should medical laboratory facilities be used for this time-consuming and somewhat difficult procedure when other diagnostic uses would provide health-giving benefit to other patients? It has been reported that some expectant mothers will fake medical histories to obtain amniocentesis and follow this up with nontherapeutic abortion (abortion on demand) if the sex of the fetus is not to their liking. Hemophilia, for example, is a sex-linked disease found only in males. The hemophilia defect cannot be detected *in utero*. If hemophilia is suspected, the standard diagnostic procedure is to karyotype the fetus (i.e., do a chromosome analysis) and determine its sex. If female, there is little or no possibility that it has bleeder's disease. If male, there is a fifty/fifty chance that it has the disease. Abortion of all male children may be the option selected to reduce to zero the risk that children will have hemophilia. Can you now understand how a potential parent may use the ruse of hemophilia to determine the sex of her fetus?

Some obstetricians are of the opinion that sexing by *in utero* diagnosis, followed by selective abortion of the unwanted sex, is morally justified for several reasons. Since abortion is legal under any circumstances, it is the couple's right to decide, and physicians are in no position to insert their own values into that choice. Further, sexual choice is especially necessary today with increasing pressure to limit family size. If a family adopts a zero population growth stance (ZPG), then it is usually preferred that they have one girl and one boy. Selective abortion on sexual grounds could provide the exercise of this option, and besides, sex selection will help defuse the population bomb by providing families their sexual preferences rather than trying several times to obtain family sex preferences. The social liberation of females will also be hastened since mothers will not be burdened for years caring for large numbers of children. A last argument suggests that the frequency of sex-linked heredity diseases may be lowered since those families harboring these genes will be aided in having fewer, healthy children.

A number of counter-positions can be offered in opposition to abortion so freely prescribed. Central to them all is the issue of the moral worth of the fetus; and this discussion is best left to another time (see Section d of this chapter, Abortion: the Issues).

There is still one more side to the issue of prenatal monitoring which returns to the question: Is all knowledge good? How much, really, do we want to know about the unborn? According to Marc Lappé, as it becomes possible to exert greater and greater control over the fetus, our attitudes toward such concepts as normalcy may be negatively affected.[9] This can foster a return to the idealized picture of humans so prevalent during Renaissance times. Aristotle defended this opinion thoroughly when he said, "let no child be brought up flawed." In both the individual and society, a denial of human frailty and fallability can reinforce still further the view that different is inferior. A rejection of the imperfect can create serious emotional trauma—a sort of self-imposed sense of guilt in those with genetic defects. The previously referenced study by Fletcher of parents undergoing amniocentesis elicited expressions like "you spend all your life looking at pictures of pretty babies and their mothers and growing up thinking that will be you. It is pretty gruesome when you're the one who is different," or, "one day it hit me: what is Johnny going to think of me . . . if something had been wrong with (him)?"[10] Further, an idealized picture of what constitutes normal can easily be translated "optimal" in the future. Again in the Fletcher study, one parent stated it like this: "We have an obligation to our children before they are born; you can't turn your back on the future." This could result in a relaxation of moral safeguards against the wide-scale application of measures like positive eugenics or selective breeding. This could lead to other kinds of quality-control being promoted when they become practicable (e.g., cloning and genetic engineering) without carefully evaluating the consequences of their use.

Even if abortion was only admitted as an option in prenatal diagnosis future family relationship may be seriously affected. Joseph Fletcher said, "Even if the diagnosis given by genetic investigation was negative you have nonetheless (at least) entertained the idea of the death of your baby. To contemplate the death of your baby in the third month of pregnancy changes very seriously the attitude we, as a society, usually have toward our babies."[11]

Still another danger with the widespread use of selective abortion is that it could become the easy and final solution to defectives instead of treatment of afflicted children. In fact, it can be argued that the option of therapeutic abortion will seriously retard if not completely halt research in these areas; in terms of cost/benefit, why spend so much on costly therapies when a much cheaper and more effective alternative is readily available? This view is a direct contradiction to the stated objectives of these researches in the first place; namely, that prevention by abortion is a necessary first stage that will be supplanted by genuine therapies developed as a result of continuing research. With abortion as the easy solution, we may never get to nor even desire the second stage.

Kass warns that we may be on the threshold of an era when defective persons will be distinguished from the rest.

> A child with genetic defect, born at a time when most of his potential fellow-sufferers were destroyed prenatally, is liable to be looked upon by the community as one unfit to be alive, as a second-class human type. He may be seen as a person who need not have been and who would not have been if someone had gotten to him in time.[12]

Kass goes on to insist that the existence of defectives can never be prevented under any circumstance since birth injuries, accidents, disease, and maltreatment all have their toll. Lumping all defective people into one class—a second or subhuman class—can have disastrous effects on our whole conception of what it means to be human.

And then there is the sticky matter of judgment! How great must the defect be to justify an abortion? Who should decide? Should there be guidelines? What effect will the decision to abort have on our collective and individual moral consciences? Are defective fetuses really "human" at all?

Amniocentesis as a diagnostic technique cannot be done until a sufficient quantity of amnionic fluid is present in the pregnant uterus. This does not occur until the fetus is into the second trimester, usually the fourteenth to sixteenth week. Add to this the minimum waiting time of 2 more weeks before results may be known, and the fetus is already well along the developmental pathway, in the middle to late second trimester or even early third trimester. The shift in focus from late detection and treatment to early detection and abortion has begun. Increasing pressure is being placed on physicians and hospitals to perform abortions early, preferably within the first or early second trimester. The time lag between diagnosis and the decision to abort is short. Technological limitations make early detection of defects difficult but the expediency of early abortions may preclude adequate testing. Could errors creep in and perfectly normal fetuses be inadvertently destroyed?

On the other hand, pushing back the time of abortion to beyond the twenty-fourth week increases the hazards of this procedure to the female, besides running into the moral objections of those with the "right-to-life" persuasion. Invariably errors will result. We can only hope that future technology will make this experience less harrowing. As with so much of our technology, we have the tools to deal with a number of situations for which we have not as yet worked out suitable moral guidelines.

VALUES PERTAINING TO PRENATAL MONITORING

1 Selective abortion of defective fetuses violates fundamental principles of justice.

2 Selective abortion of defective fetuses threatens the traditional life-preserving orientation of medicine.

3 Prenatal diagnosis is good since most often the result assures anxious parents that the fetus is normal.

4 Prenatal diagnosis saves lives by preventing nonselective abortion in cases of uncertainty.

5 Prenatal diagnosis is necessary to gain needed information in order to stimulate the development of therapeutic treatments.

6 Exposing a fetus to risk in an experiment which carries no hope of benefits to that fetus but only future fetuses is unethical.

7 Prenatal diagnosis ought not to be done for trivial reasons.

8 Selective abortion ought not to be done for trivial reasons.

9 Therapeutic abortion is valid since abortion even for non-therapeutic reasons is legal.

10 Most people prefer abortion of defective fetuses over giving birth to defective fetuses.

11 Selective abortion is justified because it procures benefits to the family.

12 The ultimate decision for both diagnosis and abortion must always be made by the parents.

13 Protection of society against physically and/or mentally defective children justifies the practice of selective abortion.

14 Defective fetuses are human in every respect and are entitled to the same legal and moral protection as other human beings.

15 The selective abortion of defective fetuses places individuals in the untenable position of having to decide how serious the defect must be to qualify, hence, they ought not to be done.

16 An uncoupling of prenatal diagnosis from selective abortion is necessary to prevent abuses of the potentially beneficial technology.

17 Prenatal diagnosis should be used in any case and for any reason when parents desire more information concerning the fetus; to do less is to deny the exercise of individual freedom as well as to reject the benefits of what modern science and technology have made possible.

18 Our perceptions of humanness will be recast in undesirable ways if prenatal diagnosis coupled with early abortion is widely used.

19 A general weakening of social, moral fiber will follow widespread implementation of prenatal diagnosis followed by selective abortion.

20 A condition of disease should never be the criterion that measures social worth.

REFERENCES

1   Tabitha Powledge and S. Sollitto, "Prenatal diagnosis—the past and the future," *Hastings Center Report* **4**, 5 (1974): 11–13.
2   Leon Kass, cited in "Genetic screening as a political and social development," by Tabitha M. Powledge, *Ethical, Social and Legal Dimensions of Screening for Human Genetic Disease*, Daniel Bergsma (ed.) (New York, and London: Stratton 1974), p. 34.
3   Barbara J. Culliton, "Anti-abortionists challenge March of Dimes," *Science* **190** (1975): 538.
4   Tabitha Powledge (in Reference 1), p. 34.
5   Karen A. Lebacqz, "Prenatal diagnosis and selective abortion," *Linacre Quarterly* **40** (1973): 109–127.
6   Amitai Etzioni, "Doctors know more than they're telling you about genetic defects," *Psychology Today* (November 1973): 28–31, 35–36, 146.
7   Barbara J. Culliton, "Amniocentesis: HEW backs test for prenatal diagnosis," *Science* **190** (1973): 537–540.
8   Morton A. Stencheuer, letter to editor, *Journal American Medical Association* **221** (1972): 408.
9   Marc Lappé, "How much do we want to know about the unborn?" *Hastings Center Report* **3**, 1 (1973): 8–9.
10 Richard Restak, "The danger of knowing too much," *Psychology Today* (September 1975): 22.
11 John Fletcher (in Reference 6), p. 35.
12 Kass (quoted in Reference 6), p. 35.

BIBLIOGRAPHY

Ashton, Jean, "Amniocentesis: safe but still ambiguous," *Hastings Center Report* **6**, 1 (1976): 5–6.
Fletcher, John, "Attitudes toward defective newborns," *Hastings Center Studies* **2**, 1 (1974): 21–32.
Rorvik, David M., with Landrum B. Shettles. *Your Baby's Sex: Now You Can Choose* (New York: Bantam, 1971).

D. ABORTION: THE ISSUES

A statement of the problem

The abortion situation in the United States is extraordinarily open-ended. The Supreme Court decision of 1973 on the question of abortion left a number of issues unresolved. While there seems to be general societal agreement that under some circumstances, a woman has a constitutional right to an abortion, argumentation continues as to what those circumstances are and how many restrictions the state may place on this right. For example, a 1977 Supreme Court decision ruled that although women may obtain abortions without fear of legal recrimination, the state is under no legal obligation to pay for them. As a result of this ruling, Medicaid funds may no longer be used by the medically indigent for purposes of obtaining an abortion. The short- and long-term consequences of this decision remain to be determined but charges of inequality and discrimination were broadcast across the land by those favoring a liberal abortion policy.

But in no area has the abortion decision inflamed the controversy between pro-choice and pro-life opinions more than whether the act of abortion itself constitutes homicide—taking the life of a human being. The increasing practice of abortion, and the growing public acceptance of abortion as an alternative to "problem pregnancies" has produced an outraged and relentless backlash from grass-root movements calling themselves the "Right-To-Life" or "Pro-Life" lobby. In its ultimate delineations, the abortion issue comes down to this: Is civilization moving backwards with the enactment of legally sanctioned liberal abortion policies or is the acceptance of such a policy the manifestation of a truly humane society where justice and individual liberty prevail?

No doubt to some readers, opening up the abortion issue yet another time is indeed a fool's errand. In their opinion all that could possibly have been said by either side has already been said, and the result of all this was that neither side convinced the other of its rightness. It would seem that the only way to keep the argument going is to debate more loudly and with more emotion repeating the old arguments over and over again. But still the question must be addressed again. The present uneasiness about the status of abortion in our country demands that some rethinking, or at least compromise, be brought into the controversy. The abortion question is far from dead and if public policy is to reflect public consensus as well as ethical considerations, then some sort of balance-striking here is required if our society desires to live comfortably with this new technology.

We have already discussed the issue of selective therapeutic abortion and although the practice is not without its critics, the public conscience is not too disturbed about the rightness or wrongness of it. Moral objections to therapeutic abortions are minimal because of several reasons: (1) congenital deformity accounts for only a small number of abortions performed; (2) the abortions are prompted by humanitarian motives; and (3) the aborted fetus is not unwanted in the sense that the pregnancy was involuntary or inconvenient to the mother—a child was really desired.

Abortions for nontherapeutic reasons, on the other hand, are another matter. Cries of murder, genocide, and discrimination on the one side, are countered by claims of right-to-privacy, quality-of-life, and population explosion on the other. Issues like these are demanding societal attention for in a very real way they are forcing us to think about deep scientific and ethical questions: What is life? What is the value of life? Are all lives equally valuable? Since in either kind of abortion, many of these same questions must be dealt with, this discussion will not differentiate between the two. There is so much overlap between therapeutic and nontherapeutic abortion that they will be considered a single topic. However, the issue of abortion and population control will be postponed until a later discussion (see Chapter 12).

The United States Supreme Court's decision of 1973 drastically changed the abortion situation in this country and has had repercussions in other countries of the world as well. A newspaper reports "the recent Supreme Court ruling was not only a victory for American women but was also a boost for European women engaged in the same battle" (*Washington Star-News*, March 2, 1973). Christopher Tietze and Sarah Lewit, both from the Population Council, recently reviewed legal abortion as a worldwide phenomenon. They point out that liberalization of abortion policies the world over has been taking place over the past ten years resulting in lower mortality rates and improved medical practice. About one-third of the world's population now live in countries with nonrestrictive abortion laws; another third in countries with moderately restrictive regulation; and a remaining third where abortion is completely illegal or is allowed only if the woman's life or health is severely threatened by continuation of the pregnancy. Changes in the United States over the past decade are part of the general international trend toward relaxation of prohibitive policies and the American position has no doubt influenced much of the shift in world opinion.[1]

Abortion legislation in the United States

Impetus to the 1973 decision originated in the late 1960s and early 1970s, brought on largely by the gap between the law and actual practice. For years, abortions had been given in many hospitals across the land, usually to those who were able to pay for them and/or who "knew the right people." The poor more frequently than not had to rely on self-induced or illegal abortions, with their uncertain consequences, or to give birth to an unwanted child. Very few cases of accused abortionists were ever tried in court in spite of the fact that state laws expressly forbade the practice as a criminal act. Opponents of abortion argued that change in abortion laws would not solve the underlying problem; rather, such services as adoption, sex information and education, contraception, an expansion of research and facilities for children with defects, and other alternatives to abortion were the way to remedy the social problem of unwanted children. Many legislatures and courts, political careers, and lives of countless individuals were deeply affected by this controversy. But for the most part, the practice of abortion was carried on out of the public eye. (It was not altogether uncommon for the daughter of an acquaintance to vacation at her sister's place out-of-town for a year or so.) It is perhaps no coincidence that up until 1970, abortion ranked as the "third largest criminal racket in the United States."[2]

The original laws in many states, most dating back to the late 1800s, were highly restrictive, forbidding abortion except for *one* therapeutic reason—"to preserve the life of the woman." A few of the original statutes held the woman herself guilty of crime if she aborted herself or submitted to an abortion.

By the beginning of 1967, about a dozen states enacted laws that provided for abortion in cases where the pregnancy posed a "substantial risk" to a woman's mental or physical health, or if the child would be born with a "grave physical or mental defect," or if the pregnancy resulted from rape or incest.

These so-called reform laws passed in the late 1960s attempted to clarify or extend the original restrictive laws. Many physicians and observers of the abortion scene saw the effect of these reform laws as making physicians "feel more secure in that what they were doing as a matter of course for years had been sanctified by the legislature."[3] Reform legislation has most often been associated with the pro-abortionist position.

However, reform laws did not eliminate the abortion problem as seen by the liberal view. For example, many women wanting abortions were being delayed as their cases were reviewed by committees, and thereby the chances of complication were increased if the abortion was subsequently granted; or, after an anxious period of waiting, they were denied the abortion altogether. To counteract this, some states introduced what were called repeal laws begining in 1970. Four states passed laws allowing abortion without specifying any reasons, thus, in effect, authorizing abortions on request. Because they did not specify grounds, the repeal laws no longer required a physician to agonize over what constitutes an indication for abortion that is medically sound and still legal. Repeal laws attempted to regulate abortions by concentrating on procedural requirements rather than biological or psychological ones. A woman could request and a physician could perform an abortion without having to give reasons as long as certain procedures were followed—for instance, if they were done in licensed hospitals by medically qualified personnel.

These laws now brought the antiabortionist forces into the fray, for they were perceived as signals of the beginning of the end of respect for life in the United States. Through the measures of massive antiabortion campaigns, appeals to voters to reject repeal amendments (e.g., as in Michigan), and court appeals, the ingredients for a full-fledged confrontation between the two camps continued to mount. Between 1969 and 1972 a phenomenal number of abortion cases were argued before all levels of the judicial system. Many of these cases were decided in favor of antiabortionist views and generally upheld the constitutionality of the original abortion laws. Further, these cases sharply dramatized the need for constitutional and/or legal clarification of such matters as privacy, the rights of the fetus, and equal protection under the law—issues laid on the table by the "new" biology and demanding commensurate innovative legal interpretations. As cases piled up in the courts and state legislatures were challenged to respond to this or that pressure group, action stalled; everyone awaited legal clarification from the U.S. Supreme Court.

The long-awaited decision was delivered on January 22, 1973, in two cases (Roe v. Wade, Texas; and Doe v. Bolton, Georgia), both by the same majority—7 to 2. The court ruled that a state cannot intervene in the abortion decision between a woman and her physician during the first three months of pregnancy. During the second trimester, when abortion is more hazardous, states if they so desire can enact legislation to protect the health of the female—for example, by specifying where abortions may or may not be performed or what methods may be used. Beyond such *procedural* requirements, the decision was still between the woman and the physician. After the fetus has reached the stage of viability, corresponding to approximately the last three months of pregnancy, the state may prohibit abortion except when it is necessary to preserve the life or health of the mother. This sweeping decision rendered all original and reform laws invalid and entirely altered the abortion picture in the United States. Overnight, we moved from being one of the most legally restrictive countries to one of the most permissive in the world on the matter of abortion.

Of the constitutional issues being debated before the ruling, the Court's decision hinged mainly on a woman's right to privacy over her own body. For the reasons that the unborn have never been recognized in the law as persons in the whole sense and that rights extended to the unborn in tort law are contingent upon live birth only, the Court argued that the protection of fetal life cannot override the woman's right to privacy as guaranteed in the Ninth and Fourteenth amendments.

A major consequence of the decision was to greatly restrict the area of legal maneuvering left to the states to regulate abortion (only during the third trimester and partially during the second) and to shift the controversy from the state to the federal level.

The countermovement of pro-life activists

However, the Supreme Court ruling has never been fully implemented.[4] A vigorous right-to-life movement has succeeded in exerting pressure on a number of state legislatures to enact new restrictive laws and on many hospitals to prevent making abortion services available. A number of states passed legislation requiring parental consent in the case of minors or husband's consent in the case of married women. Both of these were subsequently declared unconstitutional by the Supreme Court (e.g., Danforth vs. Planned Parenthood of Missouri, 1976). In at least one state, the one method for abortion—saline injection—was outlawed. Abortions are not performed in Catholic hospitals, and large numbers of non-Catholic hospitals including nonproprietary hospitals, that is, public, not-for-profit institutions.

Because of these interferences, an "abortion gap" has been experienced in the country according to the Alan Guttmacher Institute, an arm of Planned Parenthood Association of America. In the year 1974, between 400,000 and 1 million women seeking abortions were denied them. More than a third of these were poor and another third were under age 20. As stated in their study, many of the unmet abortion needs ended up in the cradle; others resulted in self-induced abortions. School drop-outs, out-of-wedlock births, and precipitous marriages also occurred.[5] In the state of Illinois, much the same picture was found. Between 33,000 and 60,000 Illinois women who desired abortions in 1974 could not obtain them because many hospitals, fearful of public pressure or legislative repercussions, were reluctant to perform the operations.[6]

This disparity between availability and desire has given rise to a new institution: the abortion clinic (or "abortion mill" as the opponents of abortion prefer to call them). Abortion clinics, as the name stipulates, are one-service, one-stop institutions. Reports of hundreds of abortions being performed each day by single clinics for fees from $150 to $500 are not uncommon. As could be guessed, the potential for abuse or dereliction is inherent in this system even when the best of intentions guide its activities.

Antiabortion forces have seized upon still another strategy to immobilize the Court's decision: the enactment of a constitutional amendment, or the so-called Human Life Amendment. Thirteen states have requested Congress to call a Constitutional Convention to consider this action (Summer, 1978). A number of constitutional amendments have been introduced into Congress. In general, most of these would extend the protection of law to human life from the moment of conception, thus outlawing most if not all reasons for abortion. Another type of amendment seeks to return abortion regulation back to the states.

The right-to-life movement is active in all 50 states. The position of the various groups that comprise it is summarized in this statement by the former president of the national Right-to-Life Committee, Mildred Johnson, M.D.:

> No one needs an abortion. Pregnancy is a normal circumstance which does not require an operation. An abortion operation is a misuse of the skills, experience, money, and prestige (of the medical profession).

Since the 1973 decision, pro-life activists have:

1 succeeded in having passed or introduced laws in most states regulating aspects of abortion, e.g., stopped the use of saline injection for second trimester abortions; enacted the California viable fetus law which legally coerces the attending physicians to use extraordinary means to sustain the life of the aborted fetus if it is within the range of viability; burial of all aborted fetuses in Rhode Island; "apron-type" ordinances; parental or spousal consent bills; etc.

2 promoted administrative regulations restricting abortions—e.g., prohibiting the use of Medicaid funds; put pressure on state hospital administrators; prohibit abortions in public hospitals; clinical regulation and licensing;

3 enacted legislation at the federal level by attaching riders to federal bills (e.g., the Hyde Amendment) prohibiting the use of federal funds for procuring abortions; Medicaid abortions have decreased by about 98 percent in 21 states (HEW statistics, 1978);

4 agitated for Constitutional reform;

5 pressed candidates for political office to publicly declare their positions on the question; supported antiabortion candidates and campaigned against those with proabortion views and probably had a significant effect on the outcome of public elections at all levels of government.

The Catholic Bishop's National Committee for a Human Life Amendment continues to lobby Congress to pass a pro-life amendment, as well as continuing to agitate for change through local parish activities.

It is apparent, then, from the deep passions generated by the abortion question that the Supreme Court decision has not laid the abortion controversy to rest. Although some legal clarification may have been given, the moral issue is still wide open. A continuation of the controversy requires that cool heads prevail—if any still remain! But no matter how the issue is faced, the contending positions on abortion can loosely be described as liberal and conservative. John Badertscher presents the following distinction between these two views:[7]

Liberal	*Conservative*
1. Values individual freedom.	1. Seeks to protect and defend some element of a given situation.
2. Favors change.	2. Is generally slow to change.
3. The really free act is the one that is chosen on the basis of reason.	3. Recognizes there must be external restraints on human action.
4. Not proabortion but pro-choice.	4. The fetus is human life and any taking of it is murder (i.e., pro-life)
5. Abortion laws fail to defend the freedom of the pregnant woman.	5. Abortion laws defend the freedom of the fetus.
6. We ought to use the possibilities which technology creates.	6. The glamorizing effect of technology blinds us to the real ethical issue involved.

7. The pregnant woman is in the best position to make judgments about herself and the fetus.	7. Societal participation requires that some aspects of human action must be restricted.
8. Abortion is determined by choice.	8. Abortion is determined by law.

Badertscher contends that any public policy that is to prove effective must somehow reconcile these two positions. But like so many arguments in the abortion discussion, the real difficulty is in deciding how much weight ought to be given to the consideration each side puts forward.

The question of humanhood

The most basic question still is whether or not a fetus is a person. This in turn poses other problems: What is the essence of a person? When does this essential element emerge? One's position on these questions will determine the abortion stance preferred. At least three different opinions have been identified by Daniel Callahan.[8] A summary of the viewpoints is included here with no attempt being made to weigh the different arguments.

I. *Human life begins at conception, hence, abortion is to be prohibited except where there is a direct threat to the life of the pregnant woman.*
Human life begins at conception when the genetic basis of the individual comes into being; it is truly human at that point because genetically it has all that is needed to be human. All that is required further is development: a physical environment to develop its body, and a social environment to develop its personality. These are life-long processes, with no essential difference between the fetal stages and those that occur after birth. A previable fetus will die if it is removed from the womb; a viable fetus will die if sophisticated high-technology care is not administered; the neonate will die if it is not properly nurtured. Suggesting that there is a line somewhere in here is foolish. Thus, establishing the time when human life begins is not a religious question, nor is it one of preference; it is settled by biology. Moreover, such a view avoids the sticky issue of "when," since any other view is arbitrary and differs with individual preference or perception. Because there is uncertainty in this matter, it is best to err on the side of safety, and recognize the humanity of the fetus right from conception. In the case of the so-called "unwanted child," where the child is viewed as a piece of property, something to own or not own as one's desires or whims dictate, it is true that we have long-since rid ourselves of this concept and for good reason—children, or any other human beings are not the property of anyone. Therefore the argument based on the "unwanted child" is as nonsensical as suggesting that "unwanted adults" ought also to be killed. Abortion makes the practice of medicine an enigma. The physician's role is to preserve life, not to take life, and is so stated in the medical ethical creed. The problems of so-called unwanted pregnancies are illegitimacy and poverty; social problems to be corrected by changing social institutions, better care for the poor, etc. The request for abortion is a symptom, not a disease; it is the solution of a society unable or unwilling to come to grips with the real issues. Medical solutions to social problems is a dangerous business to get into. Giving legal sanction to abortion places the power of the state behind decisions as to who should live and who should die. Such a society would be threatened to its very

foundations for if them, why not me, and if for this reason why not any reason that one cares or desires to invent? Unlimited availability of abortion at public expense could well be viewed by minorities as a call for genocide since it is they who have the largest number of "unwanted"births.

Summary: ethical— primacy of right to life of the fetus; protection of the defenseless

legal— right to life is the foundation of all other legal rights

social— abortion is an evasion of social responsibility; it is a threat to minorities; it can lead to destruction of the weak or unwanted

medical—corruption of the medical profession.

II. *The fetus is not yet fully human nor is it only a piece of living tissue like a tonsil or kidney that can be removed with moral impunity, hence, abortion may be allowed under carefully specified circumstances.*

There should be legal proscription against abortion except when there are bona fide medical, psychiatric, or social indicators—threat to the mental and physical health of the mother; risk of a defective child being born; or pregnancy resulting from rape or incest. Indicators should include the patient's total environment, social, economic, domestic, etc. The law should allow for differences of belief and viewpoints, but this position does not propose abortion on request. Abortion is an option of last resort when questions of human life are important. A total ban does not serve this goal for it will (1) force some women to seek and undergo illegal abortions which are degrading as well as being dangerous, or (2) force them to bear defective children or children conceived in criminal assault, or (3) impose still greater stress on an economic or domestic situation already strained. No woman should be forced to have an abortion, but no woman who has a serious reason for wanting an abortion should be denied one. The matter of a fetus being human cannot be solved by law; it is a philosophical or a religious question best worked out by the individual. Legalized abortion as a perversion of medical ethics cannot be sustained since under a liberalized abortion law no physician would be forced to perform an abortion. And besides, the physician's role, as more recently defined, encompasses the total well-being of the patient. Such a law would minimize illegal abortions and their attendant problems which is also in keeping with medical ethics as well as lessening the hypocrisy of restrictive laws in the practice of medicine; the wealthy and influential do not suffer, only the poor and the weak.

Summary: ethical— primacy of individual conscience and free choice; protection of the overall well-being of women

legal— regulation of abortion but under legally specified conditions; abortion is viewed as a medical problem; this view is a compromise between the extremes of no abortions and abortions for any reason

social— responds to needs of women with serious problems; reduces the number of degrading abortions; reduction in hypocrisy under restrictive laws; lessens discrimination

medical—abortion performed using good medical procedures are safer; grants freedom of physician to practice medicine.

III. *The fetus is a nonperson in every respect and its continued presence within the womb is completely dependent upon the discretion of the pregnant woman; therefore, abortion should be available on request with no restrictions.*

Abortion is an exercise of a fundamental right by women, the right of a woman to determine her own life. Prohibitive laws, legislated by males, are an affront to women. When human life begins cannot be decided for one by another; such decisions are arbitrary and biased; therefore, the matter should be left to individual judgment. Legalized abortion recognizes the right of a woman to have an abortion; it does not force abortion on the unwilling. Abortions based on "showing cause" are degrading in that the woman must present her case and await the judgment of others, an invasion of her privacy, humiliating, and a form of oppression. Antiabortion laws foster dangerous and illegal abortions; also they are discriminatory against all women but especially against those who cannot afford to "buy" an abortion from safe medical sources. "Indicator" laws do not meet the needs of the majority of women who seek abortions because there are usually are no compelling mental or physical health reasons for desiring one; they simply do not want a child or another child. Thus, the right of a woman to control her own sexual activity is subverted (not too many males—including male legislators—concern themselves with the consequences of the sexual act or condition their sexual behavior on the possibility that there may be untoward after-effects, so why should women?). Advocates of this position usually do not propose liberalized abortion as a contraceptive method but as a back-up only, the final means of preventing unwanted children. Unwanted children enhance suffering and block fulfillment: The woman suffers, the child suffers, the family suffers, and society suffers. Something is owed children besides mere physical life.

Summary: ethical— primacy of women to decide their own sexual behavior including procreation

social— reduction in number of unwanted children; eliminates discrimination; ends disrespect for the law; allows expression of different views

legal— government cannot interfere with the personal choices of women

medical—abortion is up to the pregnant woman or patient, and the physician as is the case in all other medical decisions (why should this one be different?); reduction in dangerous and illegal abortions.

Although these summaries are an over-simplification of various views for and against legalized abortions (there are many more), they do identify certain features which are common to most positions. A succinct comparison of the values expressed by the Supreme Court decision are these (adopted from Callahan, Reference 8):

The right of women to self-determination overshadows the rights of fetuses.

The right of women to legal freedom overshadows the right of society to make laws restricting freedom.

The possibility of determining when life begins is overshadowed by the uncertainty that such a determination can ever be made.

The role of doctors as protectors of life under all circumstances is over-shadowed by the view that they are facilitators of the quality of life which includes a woman's right to make a medical decision concerning her own body.

The role of government as protector of all human life, including that of the conceptus, is overshadowed by the exclusion of the government from the prenatal phases of the human life cycle.

It is thus seen that there are many viewpoints and interpretations on the question of abortion and each has ethical, legal, social, and medical implications associated with it. The position on abortion one will take turns on which of the above components is most important, and tensions between individuals or groups derive from the priority given each component. It's as "simple" as that. Arriving at common agreement as to which component belongs where on a scale of importance is not so simple. At least this listing of value preferences can cut through some of the emotional verbiage associated with abortion debates. Although not pointing to a solution, this listing can clear the air some, enabling a sharper focus on the real issues. For example, do the rights of women to self-determination really take priority over the rights of fetuses when these rights are in conflict? Or is it the other way around?

Advocates on either side of the question base their primary premise on the question of humanhood—when does it begin?—and here, considerable controversy rages. Adopting the position of Garrett Hardin, a biologist who has been actively engaged in the liberalization of abortion policies for a number of years, a given society defines what human is. There is no definition of human to be found in any medical or scientific text. "Personhood" as opposed to being a member of the human species is a nonscientific issue. As biological organisms, humans in possession of a set of discrete and identifiable qualifications are members of the species *Homo sapiens;* they are human. That is all the scientist can say. Personhood, on the other hand, is not a scientific question; it is a theological or metaphysical question and it clearly reflects a culture at some point in time—whatever a society ordains it to be, that is what it is. Personhood is inextricably a social construct.

In Hardin's view, life is passed on from one cell to another and from one organism to another, and in fact, it never—at least not in our experience—begins. It may end but can never begin. Spermatozoa are alive; the egg is alive; the zygote is alive; the zygote that comes after it is alive; the zygote that came before it is alive. And if you go backwards as far as you can go, all the cells and organisms are alive until practically three billion years ago, when scientists believe life first began. Life never begins—it is only passed on.

Not everyone, of course, is satisfied with so abstract a concept, preferring instead something more immediate if not more tangible to serve as a guide. Some other views are these:

Humanness begins at conception for at conception the potential to become definitively human occurs; egg and sperm do not possess the potential to become human beings; that is, a totally new set of events are triggered into action. If egg and sperm do not contact one another and the appropriate biological events do not occur, both are destined to complete their short life and die. With fertilization, an entirely new future course of development is embarked upon, that is, a point of discontinuity is reached.

Another preference selects the time of implantation into the uterine wall as the point of discontinuity. This occurs six to seven days after conception. A significant point in development is reached at this point since the probability of successful implantation is not all that high. As many as 20 to 40 percent of all conceptuses fail to implant. Consequently, it is preferable to mark this point as the real beginning of humanhood since the odds in favor of completing development go up considerably with implantations. This position would permit IUD or morning-after pills as a means of contraception since both function by preventing a conceptus from implanting. Because humanhood has not begun, there can be no moral compunction against their use.

Proceeding still further in development, some think between two to four weeks post-fertilization is the point of discontinuity on which to fix the start of humanness. At this time, cellular differentiation is sufficiently far to prevent twinning or chimeras (identical twins). The beginning of personal uniqueness is the qualifier here. Some religious opinion prefers this point also for by adopting it one avoids the issue of the "half-soul" which may be the case if the soul was imparted immediately upon conception and the developing embryo subsequently splits.

Still others suggest four to six weeks for the reason that the fetus begins to take on a human-life visage then. Psychologically one recoils at the abortion of a fetus that looks like a baby; before then there is not as much concern. This is essentially a psychological criterion.

When brain activity begins is still another widely held position. This occurs sometime around the eighth week. The reasoning here is logical: If the loss of brain activity marks the end of life, why not the beginning too? It is superficially plausible to assume this, however, since brain death is an irreversible process. In the fetus, the absence of brain waves prior to this time is only temporary.

Quickening or beginning of fetal movements has historically been the time when the presence of a fetus was definitely established. It was then that real anticipation over the imminency of birth was accepted and great joy was expressed for then the thing that is "in me is alive." It seemed natural, then, to set this time as the real beginning of humanhood, and in fact, before 1828 the abortion of a prequickened fetus was not considered a criminal offense (in New York State).

But still some are not satisfied, including the United States Supreme Court which set the time of viability as the start. At about six months, or 24 to 26 weeks, the fetus may be able to survive detached from the mother (but not from the highly sophisticated apparatus needed to assist it in its vital functions). One cannot help but wonder when the time of viability will be as the technology makes possible the survival of younger and younger fetuses.

Parturition, or birth itself, marks the beginning of a new human life according to another opinion. This requires that a breath must first be taken; stillborns are never human persons.

Some societies prefer to define an individual as human at the time of christening, which usually takes place several weeks after birth. Before the individual is taken to be christened, it is not human. The bestowal of a name, in many respects reminiscent of christening, is characteristic of societies which we call primitive and marks the time when the individual has the rights of being a member of the community. Before christening, or naming, the neonate has no such rights.

But even this is too early in some cultures. It is only after the first year of life that an individual is given a name. This practice is found in those societies where infant mortality is very high. In those societies, the name given the person establishes him or her as a rightful member of the group; names have meaning and are much too precious to waste on the reasonably high probability that the newborn will be dead before the first year. Furthermore, mourning is minimized if death occurs, as it so frequently does, in the first year.

And lastly, some—notably anthropologists—would insist that humanhood does not begin until personality begins to emerge, the product of social interaction. If enculturation is the unique feature of human evolution, why not adopt it as the identifier for those biological organisms that demonstrate culture? Does this make sense?

And there you have the major prevailing views. These views represent arbitrary positions based on preferences which usually have been worked out to defend a preconceived position. Perhaps Garrett Hardin is right. Personhood is defined by a society and no amount of scientific fact or experimentation will settle this issue.

Joseph Fletcher, medical ethicist and theologian, looking at the futility of line-drawing, suggests another tact. Since those efforts will avail nothing but enmity he proposes that we attempt to "spell out [the] which and [the] what and [the] when" of humanness.[9] Two of his papers, "Indicators of Humanhood: A Tentative Profile of Man" and "Four Indicators of Humanhood—The Enquiry Matures," have engendered a considerable amount of discussion among those concerned with this problem. In brief, his first paper presented 15 positive indicators and 5 negative criteria. These are:

Positive human criteria

1. Minimal intelligence
2. Self-awareness
3. Self-control
4. A sense of time
5. A sense of futurity
6. A sense of the past
7. The capability to relate to others
8. Concern for others
9. Communication
10. Control of existence
11. Curiosity
12. Change and changeability

Negative human criteria

1. Humans are not non- or anti-artificial.
2. Humans are not essentially parental.
3. Humans are not essentially sexual.
4. Humans are not bundles of rights.
5. Humans are not worshippers.

13. Balance of rationality and feeling
14. Idiosyncracy
15. Neocortical function

Following publication of these criteria, a number of responses led him to a narrowing of the positive list to four: neocortical function; self-awareness; the capability to relate to others; and a new one, capacity to experience happiness. To be sure, not everyone is in accord with Fletcher's approach to establishing personhood but considerable approval has been voiced in favor of neocortical function. Mentation and all other attendant human capabilities originate here; one may have reservations about the presence of humanhood without a mind.[10]

The whole effort at defining humanness or as some prefer, personhood, as a requirement for claiming a right-to-life has been, so far at least, singularly unsuccessful. It has been suggested, therefore, that the quest be abandoned. This is in keeping with the majority opinion of the Supreme Court (in the words of Chief Justice Blackman):

> We need not resolve the difficult question of when life begins. When those trained in the respective disciplines of medicine, philosophy, and theology are unable to arrive at any consensus, the judiciary at this point in the development of man's knowledge is not in a position to speculate.

Toward a solution

The practical problem is, at what time, if any, is abortion permissible? The ethicist Sissela Bok submits these guidelines for consideration. Note especially that these are not reasons for abortion, but grounds for the position that there are times when abortion may be permissible and times when it may not be allowed. Someone (the public?) should decide on these times:

> *Time* in pregnancy—early usually poses fewer problems than late (medical, psychological, emotional, and ethical problems are not nearly as great).

> *Reasons* for abortion (listed here in order from compelling to frivolous)—selective unwantedness—wanted and planned but the fetus has an identified genetic defect (the problem of second trimester diagnosis and late abortion, also the problem of how serious must the defect be must be resolved here); mother's physical and mental health; risk of suspected defect versus actual defect; unwanted—sexual assault, incest, ineffective contraception, unplanned, economic reasons, etc. As a general rule, if the pregnancy has been voluntarily begun, there is greater duty to support the fetus.[11]

In her mind, the reasons for the continuance of a pregnancy become more substantial as the unborn grows and develops. Accordingly, she accepts the position of abortion on request for the time before quickening. Between then and viability, the reasons for abortion must become more compelling. The cut-off date she would set at 18 weeks. After the time of viability, she would prohibit them, except in rare circumstances. Sissela Bok adds yet another interesting observation to the debate. The Supreme Court decision, in stressing that a woman does have the right to an abortion in the sense she may terminate the pregnancy at her own volition, does not give her the right to the death of the fetus. What Bok means is that a pregnant woman may remove her support system from the fetus as a personal right of determination over the use of her own body; but she cannot in moral good conscience wish the death of the fetus although abortion in early pregnancy carries with it fetal failure to survive. One of the implications here is that certain methods are permissible while others are not. Those that first kill the intact fetus, such as saline injection, are not morally permissible. Her concluding paragraph summarizes the general restraint she expresses:

> Abortion is a last resort and must remain so. It is much more problematic than contraception, sterilization and adoption. At the same time, there are a number of circumstances in which it can justifiably be undertaken, for which public and private facilities must be provided in such a way as to make no distinction between rich and poor.[12]

Bok's essay is one of many that remind us again how precarious the Supreme Court's position on abortion is. To reemphasize, Bok's guidelines are not applicable to an absolutist position, either pro or con.

Another way to attempt an untangling of the confusion asks the *negative* question: What reasons, if any, can justify the refusal of the state to grant permission for an abortion? Some reasons have been given and are listed below.

The state may refuse an abortion if:

The health and welfare of the mother would not be threatened (i.e., there would be no psychological or emotional scarring of the mother);

It can be shown that it is contrary to sound medical practice;

It frustrates the realization of true humanity (e.g., tends to promote individual selfishness, lack of concern for the weak, indifferent attitude toward charity, sacrifice, etc.);

It can be shown that it involves the sacrifice of the innocent (contrary to Constitutional guarantees);

It undermines family structure (e.g., it fosters a selfish spirit contrary to the virtues of family such as sharing concern for others, etc.);

Civic virtues are weakened (e.g., if individual character is weakened, immoral sexual permissiveness is increased, etc.);

It can be shown that it is murder (i.e., if innocent human life cannot be destroyed, and if fetal life is both human and innocent, then fetal life cannot be destroyed).[13]

Space does not allow for a discussion of these propositions but as many of them suggest, the burden of proof is on those who advocate a freer view on abortion. Counterpositions to some of these propositions are:

Society permits some exceptions to the taking of human life; therefore, the sanctity of life is not an absolute given (e.g., the killing of an enemy or innocent civilian in war; killing to save one's life; killing a traitor in peacetime; killing a murderer; killing an aggressor to prevent the murder of the innocent; killing in self-defense, etc.).

Can a fetus be a murder victim?—ecclesiastic, legal, and social practice suggests that a fetus is not human; consequently, feticide is not the equivalent of homicide (e.g., no baptism of a spontaneously aborted fetus if there is no identifiable matter; no extreme unction given to a dead fetus; no funeral rites nor burial certificate issued; accused abortionists, under the old laws, were not tried for murder; grief is not as intense for the dead fetus; tort law only applies to a fetus *after* birth, etc.)

A fetus is nonsentient, as far as we can determine, unable to suffer and experiences no self-awareness. It is essentially vegetating matter; although it may respond to stimuli, so do all nonhuman organisms. Simple stimulus-response is no indicator of humanness. The worth of a life grows as its *consciousness expands.*

One frequently heard argument submitted by the foes of abortion, even applied in cases of granting "indicator" abortions, is termed the thin-edge-of-the-wedge argument or the "slippery-slope" hypothesis: "First fetuses; next the senile; and next—who knows!" This association is probably unproductive, for it attempts to couple in a single equation the abortion and the euthanasia problems. The single verbal formula "the sanctity of life" cannot solve all problems of human existence, as will later be shown in the topic euthanasia. Some questions posed by the wedge school are these:

1   Can we allow abortions without risking infanticide? If we allow the taking of life before birth why not after birth?

Evidence does not suggest this, for countries that freely practice abortion do not practice infanticide (e.g., Denmark and Sweden, where exemplary health care is given newborns). In Nazi Germany, abortion was completely outlawed in 1933 and was a capital offense; Buchenwald came later, but the Nazis never relaxed the punishment against abortion. As full term approaches, there is a growing concern for protecting fetal life—the Supreme Court decision reflects this concern.

2   Can we allow abortions without cheapening the value of life?

This attitude has been named the "abortion mentality" by Sarvis and Rodman.[14] The argument goes like this: (a) an increase in abortion rate leads to (b) a decrease in the amount of guilt over abortion, and finally to (c) a growth of disrespect for life. One of the more important studies which evaluates the consequences of being an *unwanted* child showed that these children are more than twice as likely to suffer from social, emotional, and educational disadvantages as wanted children.[15] The case study was Sweden, 1939–1941, where women were denied requested abortions in the days before liberalized laws. In another study, 26 percent of the cases (out of 131) of child abuse leading to filicide (death of a child) were attributed to the child being initially unwanted. In an analysis of 23 primitive cultures, 11 of which severely punished abortion and 12 had little or no punishment for abortion, it was determined that an antiabortion stance promotes a more violent society: "Societies that prevent or punish abortion also show disrespect for human life (practice slavery), are physically violent (kill, torture, and mutilate enemies), repress the expression of physical affection and pleasure (sexual repression), and place a high value on virginity."[16] One hundred percent of the cultures that punish abortion are patrilineal while 71 percent of those who do not are matrilineal (draw your own conclusions). Although all of these are negative data, they do suggest that the proabortionist view promotes a higher regard for life.

Garrett Hardin tells this story of the nineteenth-century author Robert Louis Stevenson's visit to Polynesia: He wrote back to a friend at home that he had found a paradox. The people on those islands practiced infanticide but, said Stevenson, "love their children far more than Europeans do."[17]

3 Is there a risk of compulsory abortion?

There is some danger here (e.g., coerced abortion of medical indigents, the mentally subnormal or ADC mothers, etc.). But the battle against coercion in any form must be waged continuously, not only in matters of forced abortion but in other areas as well. What is required is an alert and aware public. The danger of compulsion is no reason for prohibiting certain options of behavior, including abortion.

This discussion has gone on for some length now. Much more could be said and literature abounds. What is becoming increasingly apparent is that the question of abortion, like that of any moral behavior, is unlikely to be resolved by religious conviction or absolutist doctrines since such convictions vary considerably among free people and are, at best, arbitrary in their formulation and implementation. The extensive debates on abortion clearly indicate that no philosophical, religious, or scientific consensus exists concerning the question of whether fetal life is human life. A more recent distinction delineates the issue still further by submitting a new category—fetushood. The fetus, in this view, is in a distinctive, unique moral class, close to but not identical with a typical human adult (see p. 164, 178). So that now we have three categories: fetushood, humanhood, and personhood! A similar lack of consensus exists concerning the moral and ethical nature of the abortive act. It should be pointed out that the U.S. Constitution specifically forbids the legislation of religious beliefs or doctrines. Advocates of a free abortion policy submit that this is precisely what the pro-life position attempts. Also, as Garrett Hardin says, in a democracy the majority must recognize that it is just as unfair for them to vote away the rights of the minority as it is for the minority to deprive the majority of its freedom. By most public opinion polls, the majority of Americans favor an elective abortion policy under some circumstances.

It would seem that a compromise between the extremes of complete freedom and complete prohibition is the preferred way out. To begin with (and here consensus is more or less assured), abortion should be considered a last resort, not an alternative to contraception, sterilization, or even adoption. Thus, although an abortion might be justifiable in some circumstances, at other times it might not be. Further, as Sissela Bok insists, it must not make any distinction between the rich and the poor. Other factors that could be weighed might be these:

1 whether or not the pregnancy was voluntarily undertaken;

2 the importance and validity of the reasons for wanting an abortion;

3 techniques to be used;

4 time in pregnancy;

5 father's wishes (rarely in conflict);

6 whether or not alternatives have been considered;

7 religious views of the parties involved;

8 other considerations (e.g., economic, domestic, demographic, sociological, etc.).

Despite the present situation in the United States, the abortion issue has not been resolved. To implement the Supreme Court's decision, if that is what is wanted by the majority, will take relentless effort. The action on both sides of the question is intense. Several recent rulings have already changed some of our thinking on this vital question. In the midst of this confusion, Garrett Hardin offers this opinion: The clock can never be turned back, times have changed; having once accepted the principle of abortion "on demand" it is doubtful we will ever again accept its prohibition. The classic example of Prohibition shows us the price for turning back time—organized crime and a widespread contempt of the law even among non-criminal elements of society. In this context, the statement has been made that we will always have abortions (as we formerly did). The only question is, Will they be legal, carried out using antiseptic procedures under sterile surroundings ensuring the good health of the woman, or will they be illegal, done in clandestine fashion by unlicensed persons under conditions which can cause disease and death?

The Supreme Court, in establishing the right to free choice in abortion, granted legal permission of elective abortion of any previable fetuses on demand, yet at the same time protected the rights of the individual who opts against abortion. In these terms the matter is prochoice, not proabortion. Medical personnel likewise are given the option not to participate in an abortion operation. Under no conditions can any pregnant woman be compelled to undergo abortion against her will, and furthermore, no physician, nurse, or hospital can be forced to take an active part in the performance of an abortion. Perhaps this is the way it should be in a free democracy such as ours.

VALUES PERTAINING TO THE ABORTION ISSUE

1 The fetus is a human being from the moment of conception; therefore, the fetus is entitled to full protection under the law.

2 The fetus is at most a member of the human species. Humanhood cannot be determined by the facts of science; rather, it is defined by society or personal judgment and derives fundamentally from a prior value position.

3 Human beings have prior claims to their own body and can make decisions concerning its use.

4 Everyone has a right to life, so the unborn person has a right to life.

5 The right to life does not allow the use of another's body even if one needs it for life itself.

6 If a woman voluntarily called a fetus into existence, she is obligated to nurture it to full term.

7 There are some cases in which the unborn fetus has a right to the use of its mother's body and therefore, some cases of abortion are unjust killing.

8 The principles of justice apply only in those cases where an individual has a right to something.

9 No person is morally required to make large sacrifices to sustain the life of another.

10 A woman may be emotionally wrecked by the thought of her child, a bit of herself whom she will never hear from or see again, being put up for adoption; therefore, she may wish the death of the fetus.

11 Legality is not the same as morality; consequently, the mere availability of abortion does not make it right.

12 Love and justice, the cornerstones of all ethics, should undergrid any decision individuals or society makes regarding abortion.

13 Women may have the right to detach their body from the fetus, but they do not have the right to the death of the fetus.

14 The principles of justice require that the law be applied equally in equal situations; therefore, the government is obligated to pay for abortions of the medically indigent.

15 Feticide is not the same thing as homicide since the fetus is not a person.

16 The state may proscribe abortion if it can be shown that the common good is threatened.

17 There is the ever-present danger that if society allows abortion it will lead to greater social abuse, including a cheapening of the value of life.

18 In the justice as fairness principle, the most defenseless should be accorded greater priority in situations of conflict; hence, fetal right must over-shadow the female's (or society's) rights.

19 The right to life is not an absolute one; therefore, there are ethically valid reasons for withdrawing it from a fetus.

20 Just abortion laws maximize the real choices open to women.

21 Abortion is a symptom of much deeper problems in society and it should not be used to solve those problems.

22 Neither the fetus nor a child is the property of anyone; therefore, it cannot be discarded simply because it is not wanted.

23 No woman who has a serious reason for wanting an abortion should be denied one.

24 Since life is more than sheer physical survival, the only children who are born should be wanted children.

25 Genuine equality of sexes demands that women be given full control over the biological function of childbearing.

REFERENCES

1 Christopher Tietze and Sarah Lewit, "Legal abortion," *Scientific American* **236**, 1 (1977): 21–27.

2 Betty Sarvis and Hyman Rodman, *The Abortion Controversy*, 2nd ed. (New York and London: Columbia University Press, 1974), p. 53.

3 Sarvis and Rodman (in Reference 2), p. 43.

4　Tietze and Lewit (in Reference 1), p. 22.

5　Patricia McCormack, "National report finds 'abortion gap'," Champaign-Urbana *News-Gazette* (Oct. 9, 1975).

6　"Report says abortions hard to obtain," Champaign-Urbana *News-Gazette* (Dec. 12, 1975).

7　John Badertscher, "Religious dimensions of the abortion debate," *Studies in Religion* 6, 2 (1977): 177–183.

8　Daniel Callahan, "Abortion: a summary of the arguments," in *Aspects of Population Growth, the Commission on Population and the American Future, Research Reports,* Vol. 6 (Washington, D.C.: U.S. Government Printing Office, 1972), pp. 253–259.

9　Joseph Fletcher, "Indicators of humanhood: a tentative profile of man," *Hastings Center Report* 2, 5 (1972): 1–4. "Four indicators of humanhood—the enquiry matures," *Hastings Center Report* 4, 6 (1974): 4–7.

10　Marjorie Grene, "To have a mind. . . .," *The Journal of Medicine and Philosophy* 1, 1 (1976): 177–199.

11　Sissela Bok, "Ethical problems of abortion," *Hastings Center Studies* 2, 1 (1974): 33–52.

12　Sissela Bok (in Reference 11), p. 52.

13　Ralph B. Potter, Jr., "The abortion debate," in *Updating Life and Death,* Donald R. Culter (ed.), (Boston: Beacon, 1969), pp. 85–134.

14　Sarvis and Rodman (in Reference 2), p. 141.

15　James W. Prescott, "Abortion or the unwanted child: a choice for a humanistic society," *The Humanist* 35, 2 (1975): 11–15.

16　James W. Prescott (in Reference 15), p. 14.

17　Garrett Hardin cited in "Moral aspects of obstetrical practice," by John Fletcher in *Ethical Dilemmas in Current Obstetric and Newborn Care* (Columbus, Ohio: Ross Laboratories, 1973), p. 71.

BIBLIOGRAPHY

Camenisch, Paul F., "Abortion: For the Fetus's Own Sake?" *Hastings Center Report* 6, 2 (1976): 38–41.

Hardin, Garrett, "The evil of mandatory motherhood," *Psychology Today* (Nov. 1974): 42–43, 46–50, 147–148.

Hardin, Garrett, *Mandatory Motherhood* (Boston: Beacon, 1974).

Lappé, Marc, "The moral claims of the wanted fetus," *Hastings Center Report* 5, 2 (1975): 11–13.

Legalized Abortion and the Public Health, Report of a study by a Committee of the Institute of Medicine (Washington: National Academy of Sciences, 1975).

Steinfels, Margaret, et al, "Is Abortion a Religious Issue?" Three articles. *Hastings Center Report* 8, 4 (1978): 12–23.

Thomson, Judith Jarvis, "A defense of abortion," *Philosophy & Public Affairs* 1, 1 (1971): 47–66.

E. EXPERIMENTATION USING THE HUMAN FETUS AS RESEARCH MATERIAL

Kinds of fetal research

Fetal research has been a traditional form of medical inquiry carried on without public dissent until the issue of abortion was interjected into the practice. The Supreme Court decision of 1973 made readily available a large amount of research material in the form of nontherapeutically aborted fetuses. From the investigators' point of view at least, the healthy tissues of these aborted fetuses are to be preferred over those which in some ways may be defective, the products of spontaneous abortion or abortions induced for medical reasons. The use of fetuses obtained from elective abortions has the added feature that the timing of experiments can be better controlled since the research subject (the fetus) is not spontaneously aborted or health reasons do not compel the removal of the fetus.

Public concern has arisen because of the research on these aborted fetuses or on fetuses to be aborted. Consequently, we are forced to deal with the ethical and legal issues of fetal research in much the same context in which we deal with the ethical and legal issues of abortion, for implicit in whatever policies or legislation is enacted regarding fetal research is the question: Is the fetus a human subject? If the answer is affirmative, then as a human person the fetus is entitled to all the protections and safeguards guaranteed every citizen by constitutional law (see also Chapter 7). The alternative view contends that since a previable fetus is not a person whom the law is under obligation to protect, then one is relatively free to carry out any experimentation that is likely to yield beneficial results for society.

There is hardly any question that a lowering of infant mortality and a lessening in morbidity can be attributed directly to research on the fetus and the neonate. Examples are improved management of Rh disease and respiratory distress syndrome, two achievements that could only have been accomplished by conducting experiments with the human fetus and the newborn. Our prevailing concern with the health-debilitating effects of a growing number of chemicals in the environment including the fetal environment, emphasizes another area where more extensive research involving fetuses attracts the interest of scientists. Pharmacological research—the effect of drugs on humans—is still another area where much knowledge remains undiscovered. Endocrine research and its contribution to fetal welfare and survival need further study and evaluation. The development of prenatal diagnostic techniques, studies of fetal behavior, nutrition studies, improvement of abortion techniques, development of better procedures for facilitating delivery— these are a few of the many questions motivating this kind of research. Using animal studies to investigate many of these problems is useful but it has limitations. The final test must still be done on the organism in question—in these instances, the human fetus.

At least six major categories of fetal research can be distinguished:[1]

1. Research involving (a) live or (b) dead fetuses.
2. Research involving fetuses (a) *in utero* or (b) *ex utero*.
3. Research involving (a) induced abortion or (b) spontaneous abortion.
4. Research involving (a) previable or (b) viable fetuses.
5. Research which is (a) therapeutic or (b) nontherapeutic for fetuses.
6. Research involving varying degrees of risk to the fetus: (a) low, (b) moderate, (c) serious.

Chronologically speaking, the use of live fetuses is most often done at four stages of fetal life:[2]

1. When the fetus is *in utero* and will remain *in utero* for at least one week.

2. When the fetus is *in utero* and delivery or induced abortion is anticipated within a few hours or days.

3. During an abortion procedure (the procedure has begun but the placental bond is still intact).

4. When the fetus is *ex utero*, that is, after surgical separation of the fetus and mother.

The fetal research controversy

The concern encountered in any of these stages is not only a scientific one but an ethical one as well—it involves protection of "one of the most helpless creatures in our society" on the one hand, while on the other hand, permits research that can potentially benefit untold numbers of future fetuses who will, as a result of these experiments, have a better chance to develop into human infants or survive early infancy. If children have the right to be born well as previously claimed, then fetal research is one way to develop the knowledge that will ultimately lead to only well-born children. (It is of interest to note in this context that the foes of fetal research also oppose elective abortions. Yet continued fetal research is defended by some on the grounds that it has the potential to make most abortions obsolete.) Knowledge to control the reproductive process more effectively as well as to insure that "normal" babies will be born obviates the need for continued and extensive fetal experimentation. A number of positions have been advanced for and against fetal research:

1. Nontherapeutic research on fetuses should not be allowed under any circumstances.

2. Any type of experimentation, therapeutic or nontherapeutic, may legitimately be performed using fetuses.

3. Nontherapeutic research should be done on fetuses only to the extent that such research is permitted on children or on fetuses going to full term.

4. Greater latitude should be allowed for nontherapeutic research on fetuses to be aborted than for research on children or on fetuses carried to full term; however, certain types of experiment should never be done (e.g., the perfusion of excised fetal heads).

5. *Ex utero* experimentation should not be permitted on an aborted fetus which does not have as its primary aim the enhancement of the life systems of that fetus; application of artificial life-sustaining equipment for the sole purpose of experimentation should not be done (e.g., fetal incubator).

Professor Richard Wasserstrom, a UCLA philosopher, provides a taxonomy of different views regarding the status of the fetus which fixes one's primary position on the issue of fetal research.[3]

1. The fetus is in most, if not all, morally relevant respects like a fully developed, adult human being. The fetus comes under the same curtain of protection that any adult human experimental subject enjoys (see Chapter 7).

2. The fetus is in most, if not all, morally relevant respects like a piece of tissue or a discrete human organ. Here, fetal experimentation of almost any kind is permissible.

3. The fetus is in most, if not all, morally relevant respects like a higher animal, like a dog or a monkey. Although clearly not a person, the fetus deserves consideration similar to that shown animals in live experimentation; for example, the avoidance of cruelty or unnecessary suffering.

4. The fetus is in a distinctive, relatively unique moral category, close to but not identical with a typical human adult. In this view, the fetus is higher than the animals but lower than postnatal humans; the status here is similar to that of the mentally deranged or a slave. Fetal experimentation here is problematical at best and must be carefully evaluated and regulated.

No single position described above commands majority consensus.

The controversy over whether fetal research should be allowed or under what conditions it ought to be allowed peaked with the signing into law of the National Research Act on July 12, 1974. Among other things, this law declared a moratorium on all fetal research, except that research intended to promote the survival of the fetus, until such time as the issue could be clarified. Specifically, the act made provisions for a study commission—the National Commission for the Protection of Human Subjects of Biomedical and Behavioral Research—one of whose tasks was to determine the nature, extent, and purposes of research involving living fetuses and to consider alternative means for reaching those purposes. Further, the Commission was to draw up regulations governing fetal research for submission to the Department of Health, Education, and Welfare (HEW). A stipulation of the act required that these recommendations must be implemented by the Secretary of HEW as policy or he/she must explain in writing to the public the reasons for not doing so. (Precedent was set here in that this was one of the few times that a national commission's recommendations had some impact on federal policy)

The commission of eleven members, representing a number of different areas of specialization, including medicine, law, and ethics (see *Bioscience*, reference 4, for a listing of membership), held a series of public meetings and study sessions during the winter and spring of 1975. It grappled with questions like the following:

When is high-risk research justified?

How does the status of a fetus to be aborted differ from that of a fetus going to full term?

Does a fetus feel pain?

Can a fetus to be aborted be harmed?

What responsibility must be taken and by whom for a fetus born alive but damaged by research?

Which takes precedence when the rights of the mother conflict with the rights of the fetus?

Is there ever a time when risks can be imposed on a nonconsenting subject?

Some ethical positions on fetal research

Eight philosophers and ethicists prepared position papers for the commission which outlined the major ethical issues concerning research with fetuses. A summary of each paper follows:[5]

Sissela Bok (Teacher of bioethics at Radcliffe Institute and Harvard University)

> The fetus is a person and research on it without its consent and not for its benefit is an affront to its humanity; research on the fetus may lead to other categories of research on the defenseless (e.g., the mentally handicapped, the terminally ill, comatose patient, etc.); fetal research may be permitted if (1) the information to be gained is not obtainable by any other means, (2) it is carried out using previable fetuses—the first 18 weeks of gestational age and under 300 grams in weight (recall Bok's position on abortion discussed on p. 169, and (3) careful safeguards are utilized. Dr. Bok would permit research on a fetus scheduled for abortion provided the mother consents and the research has been properly reviewed and approved by a research committee.

Joseph Fletcher (Medical ethicist, University of Virginia Medical School)

> Consequences determine rightness or wrongness; therefore, if fetal research benefits others, especially children, then it is permissible. The fetus is not an actual person, ethically or legally, until it is born alive and lives entirely outside the mother's uterus supported by its own cardiovascular system. Fetal experimentation may be carried out in these situations: (1) the use of a dead fetus *ex utero* with or without the mother's consent; (2) the use of a live fetus, viable or inviable, if survival is not wanted and there is maternal consent; and (3) the use of a live fetus *in utero* if survival is not wanted and there is maternal consent. Restricting fetal research by legislation is unethical unless the ethics on which the legislation itself is based are fully explained.

Marc Lappé (Director, Office of Health, Law, and Values, State of California)

> Fetuses both *in utero* and *ex utero* have a right to protection; these rights are compromised by the abortion act—the abortion procedure used should minimize health-debilitating effects on the mother while expeditiously expelling the fetus and rendering it incapable of future survival. Research on *in utero* fetuses is justified if and only if it is intended to benefit other fetuses and there is no risk of harm to the fetus or the mother. Nonviable fetal research should be restricted to dead fetuses.

Richard A. McCormick (Professor of Christian Ethics, Georgetown University)

> Starting from the premise that all humans, including children, have an obligation in social justice to contribute to the benefit of the human community, we can extend the same obligation to the fetus. Fetal research, therefore, is morally permissible if maternal proxy consent is given, abortion is *not* contemplated, the risk or discomfort to the fetus is not discernible, and the results of the experiment cannot be obtained in any other way. Because most abortions are immoral, experiments on abortants are also morally objectionable because they derive from a prior wrong (see, The Principle of Double Effect, p. 62). Since

this principle is not feasible in our morally pluralistic society, the following guidelines should be followed: (1) the research must be necessary; (2) the researcher bears the responsibility of showing its necessity; (3) there must be no discernible risk for the fetus or mother, or if the fetus is dying, there must be no added pain or discomfort; (4) the scientist bears the responsibility of showing no risk; and (5) adequate review boards must supervise all aspects of the research to insure compliance.

Paul Ramsey (Christian ethicist, Princeton University)

Fetal viability should not be confused with life—a fetus may be alive but not viable; the line between the living, the nonviable, and the viable fetus is indistinct and great care should be exercised not to enter a viable fetus by mistake. Fetal research is reluctantly allowed but under specified conditions: (1) the procedures should not deliberately do harm to the fetus for any reason; (2) if the research carries known or uncertain risks even if the fetus is to be aborted, then it must not be done; (3) respect for the dignity of life must never be compromised whatever the age, circumstances, or expectations of life of the subject (the Supreme Court decision did not remove the moral obligation of protecting life from harm even if the harm is less than abortion); (4) *ex utero* maintenance of life should not be done except to enable that aborted fetus to survive; and (5) the same ethical standards that apply to research on the defenseless (e.g., the unconscious, the comatose, children, etc.) should be subscribed to in fetal research—nontherapeutic research which involves discernible risk, undue discomfort, or inconvenience is thus precluded. (Paul Ramsey's *The Ethics of Fetal Research*—see bibliography—is an eloquent elucidation of his views and has become one of the standards in the field of fetal research.)

Seymour Siegel (Theologian and Ethicist, Jewish Theological Seminary, New York)

The fetus is not the same as an infant since it has no life independent of its mother; the fetus has real but limited rights of protection (e.g., it cannot threaten the life of another). *In utero* research is permissible if (a) it is harmless to the fetus, (b) it helps the mother, or (c) it is designed to help other fetuses. The *ex utero* fetus has more rights than an *in utero* fetus, hence prolongation of its life is prohibited unless the research is intended to enhance the survival of that fetus. Maternal consent supplemented by a special review board is required.

Leroy Walters (Director, Center for Bioethics, Georgetown University)

Nontherapeutic research on the fetus should be permitted only to the extent that such research is permitted on children or on fetuses that will be carried to full term; parental consent may properly allow this research since the good of the child is the motivation. There is an essential continuity between previable, viable, and neonate life and this view recognizes the equality of all three categories; hence, nontherapeutic research is allowable if it involves no or only minimal risks to the subjects and includes both fetuses to be aborted and live fetuses which have been aborted.

Richard Wasserstrom (Professor of Law and Philosophy, UCLA)

The fetus is in a unique moral category, not human but very close to one; the fetus has value because of its potential to become a fully developed human being; because research on the fetus may impair this potential-to-become, no research should be permitted *in utero* if it involves a substantial risk to the fetus. This restriction applies to fetuses to be aborted also since the decision to abort may be revocable. *Ex utero* experimentation is permissible providing (1) the mother consents before abortion; (2) a review board has ascertained prior to the experiment that the research is for essential knowledge not available in any other way; (3) the medical personnel attending the woman are not connected to the experiment in any way; and (4) the fetus is not viable in any way.

Other positions in opposition to fetal research expressed the fear that science would become too dependent on the products of an abortion and that society would be less inclined to try to find alternatives to abortion. An objection that raised major concern had to do with the dangers to the fetus if, after a research procedure had been performed, the mother changed her mind and decided to allow the fetus to come to full term. There is the genuine possibility that she would then give birth to a child who is unnecessarily injured. It would seem morally unjustifiable to bring a child into the world with defects or disabilities that had been intentionally induced.

The commission considered research on living fetuses in a variety of circumstances, and in every case, they emphasized the need for careful evaluation of a proposed experiment for both its medical and *ethical* soundness. Also in every case, the commission placed high priority on informed consent. A pregnant woman has absolute veto power over *in utero* research whether it be therapeutic or nontherapeutic.

Federal policy on fetal research

The guiding principle that formed the basis for subsequent recommendations became known as the Brady Principle after Joseph V. Brady, a commission member from Johns Hopkins University. It held that there was "no difference in the status of a fetus to be aborted and a fetus going to full term until abortion *procedures* had actually started." It was the aim of this principle to preclude any possibility that the pregnant woman may withdraw her consent to an experiment which could leave her with a damaged fetus. Also, this would minimize any coercion connected with the abortion act itself in the rare event she chose not to proceed with the experimental procedure just prior to its enactment. The possibility of bearing an injured fetus might affect her decision not to abort and thus limit her freedom to choose. The report of the commission was made public on May 1, 1975, and contained the following ten recommendations:[6]

1. *Therapeutic research directed toward the fetus* may be conducted or supported, and should be encouraged, by the Secretary, DHEW, provided such research (a) is within appropriate medical standards, (b) has received the informed consent of the parent(s), and (c) has been approved by existing review procedures with adequate provision for the monitoring of the consent process.   (Adopted unanimously.)

2. *Therapeutic research directed toward the pregnant woman* may be conducted or supported, and should be encouraged, by the Secretary, DHEW, provided such research (a) has been evaluated for possible impact on the fetus, (b) will place the fetus at risk to the minimum extent consistent with meeting the health needs of the pregnant woman, (c) has been approved by existing review procedures with adequate provision for the monitoring of the consent process, and (d) the pregnant woman has given her informed consent.   (Adopted unanimously.)

3. *Nontherapeutic research directed toward the pregnant woman may be conducted* or supported by the Secretary, DHEW, provided such research (a) has been evaluated for possible impact on the fetus, (b) will impose minimal or no risk to the well-being of the fetus, (c) has been approved by existing review procedures with adequate provision for monitoring of the consent process, (d) special care has been taken to assure that the woman has been fully informed regarding possible impact on the fetus, and (e) the woman has given informed consent.

(Adopted unanimously.)

It is further provided that nontherapeutic research directed at the pregnant woman may be conducted or supported only if the father has not objected, both where abortion is not at issue (adopted by a vote of 8 to 1), and where an abortion is anticipated (adopted by a vote of 5 to 4).

4. *Nontherapeutic research directed toward the fetus in utero* (other than research in anticipation of, or during, abortion) may be conducted or supported by the Secretary, DHEW, provided (a) the purpose of such research is the development of important biomedical knowledge that cannot be obtained by alternative means, (b) investigation on pertinent animal models and nonpregnant humans has preceded such research, (c) minimal or no risk to the well-being of the fetus will be imposed by the research, (d) the research has been approved by existing review procedures with adequate provision for the monitoring of the consent process, (e) the informed consent of the mother has been obtained, and (f) the father has not objected to the research.   (Adopted unanimously.)

5. *Nontherapeutic research directed toward the fetus in anticipation of abortion* may be conducted or supported by the Secretary, DHEW, provided such research is carried out within the guidelines for all other nontherapeutic research directed toward the fetus in utero.   (Adopted unanimously.)

Such research presenting special problems related to the interpretation or application of these guidelines may be conducted or supported by the Secretary, DHEW, provided such research has been approved by a national ethical review body.   (Adopted by vote of 8 to 1.)

6. *Nontherapeutic research directed toward the fetus during the abortion procedure and nontherapeutic research directed toward the nonviable fetus ex utero* may be conducted or supported by the Secretary, DHEW, provided (a) the purpose of such research is the development of important biomedical knowledge that cannot be obtained by alternative means, (b) investigation on pertinent animal models and nonpregnant humans (when appropriate) has preceded such research, (c) the research has been approved by existing review procedures with adequate provision for the monitoring of the consent process, (d) the informed consent of the mother has been obtained, and (e) the father has not objected to the research; and provided further that (f) the fetus is less than 20 weeks gestational age, (g) no significant pro-

cedural changes are introduced into the abortion procedure in the interest of research alone, and (h) no intrusion into the fetus is made which alters the possibility of survival. Such research presenting special problems related to the interpretation or application of these guidelines may be conducted or supported by the Secretary, DHEW, provided such research has been approved by a national ethical review body.   (Adopted by a vote of 8 to 1.)

7. *Nontherapeutic research directed toward the possibly viable infant* may be conducted or supported by the Secretary, DHEW, provided (a) the purpose of such research is the development of important biomedical knowledge that cannot be obtained by alternative means, (b) investigation on pertinent animal models and nonpregnant humans (when appropriate) has preceded such research, (c) no additional risk to the well-being of the fetus will be imposed by the research, (d) the research has been approved by existing review procedures with adequate provision for the monitoring of the consent process, and (e) informed consent of either parent has been given and neither parent has objected.   (Adopted unanimously.)

8. *Review Procedures.* Until the Commission makes its recommendations regarding review and consent procedures, the review procedures mentioned above are to be those presently required by the Department of Health, Education, and Welfare. In addition, provision for monitoring the consent process shall be required in order to insure adequacy of the consent process and to prevent unfair discrimination in the selection of research subjects for all categories of research mentioned above. A national ethical review, as required in recommendations 5 and 6, shall be carried out by an appropriate body designated by the Secretary, DHEW, until the establishment of the National Advisory Council for the Protection of Subjects of Biomedical and Behavioral Research. In order to facilitate public understanding and the presentation of public attitudes toward special problems reviewed by the national review body, appropriate provision should be made for public attendance and public participation in the national review process.

(Adopted unanimously, one abstention.)

9. *Research* which is supported by the Secretary, DHEW, to be *conducted outside the United States* should at the minimum comply in full with the standards and procedures recommended herein.   (Adopted unanimously.)

10. *The moratorium* which is currently in effect, as a result of section 213 of the National Research Act, P.L. 93–348, *should be lifted immediately,* allowing research to proceed under current regulations; and all the foregoing recommendations of the Commission should be implemented as soon as the Secretary, DHEW, is able to promulgate regulations based upon these recommendations and the public response to them.   (Adopted by a vote of 8 to 1.)

These recommendations offered by the commission opt for a middle position between outright ban and complete freedom for fetal biomedical research. The commission advocates a system of social controls designed to limit the scope of experimentation as well as suggesting curbs to prevent abuse.[7]

An interesting and precedent-setting recommendation provides for the establishment of a national ethical review body to handle situations that cannot be dealt with adequately at the local level by institutional review committees. Further, it provides that the activities of the national ethical review committee be public. Here, for the first time, we see an opening up of the decision-making process to the inspection of society. Still another unusual but most significant aspect of the whole commission effort is that it deliberately and consistently tried to apply philosophical and moral principles to public policy, demonstrating the proposition that ethical and moral considerations can be fused with public policy in formulating policy for using the "new" biology.

Although the recommendations for conducting fetal research would seem to have been formulated, in practice those in this area of research are particularly wary of all fetal experimentation. The much discussed Edelin case[8] in Boston as well as the almost militant activities of pro-life groups across the country have greatly increased the wariness of scientists in this area of research. According to some opinion, fetal research has all but been brought to a halt—an unanticipated reaction to the Commission guidelines. It remains to be seen whether the new guidelines can change the present climate, which interferes with any kind of fetal research, even therapeutic research, and satisfactorily answer the attacks of the critics. In the words of Commission Chairman John Ryan of Harvard Medical School, "the issue is to create an environment where the kind of research we all accept as beneficial is not inhibited."

VALUES PERTAINING TO FETAL EXPERIMENTATION

1   The objective of all fetal research is the acquisition of biomedical knowledge; therefore, any fetal experimentation is good and ought to be supported.

2   Fetal experimentation is justifiable only where its aim is immediately therapeutic and so should be limited.

3   All nontherapeutic fetal experimentation is morally inadmissable, hence it ought to be banned.

4   The fetus as a human person has primary rights to respect for life and protection against harm, neither of which is consistent with nontherapeutic fetal research.

5   Consent for experimentation must be given before any research can proceed, including fetal research.

6   Proxy consent in cases of unwanted pregnancies is meaningless in view of the fact that the party(s) giving the consent has made a prior decision to reject the fetus, forfeiting thereby any claims to the fate of the fetus.

7   The dignity of present human life is compromised for hypothetical benefits of future human beings in fetal experimentation.

8   Two moral wrongs do not make one moral right.

9   The risk of brutalization (a lowering of respect for human life) is inherent in procedures which treat the fetus as a research tool.

10   Fetuses should never be used as means just as people, whatever their age, should not be used as means.

11   The previable fetus has no claim to the primary rights normally associated with humanhood.

12   Nontherapeutic research must be of such a kind that the fetus would not object

to it were it cognizant (that is, the experiment carries minimal or no risk of harm to the fetus).

13 Institutional safeguards and/or review boards must supervise all aspects of fetal research.

14 To minimize the affront to human dignity, fetal experiments should be undertaken only as part of a single operative procedure.

15 The general public has a compelling interest in being effectively represented on ethical and human experimentation institutional review committees.

16 The principle of equity requires that women selected for purposes of nontherapeutic research should be taken equally from all social classes.

17 For all practical purposes, the Supreme Court decision of 1973 settled the issue in favor of fetal experimentation.

18 Fetal research is necessary to develop knowledge that would ultimately lead to well-born children.

REFERENCES

1 Leroy Walters, "Fetal research and the ethical issues," *Hastings Center Report* 5, 3 (1975): 13–18.
2 Leroy Walters (in Reference 1), p. 13.
3 Richard Wasserstrom, "The status of the fetus," *Hastings Center Report* 5, 3 (1975): 18–20.
4 "Commission sets guidelines for experimentation," *Bioscience* 25, 6 (1975): 360.
5 "The National Commission for the Protection of Human Subjects of Biochemical and Behavioral Research, research on the fetus: report and recommendations," *Federal Register* 40 (1975): 33526–33551.
6 (In Reference 4), p. 397.
7 Stephen Toulmin, "Exploring the moderate consensus," *Hastings Center Report* 5, 3 (1975): 31–35.
8 Barbara J. Culliton, "Abortion and manslaughter: a Boston doctor goes on trial," *Science* 187 (1975): 334–335 and *Science* 187 (1975): 814–816.

BIBLIOGRAPHY

Hasting Center Report 5,3 (1975). Other articles in the special issue devoted to fetal research:
    "Abortion and Research" by Marc Lappé.
    "A Bias for Life" by Seymour Siegal.
    "Research, Casual or Planned" by Sissela Bok.
    "Fetal Research, Morality and Public Policy" by Richard A. McCormick.
    "Pragmatists and Doctrinaries" by Joseph Fletcher.
Hastings Center Report 5, 5 (1975). More on fetal research; articles included are these:
    "Compelled to Disagree" by David W. Louisell.
    "Important Elaborations" by Karen Lebacqz.
    "A Good Beginning" by Richard A. McCormick and Leroy Walters.
    "The (Supreme) Court and the Commission" by Paul Menzel.
Powledge, Tabitha, "Fetal experimentation: sorting out the issues," *Hastings Center Report* 5, 2 (1975): 8–10.
Ramsey, Paul, *The Ethics of Fetal Research* (New Haven and London: Yale University Press, 1975).

F. NEONATAL EUTHANASIA

The problem

Of the babies born in the United States every year, ninety percent arrive perfectly healthy. But the remaining 30,000 or so are not unequivocally human and someone must decide whether or not to keep these neonates alive. The moral question is this: Is it perhaps the ultimate kindness to let the severely defective child die naturally, or more beneficently, to hasten its death?

In former times, this issue posed no moral problem, for nature's solution was simple and direct—imminent and usually rapid death. But developing medical technology can often prolong the life of the defective newborn indefinitely. New surgical techniques and procedures such as the ventriculoatrial shunt introduced in 1958 to control hydrocephalus have allowed neonates to surmount obstacles which in times past were almost always fatal. Remarkable progress has occurred in resuscitating infants with respiratory problems, ministering to infants with Down's syndrome, cerebral dysfunction, congenital heart malformations, cerebral palsy, spine defects, cleft palate/cleft lip, minimal to severe motor problems, low birth weights, and a number of other genetic and congenital disorders. Infants born with these have a significant new lease on life due to the advance of medical science. More and more babies who only a few years ago would have died within days or, at the longest, weeks or months are being saved. Between 1940 and 1970, a 58 percent decrease in the infant death rate in the United States was observed.[1] Neonatal intensive care units have contributed mightily to this increase in newborn life expectancy.

But this leap in the survival rate is a mixed blessing. Mere survival of the congenitally handicapped does not at all predict a productive and happy future life. As theologian Richard A. McCormick asks: "Granted that we can easily save the life, what kind of life are we saving?"[2] At some point, the forced prolongation of such life becomes questionable. The severely brain-damaged, if they survive, frequently become wards of the state ending up in foster homes or in institutions that are still aptly described as "snake pits." The fate of the grossly immature newborn whose respiration, body temperature, acid-base balance, and nutrition are maintained by artificial devices in the intensive care unit more shielded from the public eye than any other hospital ward turns on decisions that can have lifetime effects. Degrees of physical and mental retardation are not uncommon among the survivors. The newborn child with a large myelomeningocele repaired by the skill of the neurosurgeon may well end his/her short life in some institution, paraplegic, perhaps blind, soiled, and utterly helpless. Many of the newborns, according to physicians Duff and Campbell, have "almost no capacity to be loved. They are cared for in facilities that have been characterized as hardly more than dying bins." Some malformations are simple and easily corrected. Others are a challenge to the ingenuity of the medical practitioner. Patients may undergo numerous operations, spend untold months in the hospital, catheterized, x-rayed, transfused, and punctured—subjected to a whole list of unplesantries, and still end up cripples, mentally and/or physically. The economic resources of the family are strained, the welfare of other children becomes involved, and the family's physical and emotional capacity to cope is stretched sometimes to the breaking point.

On the larger front, obligations to the species again attracts the attention of some. The questions are put: Can we forever and indefinitely circumvent the regulatory mechanisms of evolution? Does an unchecked accumulation of undesirable genes constitute a danger to the species? The wherewithal exists to treat patients even though this means in many cases limited survival—only to or through adolescence, accompanied by much suffering, and at great expense. At least one opinion insists that we must find more effective substitutes for natural selection.[3] Genetic counseling and voluntary sterilization are possibilities here.

Still another issue is forced: Can we as a society stand the expense of a large number of grossly defective children? The obvious economic burdens of prolonged care and institutionalization on the family, insurance companies, and the public treasury have been expressed before (see Section a of this chapter: The ethics of genetic responsibility). Our affluent society may be able to stand the expense but for how long? We have a large number of unmet health needs right now—what will be the condition of national resources when a national health insurance is implemented? (See Chapter 9.)

Not only should actual dollar costs and resource allocation be part of the expense society is being called upon to bear but psychological and sociological costs enter here, too. At this point in our history we know next to nothing about the impact that large numbers of defective and retarded persons might have on our social fabric: our culture, our political institutions, and our schools. If it is affirmed that we have a duty and responsibility in caring for these persons, then our social institutions must be restructured to accommodate them. Simply putting the deformed out of sight in custodial care institutions does not speak very highly of a society which freely subscribes to and encourages the principles of love, justice, and humanity.

These are but a few of the problems arising from this new technology. It appears that in more ways than one, modern medicine has conquered death at the cost of a Pyrrhic victory. Because of the sheer numbers of surviving infants with gross abnormalities, the ethical dilemmas involved with saving the severely damaged can no longer be avoided in the vain hope that they will go away. Collective irresponsibility, so often the approach to vexing problems, will not work here. Society must take a closer look at the concept of life in its absolute sense. Leon Eisenberg poses the question for us in clear terms: ". . . we are beginning to ask, not *can* it be done, but *should* it be done?"[4]

The solution

Neonatal euthanasia, the elective death of the badly damaged newborn, is seen by many as the only viable solution to this tragic scene. In electing this course of action the attending physician has several alternatives available. He or she can, in consultation and with the consent of others, end the life of the infant quickly and painlessly by administering a lethal drug; or can, in consultation and with the consent of others, allow the newborn to starve. This alternative has been used in circumstances where one defect is accompanied by deformities in the digestive tract. For example, in Down's syndrome and duodenal atresia, a simple surgical procedure can permanently correct the intestinal blockage, but without it the infant will be unable to absorb nourishment and will starve to death within eight to fifteen days. Several well-publicized instances of this happening has injected a caution in the use of this procedure (see Reference 5). Lastly, the physician can, in consultation and with the consent of others, not treat the defect at all, providing only water, nourishment, and relief from pain until "nature takes its course."

Of these options, the first belongs in the category of active euthanasia—the willful taking of a life through direct action; the second and third are classified as passive euthanasia—neither causing death directly but not preventing it either (see Chapter 6 for a more complete discussion of euthanasia.) Active euthanasia, whatever the motivation of the parties involved, is by legal definition a criminal act. Passive euthanasia is legally (and morally) questionable in some instances. Among pediatricians who responded to a questionnaire in regard to the use of active euthanasia for an anencephalic newborn only one percent said that they would be likely to give a lethal dose of medication; three percent said they might do so.[6] These findings could be variously interpreted as a moral distaste for using active measures, or a fear of legal recrimination, or concern over malpractice suits. However, the utilization of passive measures is quite a different matter.

Joseph Fletcher labels passive euthanasia as a *fait accompli* in medical practice today.[7] It is an accepted medical procedure at both ends of the life cycle. There are problems with this course of action when it is applied to deformed infants: (1) the dying process can last for months at the cost of much parental suffering and expense; and (2) the child may actually survive the initial fatal diagnosis only to be afflicted with severe handicaps. The anguish of waiting for the inevitable to occur can be traumatic. One physician noted that the waiting period for one infant lasted three months at a cost of $85,000 to the family. The parents' suffering during this time was also noted:

> Having seen children with unoperated meningomyeloceles be around the ward for weeks or months untreated, waiting to die, one cannot help but feel that the highest form of medical ethic would have been to end the pain and suffering.[8]

Leaving a severely malformed infant to die untreated does not necessarily ensure their speedy death. Some live for years in wretched, severely handicapped states.

Euthanasia may be of two kinds—voluntary or involuntary. In the first case, the patient consents to whatever course of action is elected; in the second, the act is performed without the patient's knowledge and/or permission. Neonatal euthanasia is always involuntary. And this is the crux of the ethical issue—others must make a life and death decision *for* the neonate. It is an unquestionable assumption that we desire to be ethical in our motives and actions in regard to the grossly malformed newborn. For motives to be ethical, they must determine what is good and in the best interests of the affected infant. These actions must comply with moral directives in order to insure justice to those who have no voice in the matter.

Medical criteria in decision-making

Since physicians must make a life and death choice in determining their course of action in regard to the grossly deformed newborns, it is instructive to note some of the criteria that have been used in some instances for deciding who is to be treated and who is not. The primary decision to commence treatment is based primarily on the life expectancy of the child and the level of impairment it will have to bear if long-term survival results. John Lorber, a medical authority on the treatment of meningomyelocele, believes that it is possible to determine the minimum degree of handicap that the individual would have; this is in contrast to some who insist that such a diagnosis is impossible. Lorber suggests that the best time to select infants for passive euthanasia is soon after birth when parental emotional attachment is least. Along with the presence of spina bifida,* his criteria for selecting those who are not to be treated include:[9]

1. Gross paralysis of the legs
2. Thoracolumbar and thoracolumbosacral lesions
3. Kyphosis or scoliosis
4. Grossly enlarged head
5. Intercerebral birth injury
6. Other gross congenital defects—e.g., cyanotic heart disease, ectopia of the bladder, and mongolism

Dr. D. W. Hide notes that along with the presence of meningomyelocele he uses the following to decide against treatment:[10]

1. Baby's weight
2. Size of head
3. Degree of paralysis
4. Presence of other abnormalities
5. The health of the parents

Selective treatment over full treatment has made possible a greater percentage of survival; the quality of the survivors was decidedly better in the selective approach.

The use of criteria for selection has brought about many vexing problems to physicians, parents, and the greater community. Dr. Raymond Duff, a pediatrician at the Yale–New Haven Hospital, describes the procedures they follow in decision-making. The Yale–New Haven approach focuses on family participation throughout. Duff argues that since it is primarily the families who must live with and are affected by the decisions, it is they who must make the ultimate decision; the health profession and society should only provide input or set guidelines to assist in the decision.[11]

The ethical issues

It is apparent that no general consensus exists on what to do with the severely damaged newborn, even among the medical specialists. Among the perplexing and unanswered questions are these:

---

* spina bifida: defect in the spinal column, in which spinal arches are absent allowing spinal membranes and/or spinal cord to protrude through.

meningomyelocele: protrusion of the membranes and spinal cord through a defect in the vertebral column.

scoliosis: lateral curvature of the spine.

kyphosis: abnormal curvature of the spine with convexity backward.

lesion: pathologic change in tissue.

Who speaks for the newborn?

What about the guilt feelings of the parents?

What effect might allowing the infant patient to die have on the healing profession?

Are the wishes of the parents to be honored or are there overriding issues here?

Should the state involve itself in such matters?

Is neonatal euthanasia too easy a solution? Isn't there another way for society to respond?

How do we handle the serious emotional conflicts of the attending medical personnel—the nurses and attendants?

Who is responsible for the congenitally deformed infant?

Is allowing the "unfit" to die the "cork in the bottle" that unleashes the possibility of using any flimsy circumstance for eliminating the undesirable (the so-called Nazi experience)?

Above all, what effect can the practice have on our conceptions of humanness, for example, selflessness, concern for the weak, and charity to sacrifice?

The answers to these questions presuppose values and notions of what is right and what is wrong. In trying to identify and rank order them, considerable disagreement is expressed. The basic ethical issue is this:

Are we to live and act by a "sanctity-of-life" ethic or a "quality-of-life" ethic?[12]

If the former is our answer, we assign life a first-order value and all other values must be subordinate to it. The right to life must take prior claim over all other concerns, the biological damage of the infant notwithstanding. Costs and benefits are not added up; the judgment is based solely on justice and fairness. If there is to be any limit placed on these rights, it must be done only by due process either through the legislative and/or the judicial systems of the state, not by individual choice where bias, convenience, economic security, or other noncompelling reasons can arbitrarily remove these rights which protect all life. It can be argued that we put ourselves in a dangerous position when society accepts the principle that any one individual, infant, child, or adult is too useless, too unproductive, or too costly to protect with full legal and moral rights. There must remain a clear prohibition against killing of any kind.

The sanctity-of-life position, however, is not a single view but rather can be subdivided into two categories. On the extreme are those who insist that every effort should be made to save every life. Life is inherently good even if it is only biological life. "It is better to be alive than not alive" is the major ethical axiom here. The second representation of the sanctity-of-life principle submits that although human life is valuable, nonetheless human physical life is relative to other values. It is morally troublesome to identify what these values are such that if they are missing, moral claim to human life in this world is invalid. The danger of error here is great for it may be a very thin line between the weak and the dependent and those persons who are flatly unwanted for whatever reason. Also, this view would distinguish between active and passive neonatal euthanasia. There is a profound distinction between killing and allowing to die. Even the infirm must be granted the dignity of humanhood if "we wish to preserve a society in which the weak are protected and life is everywhere reverenced."[13] In this second view, neonatal euthanasia may be permissible under restricted and severe conditions, but its practice must be motivated by charity, love, and justice and not by a callous rejection of the unfit.

The quality-of-life ethic holds that neonatal euthanasia is correct if the foreseeable consequences of the action contribute to an enhancement of human well-being. This is again recognized as a consequentialist view. Rather than accepting the maxim that all life is good, the concern here is with what is the good life. Biological life is a relative value that takes meaning only when it is used to contribute to the betterment of an individual's condition. To the question, should life be preserved at all costs?— the answer must be based on the relative state of that life.

Fletcher provides us with the practical elements for decision-making in the case of neonatal euthanasia:[14]

1. The extent to which parents are (or can be) counseled
2. Parent's attitude toward the defects
3. Severity of the defect
4. Economic resources of the family
5. Welfare of other children involved, as well as the parent's physical and emotional capacity to cope

To these might be added the additional factors of cost to society if they must assume the burden of care as well as the allocation of other societal resources (e.g., intensive medical care, highly trained medical personnel, etc.) These all raise serious qualification problems since the elements to be judged are primarily subjective. For example, comparing psychic stress on parents to the dollar costs of care may be utterly impossible.

Fletcher adds still another defense to the quality-of-life stance where he argues that if it is defensible to interrupt fetal life by elective therapeutic abortion when a gross anomaly is detected in prenatal diagnosis, then can't the same grounds of mercy and beneficence be allowable in regard to defective newborns? In the case of therapeutic abortion, the judgment is made that in certain cases it is better that a life not be lived; there are benefits to the fetus, the mother, the family, and society if an abortion is performed. The same set of circumstances applies to the defective neonate as well and it is only a moral quibble that we attempt to distinguish the two. It is the same yardstick that is being used.

A considerable amount of confusion still remains as to what is the correct moral course. Whatever line of reasoning is followed, common sense tells most of us that somewhere a line must be drawn beyond which life lacks the qualities that we perceive to be human. The question is: Where is that line?

At a conference held in California in 1975, "Ethical Issues in Newborn Intensive Care," a group of physicians, lawyers, social workers, ethicists, economists, and laypersons studied that question. In general, the conference concluded that there are indeed circumstances in which it is permissible to let a neonate die. It was further suggested that a moral policy be codified which could function as a mechanism for making the decision of life or death. Such a moral policy should be based on these values:[15]

1. Every baby born possesses a moral value entitling it to the medical and social care necessary to effect its well-being.

2. Parents are principally *responsible* for all decisions regarding the well-being of their newborn children.

3. Physicians have the *duty* to take medical measures conducive to the well-being of the baby in proportion to their fiduciary relationship with the parents.

4. The state has an *interest* in the proper fulfillment of responsibilities and duties regarding the well-being of the child.

5. The responsibility of the parents, the duty of the physician, and the interests of the state are conditioned by the medico-moral principle, "do no harm, without expecting compensating benefits for the patient."

6. Neither physicians nor parents are obliged to initiate or to continue actions which do harm to the well-being of a newborn infant (e.g., prolonged life beyond infancy with excruciating pain and with minimal potential of participating in human experiences).

7. In cases of disagreement between parents and physician, legal judgment should weigh heavily the prognosis regarding quality of life and the injunction, "do no harm."

8. If an infant is judged beyond medical intervention and if it is judged that its continued brief life will be marked by pain and discomfort, it is permissible to hasten death.

9. If it is necessary to discriminate between several infants (lack of resources), it is ethical to recommend that therapeutic care for an infant with poor prognosis be terminated in order to provide care for an infant with a better prognosis.

These guidelines are construed by their framers as conservative, attempting a middle course between a too-easy attitude which allows for an almost inconsiderate destruction of human life and a too-firm one which insists that all must be saved.

The facts of the issue are rapidly coming in. Handicapped newborns often place crushing ethical, emotional, social, and economic burdens on parents, physicians, families, and society. Although to parents, it is quite inconceivable that their children will be born defective, to physicians, the kind of life-and-death decision involved here is commonplace in most hospital delivery rooms. Many doctors simply decide on their own that death is the best option, reporting to the parents that the fetus was stillborn. But Campbell and Duff are calling for another way. The potential for error, the fear of malpractice suits, the lies and dishonesty often employed to cover up these tragic occurrences, the increasing pressure from pro-life groups, and the like require a different approach. They are calling for a public and open debate: "The public has got to decide what to do with vegetated individuals who have no human potential. We doctors can't solve these problems alone."[16] Which way society elects to go on this issue has not yet been decided.

VALUES PERTAINING TO NEONATAL EUTHANASIA

In addition to those listed above, the following values are added:

1 The right to life is a moral absolute; hence, there can be no justification for refusing to treat the grossly deformed newborn.

2 The quality of life is to be preferred over sheer survival; therefore, it is better that some lives be terminated early.

3 The danger of labeling individuals as unfit be they fetuses, infants, or adults opens the door to social and political abuse.

4 The greatest-good principle validates certain life and death judgments in the matter of infant euthanasia.

5 The principles of charity, love, and justice must motivate our behavior in all situations requiring value judgments, including our concern for the defective newborn.

6 The principle of truth telling should guide the flow of information between the medical professional and the parents regarding the status of the newborn.

7 It is part of society's greater responsibilities to provide aid and assistance to those in need, including the grossly deformed infants.

8 There is a distinct moral difference between active intervention, or positive euthanasia, and allowing the patient to die, or passive euthanasia.

REFERENCES

1 M. E. Wegman, "Annual Summary of Vital Statistics—1970," *Pediatrics* 48 (1971): 979.

2 Richard A. McCormick, "To Save or Let Die," *Journal of American Medical Association* (July 8, 1974): 174.

3 Wolf W. Zuelzer, "Ethical Dilemmas—Relationship to Pediatrics," in *Ethical Dilemmas in Current Obstetric and Newborn Care:* Report of the Sixty-Fifty Ross Conference on Pediatric Research (Columbus, Ohio: Ross Laboratories, 1973), p. 19.

4 Leon Eisenberg, "The Human Nature of Human Nature," *Science* 176 (1972): 123.

5 James M. Gustafson, "Mongolism, Parental Desires, and the Right to Life," *Perspectives in Biology and Medicine* 16, 4 (1973): 529–557.

6 Diana Crane, "Physician's Attitude Toward the Treatment of Critically Ill Patients," *Bioscience* 23 (Aug. 1973): 472.

7 Joseph Fletcher, "Ethics and Euthanasia," *American Journal of Nursing* 73 (1973): 78–82.

8 John M. Freeman, "Is There a Right to Die—Quickly?" *Journal of Pediatrics* 80 (1972): 905.

9 John Lorber, "Early Results of Selective Treatment of Spina Bifida Eystica," *British Medical Journal* 4 (1973): 201.

10 D. W. Hide, H. P. Williams, and H. L. Ellis, "The Outlook for the Child With Myelomeningocele," *Developmental Medicine and Child Neurology* 14 (1972): 307.

11 Raymond S. Duff and A. G. M. Campbell, "Moral and Ethical Dilemmas in the Special-Care Nursery," *New England Journal of Medicine* 289 (1973): 890–894.

12 Joseph Fletcher, "Moral Aspects," (in Reference 3), p. 70.

13 Margaret Farley, "The Importance of Moral Quibble," *Hastings Center Report* 5, 2 (1975): 6.
14 Joseph Fletcher (in Reference 3), p. 70.
15 Barbara J. Culliton, "Intensive Care for Newborns: Are There Times to Pull the Plug?" *Science* 188, 4184 (1975): 134.
16 Raymond G. Duff, in "Shall This Child Die?" *Newsweek* (Nov. 12, 1973), p. 70.

BIBLIOGRAPHY

Ethical Dilemmas in Current Obstetric and Newborn Care (Columbus, Ohio: Ross Laboratories, 1973).
Hearings Before the Subcommittee on Labor and Public Welfare, United States Senate: Examination of the moral and ethical problems faced with the agonizing decisions of life and death (neonatal euthanasia); 93rd Congress, June 11, 1974 (Washington, D.C.: Government Printing Office, 1974).
Heifetz, Milton D., "The tragic newborn," in *The Right to Die*, Milton D. Heifetz with Charles Mangel (New York: Putnam, 1975).
Jonsen, Albert R., and G. Lister, "Newborn intensive care: the ethical problems," *Hastings Center Report* 8, 1 (1978): 15–18.
Kelsey, Beverly, "Which infants shall live? Who should decide?" *Hastings Center Report* 5, 2 (1975): 5–8.
Smith, David H., "On letting some babies die," *Hastings Center Studies* 2, 2 (1974): 37–46.
Spina Bifida: Three articles in *Hastings Center Report* 7, 4 (1977): 10–19.
    Rosalyn Benjamin Darling, "Parents, physicians and spina bifida"
    Robert M. Veatch, "The technical criteria fallacy"
    Robert Reid, "Spina bifida: the fate of the untreated"
Steinfels, Margaret O'Brien, "New childbirth technology: a clash of values," *Hastings Center Report* 8, 1 (1978): 9–12.

G. STERILIZATION

Sterilization—a study in confusion

The practice of nontherapeutic sterilization in this country and the world presents an interesting study in contradiction. On the one hand are those who voluntarily request the surgery be performed on them but are unable to secure it; on the other, there are charges that the procedure is executed on women, especially the poor, the blacks, and the mentally incompetent, against their will. Responding to the first claim, defenders of nontherapeutic sterilization call for less stringent restrictions so that the service can be more readily available in suitable circumstances; the other side insists on more effective restrictions to curb the growing incidences of abuse. Both critics and advocates agree that the matter of individual freedom is the major ethical issue here—persons should be able to select that course of action they judge to be appropriate relative to their own procreative behavior. Let's examine this issue further.

Nontherapeutic sterilization has been tainted with a bad name for some time; it continues to suffer from a variety of negative associations, many of which were widely publicized in the popular media. The classic case in point is the forced sterilization of the Relf girls, two blacks aged 14 and 12 in Montgomery, Alabama in 1973. (A multimillion dollar settlement was awarded them four years later.) Sterilization first came to major public attention in this country as a eugenic, nonvoluntary procedure. The objective of these eugenic programs was to forcibly prevent the unfit—variously defined—from reproducing. The usual candidates were the insane, the feeble-minded, and to some extent, criminals. Compulsory sterilization laws were enacted by approximately half the states and are still on the books in some of them but they are rarely enforced. And in fact, the Supreme Court in 1942 judged one of these statutes to be unconstitutional as being inconsistent with the Ninth and Fourteenth Amendment rights. There are substantial grounds for questioning their validity today if one cares to challenge them. For the most part, they remain as anachronisms from a by-gone day. (See Reference 1: Sarvis and Rodman and Beckwith for a discussion of the abuses of sterilization in the early part of this century.) The use of compulsory sterilization in Nazi Germany in the 1930s for genocidal purposes is another mark against the practice of sterilization and in many people's minds the very word itself is associated with Hitler's terror.

But voluntary and compulsory sterilization are at opposite ends of a spectrum. Although the two are frequently lumped together in the public eye, it would seem wise to use a different name for the first and avoid, thereby, the unpleasant connotations of the second. Some terms that have been suggested are "surgical contraceptions" or "voluntary infertility."[2] The authors Pilpel and Ames (in Reference 2) point out that by using these or similar designations, a different idea could be communicated to those who are suspicious of sterilization, namely, that it is one way to exercise freedom of choice in the matter of having children.

Perhaps, though, this is an ungrounded fear for as more recent data suggest, voluntary sterilization has become the foremost means of fertility control worldwide.[3] The Agency for International Development of the United States Government estimated that 65 million couples throughout the world were using male or female sterilization for birth control at the start of 1976. The total included 8 million couples in the United States where by now in the late 1970s, surgical sterilization has forged ahead of oral contraceptives as the foremost means of controlling fertility. The increasing number of sterilizations performed are in all probability indicative of a new attitude on the part of the general population, and in fact, eighty percent of the Americans in a Gallup poll voted for its acceptance.

But still problems exist. Although voluntary sterilization is legal in all fifty states, there remains a climate of uncertainty connected with its practice. State laws vary considerably in their stance on the question and in some instances actually work against effective implementation of the procedure in hospitals, by physicians, and with health insurance companies. For example, a number of state laws allow medical facilities and health personnel to exempt themselves from performing the procedure and prohibit discrimination against them if they refuse to participate. On the other hand, in a state court judgment resulting from a suit brought by the Association for Voluntary Sterilization against a Massachusetts city hospital, it was ruled that a publicly supported hospital could not refuse to perform sterilizations. The professional reservation of voluntary exclusion is consistent with the present standards of the American College of Obstetricians and Gynecologists which specify that "surgical sterilization can be performed on anyone who is legally capable of giving permission to operate upon her . . . , each hospital must establish its own regulations concerning sterilization . . . , and these should be developed by members of the department of obstetrics and gynecology and approved by the medical staff and appropriate governing body."[4] The last provisions in these specifications are the source of uncertainty for they provide support for the many hospitals and physicians who desire to refrain from performing the operation. Catholic hospitals refuse to provide the service and many private hospitals are reluctant to do so. A few states have enacted laws that set specific conditions covering such aspects as counseling of patients, medical consultation requirements, consent of the spouse, age of the patient, and the like.

It appears that among the several deterrents to voluntary sterilization, the greatest is "the reluctance of doctors to get involved with it although the procedure (is legal). Those doctors who are willing find themselves swamped with requests."[5] The Association for Voluntary Sterilization listed only 2000 cooperating physicians nationwide in 1974. In many states, although the practice is permitted, the legal guidelines governing the procedure have not been settled. Physicians and health agencies worry constantly about the increasing number of malpractice suits. In at least one recently reported case, it was ruled that the patient of a sterilization that had failed could sue the hospital and the attending physician.[6] Recalling the earlier mentioned example of convicts requesting sterilization (Chapter 2), the San Diego County Medical Society cautioned a physician-member against proceeding with the planned operation. The charge of criminal "mayhem" was feared. The original legal meaning of mayhem was the deliberate infliction of injury on oneself or another which had the result of interfering with that person's potential to serve the king.[7] Whether the rationale applies to the case of sterilization is conjectural but physicians continue to worry about it. What is no doubt needed is for some statutory assurance that voluntary sterilization is legal and that physicians may not be held liable for negligence as in any other medical procedure where the treatment is satisfactorily performed.

What can be said for physicians holds true for hospitals as well. Here, too, local reservations may preclude the availability of sterilization. The ever-present fear of retribution by an antagonistic state legislature through a reduction in public funding serves as ample motive for some to go slow here. The age-parity formula was common in times past; it may still be used in some instances or in some institutions. This formula calculated the female's qualifications as a candidate for sterilization. The patient's age times the number of living children had to equal between 100 and 120 for her to be considered eligible. Of course, many young women with few or no living children could never qualify. As a means of controlling the number of children desired, including none, sterilization was simply beyond the young when this principle was applied.

The whole matter of age requirements has led to some discrimination. Although there are relatively few minors interested in permanent sterilization, its growing acceptance as a safe method of contraception coupled with the increasing desire to remain childless, plus the movement for sexual equality and the inclination for non-marital relationships as a life-style, will make its use more and more commonplace. Although most state laws do not even face the issue of minors, most doctors play it safe and insist that the patient be at least 21, be married and have the spouse's consent, or have parental consent. One can question whether or not freedom of choice is being infringed upon here.

Some medical institutions permit only what they call therapeutic, as opposed to contraceptive, sterilizations. There is a weak distinction between the two; refusing a simple and nonhazardous sterilization to persons requesting it, simply because they have not had "enough" children, is arbitrary at best, discriminatory at worst. No state law prohibits hospitals from distinguishing between therapeutic and contraceptive sterilizations.

Requiring a spouse's consent raises still another barrier. The approval in writing of a spouse is a frequent requirement. Some states allow for waivers such as in cases of separation, divorce, or abandonment. It has been questioned whether a spouse's consent should be required at all. Where a marriage is healthy, the decision for sterilization is no doubt arrived at mutually. Where this is not so, the unilateral decision by one parent not to bring more children into a fragile family should be even more respected. The unmarried or the no-longer-married person presents still another instance that clouds the availability of a voluntary sterilization.

Some hospitals require a waiting period after the consent is given and the performance of the operation. This requirement imposes an additional frustration for some. The stipulation is to preclude the possibility that the person may change his/her mind after the procedure is completed. Times of from 72 hours to 30 days have been used. A special problem is encountered with those women desiring sterilization immediately following the birth of a child or after an elective abortion—a time when the operation is most easily done. A waiting period requirement necessitates a second visit to the operating room and the attendant risks of added surgery and anesthesia as well as the extra inconvenience. Whatever the sex, and whatever the circumstance, a waiting period does require a minimum of two visits to the doctor. At least one state, Missouri, requires that a certificate be filed with the state registrar by the physician and/or hospital during the waiting period declaring the intention for sterilization.

Lastly, there is considerable confusion in insurance coverage. Commercial health insurance companies frequently exclude sterilization unless it is related to illness or injury. As a single procedure, it is considered an exclusion. Proof of medical necessity, waiting periods of varying length, and the omission of certain procedures are still policies practiced by insurance companies that may cause hesitation by the patient.[8] Medicaid, a government-sponsored health program for the poor, covers voluntary sterilization in 38 states. There are some serious legal and ethical problems associated with its administration that will be discussed shortly. Blue Cross usually pays the direct cost if it is a "medical necessity" but may not include the costs of x-rays if any are required. Blue Shield plans do not as a rule include sterilization in group plans although they may be included upon request. Commercial health plans vary—some pay the costs, some don't; some may accept them with the qualification that they must be "related to illness or injury."

In voluntary sterilization, we have an issue that is certainly enigmatic as well as being unique. Here, agreement by the general public has been expressed in favor of the practice; most of the other issues we have encountered so far are still awaiting this kind of consensus. But the roadblocks in the way of effective implementation of the practice may serve to discourage more active participation. This is certainly an issue on which we have done an about face. Can this be interpreted as an instance where the ethical and/or moral position of the minority deprives the majority of its freedom to choose? Who decides what is permissible for the public at large? How does one enforce provisions designed to benefit the majority which are blocked by special interest groups regardless of their motivation? It does seem that we have a unique problem in voluntary sterilization.

The Association for Voluntary Sterilization (AVS), founded in 1937, has taken on the role of advocate "to make voluntary sterilization freely available to all Americans, age 21 years or over, with children or without children, married or single." The AVS is actively engaged in promoting legal action against hospitals, public and nonsectarian, that deny sterilization procedures. Successful suits, including the earlier-mentioned Massachusetts one, have been brought by AVS to promote their objectives. They have expanded their operations to the international community and the IPAVS (International Project of the Association for Voluntary Sterilization), founded in 1972, now administers a multimillion dollar AID grant (Agency for International Development, an arm of the federal government) aimed to encourage voluntary sterilization in countries abroad. Voluntarism is stressed throughout, and in all IPAVS projects individuals seeking sterilization must receive counseling first, which describes the risks and benefits including the irreversible nature of the operation and the requirement of a signed consent form. It would thus seem that in the AVS and its offspring, the IPAVS, we have a model that may be applicable to the formation of a larger policy at both the national and the international level regarding voluntary sterilization.

The compulsory sterilization issue

The issue of involuntary or compulsory sterilization presents us with a different set of concerns. Some people see the role of sterilization as a means to prevent the poor or other "undesirables" from over-breeding. A minority, some of them state legislators, are proposing laws requiring the sterilization of welfare recipients and mental incompetents in order to relieve what is perceived to be the unjust burden carried by the taxpayer and the state in caring for their numerous children. One physician-gynecologist has written:

> People pollute and too many people crowded too close together cause many of our social and economic problems. These, in turn, are aggravated by involuntary and irresponsible parenthood. As physicians, we have obligations to our individual patients, but we have obligations to the society of which we are a part. The welfare mess, as it has been called, cries out for solutions, one of which is fertility control.[9]

Compulsory sterilization, implied or direct, cannot be shrugged off as an isolated practice in a few hospitals. Since the disclosure of the Relf case, a large number of other instances of uninformed sterilizations have been discovered, most of them on black teenagers or women on welfare. In a large-scale study cited by Sarvis and Rodman, the following situation was reported:

> Some women desiring an abortion were required to have a simultaneous operation as a condition of approval of the abortion in from one-third to two-thirds of (the) teaching hospitals (studied) in different regions of the country. This practice was most common in the Mountain States, the Far West, Canada, and the lowest in the New England and

Plain States. In all, 53.6% of teaching hospitals made this requirement for *some* of their patients.[10] (Emphasis added.)

In a women's teach-in in Detroit, the following was expressed by a black woman:

> The real reason that many low-income women and minority group women are refusing to have abortions or other operations is that they are afraid of what will happen to them. I know one woman who died needing an appendix operation and she was afraid to go for the operation. Women are afraid they will come out sterilized or with parts of their body missing.[11]

In late November of 1974, three Mexican-American women from Los Angeles filed claims for $2 million each against Los Angeles County and the University of Southern California Medical Center, contending that they were sterilized without proper consent. The women, aged 24, 26, and 32, claimed that their signatures on consent forms were obtained while they were in pain and under sedation immediately before undergoing childbirth by caesarean section. Two of the women were led to believe that the sterilization was only temporary; the third was unaware she had been sterilized at all and continued to wear an IUD for two years after until she learned she was sterilized.[12]

Case after case could be recited repeating essentially the same thing—eighteen women, poor and black, in South Carolina had to agree to sterilization to have their babies delivered; laws have been proposed that welfare benefits be taken away or even prison sentences imposed if mothers bearing illegitimate children did not undergo sterilization; and the like. All of these are examples of what has been given the personally degrading designation, the package deal: abortion or delivery and sterilization—you cannot get one without the other. A recent study by Ralph Nader's Health Research Group found that such pressuring of poor and black women to consent to sterilization is a widespread practice in American hospitals.

The now widely known sterilization of the Relf girls is an instance where no pregnancy was involved and is representative of but another eugenic practice using involuntary sterilization. Here the girls, who were of welfare parents mildly retarded, were led to believe that they were to be given shots and the mother signed the consent form on this assumption.

The Ralph Nader Health Research Group investigated the issue of abuse in sterilization procedures. Their report, entitled *Surgical Sterilization: Present Abuses and Proposed Regulations*, identified three factors that contribute most to the regret that follows sterilization:

1. being very young.
2. deciding under duress.
3. procedures were suggested by the physician rather than the patient.

Again, the latter two categories lend themselves to easy exploitation and/or discrimination of welfare patients and the poorly educated.

Statistics on sterilizations performed are incomplete. The North Carolina State Eugenics Board reports that between 1960 and 1968, 1620 persons were sterilized in North Carolina—1583 were female, 1023 were black, 55.9 percent were under 20 years of age. HEW says that 25,000 adults were sterilized in federally funded birth control clinics from mid-1972 to mid-1973.[13]

According to the Alan Gutemacher Institute, an estimated 63,000 sterilizations each year are subsidized by the federal government for low-income families.[14]

Until 1974, there were no federal standards for assuring voluntarism. In that year, the suit of the Relf girls, requesting damages of $5 million, led to a revision in federal policy concerning government-financed sterilizations. Responding to a growing controversy, HEW, in February of 1974, issued a set of guidelines regulating sterilization procedures if government funds are involved. The regulations require written consent following a "fair" explanation of the sterilization procedure, including its irreversible nature. A 72-hour waiting period is required between the time of consent and the operation. A statement declaring that there will be no loss of welfare benefits, either real or implied, must accompany the explanation. Furthermore, sterilization must be approved by a five-member review committee appointed by "responsible authorities of the (federally aided) program or project" with two of the members being representatives of the population served by the project. If the request is to sterilize a minor or mentally incompetent person, a court must determine that the operation is "in the best interest of the patient."[15] These guidelines also apply to any sterilization financed by Medicaid or Social Security. A subsequent district court injunction permanently enjoined the government from sterilizing any minors as well as mentally incompetent persons.

Critics of the HEW regulations have raised their arguments, in part, by filing a suit in New York.[16] They contended that the occurrence of abuse is vastly overestimated and that the medically indigent are being denied sterilizations on the basis of arbitrary judgments by physicians and hospitals. Besides, coercion, if there is any, cannot be prevented by government regulations. Furthermore, there should be no minimum age and no parental consent required. Doctors want complete discretion in performing sterilizations on their Medicaid patients.

The defenders of the regulations insist that abuses do in fact continue to occur, in spite of government guidelines. Also, the federal government has failed to enforce the regulations. A recent survey revealed that minors and mentally incompetent persons are still being sterilized.[17] Rather than a loosening of the guidelines, more rigidity was being called for.

This part of the sterilization controversy also remains unresolved and as Patricia Donovan suggests, the U.S. Supreme Court will again be called upon to determine what restrictions may be imposed on the sterilization of the poor without infringing on their constitutional rights.[18]

The problem of the sexually active, but mentally retarded, persons presents society with still another vexing problem. Do they have rights to procreative freedom? Should the institutionalized mentally retarded be sterilized if there is a risk that they may procreate either while in the institution or on the outside? (Many of the mentally deficient are especially vulnerable to sexual exploitation.) Can they marry and have children of their own? A California couple, mentally disabled, planned marriage in spite of their parents' objections. Publicity concerning their circumstance raised the question, have mentally retarded the right to a sex life?[19] Ought sterilization be made available, even be mandatory, for people who are sexually active but are unable to care for a child? How valid is informed consent when the signer is mentally incompetent? Do the mentally incompetent have Constitutional rights like anyone else? Are there moral considerations here, too? How should the legal system respond in this instance?

The Ralph Nader Health Research Group submits these guidelines for minimizing the risk of abuse in any sterilization:

1. All sterilizations should be considered permanent.
2. Age should be an important factor—women over 30 are less likely to regret the operation than those under 30; other alternatives should be explored including early termination of unwanted pregnancy.
3. Is sterilization being chosen under stress? Financial, emotional, and situational consideration should be covered; also the possibility that these may not exist at some future times.
4. There are very few reasons for needing a sterilization—if a doctor suggests one, obtain a second opinion.
5. Do not make hasty decisions; a 30-day wait period is not too long for so permanent a decision.

Whether any or all of these can reduce the ethical, political, emotional, and social hazards associated with sterilization remains to be ascertained.

Sterilization as a political weapon

One final area of concern needs to be opened up—the use of sterilization as a political weapon in foreign countries. It is not uncommon for the accusation of genocide to be hurled by ethnic minorities or other socially depressed groups when revelations of coerced sterilizations surface. Certainly in our country it has been expressed on a number of occasions. Overseas the charge is also heard. Latin America with its high birth rates seems especially vulnerable. Two Puerto Rican doctors reported that there is mass sterilization going on in their country, with U.S. support. The deception being used in prosterilization programs is to focus on the advantages only and not on the psychological, behavioral, or economic effects. A Puerto Rican Catholic archbishop claims that his country is being used as a laboratory for testing the effectiveness of sterilization to control population growth. According to him, 300,000 fertile-aged persons have been sterilized, many without their knowledge. A Mexican front page headline read, "Genocide in Puerto Rico," and it went on to draw the analogy between that program and Hitler's forced sterilization efforts.[20] A personal communication with a former Peace Corps worker in Latin America informed this author that the scare, whether true or not, is perceived to be very real by native populations. He reported an instance where parents refused to send their children to school, some for several weeks, because rumor had it that they would be sterilized if they attended class.

Forced sterilization as a political weapon remains a particularly sensitive point. No one should minimize the significance of this abuse nor should efforts to force sterilization be tolerated. Here, the admonition "eternal vigilance is the price of liberty" must ring true! (A discussion of compulsory sterilization and population control will be found in Chapter 12.)

The ethical side of the sterilization question

This section began with the ethical proposition that individuals should be able to select that course of action *they* judge to be appropriate relative to their own procreative desires. We have looked at the complexities of the sterilization issue and noted the difficulties related to its solution, how to protect people from possible abuses of sterilization while making it available when freely chosen. Many of the ethical positions raised in earlier discussions in this text find application here for in the final analysis it must be asked, How far do individual rights extend in terms of procreative behavior? Again, on the one side will be those who insist that all life is sacred and God-given; hence, any human interdiction that degrades that gift is to be rejected. Any form of sterilization, in this view, is bad since it is a contradiction of natural law. This is the position of some religious groups, including the Roman Catholic Church and some pro-life activists. They oppose any state or federal aid for sterilization as well as rejecting it as a medical practice unless there are sound medical indicators. Furthermore, doctors who perform sterilizations for nonmedical reasons may be doing good; but they are not doing medicine. The distinction between the true and false ends of medicine are again germane to the sterilization issue.

On the other side are the consequentialists who again see the "greatest good" as a necessary condition for any decision. It is hard to argue that unlimited reproduction is good, whether it be by the general population, or welfare recipients who "year-after-year turn them out one and two at a time" only to be supported by welfare programs; or the mentally incompetent who are certainly in a poor position to care for children. Sterilization in any of these instances qualifies as a greater good.

And then there is the third position which insists that freedom to choose must be guarded at all cost. Under no circumstances should anyone ever be coerced into accepting sterilization, but its ready availability should be there for those who freely choose it.

No listing of values will close this section since most, if not all, of the values would be a repetition of those already included in the sections of this chapter. Rather, reflect on this:

> The new reproductive technologies have placed at humankind's disposal an enormous potential to improve the human lot. But in order to achieve this it must make profound and humane decisions—decisions that are at the same time moral, ethical, political, economic, personal, social, religious, and emotional.

Lying at the root of these judgments is the most primary question of all:

> *Can one prescribe for another a life worth living?*

What is your opinion on this most philosophical question which has at the same time tremendous pragmatic overtones?

REFERENCES

1   Betty Sarvis and Hyman Rodman, *The Abortion Controversy*, 2nd ed. (New York and London: Columbia University Press, 1974), pp. 176–178, and Jonathan Beckwith, "Social and political uses of genetics in the United States: past and present," in *Ethical and Scientific Issues Posed by the Human Uses of Molecular Genetics*, Marc Lappe and Robert Morison (eds.) (New York: New York Academy of Science, 1976).
2   Harriet F. Pilpel and Peter Ames, "Legal obstacles to freedom of choice in the areas of contraception, abortion, and voluntary sterilization in the United States," in *Aspects of*

Population Growth Policy, Vol. 6 (Washington: U.S. Government Printing Office, 1972), p. 71.

3 R. T. Ravenholt, "Winning the battle against overpopulation," *Futurist* 10, 2 (1976): 64–68.

4 Harriet F. Pilpel and Peter Ames (in Reference 2), p. 73.

5 Susan L. Peck, "Voluntary sterilization: attitude and legislation," *Hastings Center Report* 4, 3 (1974): 8–10.

6 "Ask to sue as vasectomy, abortion fail," *Chicago Sun-Times* (April 19, 1977).

7 Harriet F. Pilpel and Peter Ames (in Reference 2), p. 71.

8 Susan L. Peck (in Reference 5), p. 8.

9 Cited in Peck (in Reference 5), p. 7 (original reference in *Contemporary Obstetrics and Gynecology* 1 (1973): 31–40.

10 Betty Sarvis and Hyman Rodman (in Reference 1), p. 177.

11 Betty Sarvis and Hyman Rodman (in Reference 1), p. 178.

12 Al Huebner, "Dare call it genocide," *Science for the People* 7, 2 (1975): 7, 20–21.

13 Judith Coburn, "Sterilization regulations: debate not quelled by HEW document," *Science* 183 (1974): 935–939.

14 "Another look at sterilization," *ZPG Newsletter* 9, 2 (1977): 1–2.

15 Judith Coburn (in Reference 13), p. 936.

16 Patricia Donovan, "Sterilizing the poor and incompetent," *Hastings Center Report* 6, 5 (1976): 7–8.

17 Patricia Donovan (in Reference 16), p. 7.

18 Patricia Donovan (in Reference 16), p. 8.

19 Betty Liddick, "Have mentally retarded the right to sex life?" *Champaign-Urbana News-Gazette* (June 29, 1975).

20 "Sterilization persists as political issue in Latin America," *Hastings Center Report* 5, 1 (1975): 2.

BIBLIOGRAPHY

Gaylin, Willard, et al., "Sterilization of the Retarded: In Whose Interest?" Four articles. *Hastings Center Report* 8, 3 (1978): 28–41.

McFadden, Charles, "Sterilization," Chapter 13, in *Medical Ethics* (Philadelphia: F. A. Davis, 1967).

McGarrah, Robert E., and Susan L. Peck, "Voluntary female sterilization: abuses, risks and guidelines," *Hastings Center Report* 4, 3 (1974): 5–7.

H. CLONING

Cloning—A futuristic problem

The problems that have been discussed heretofore in this chapter might be termed proximate or nearby ones. They express real-life concerns calling out for solution, if not immediately, then in the very near future. And what has been cited are only a few of the more pressing problems. It is hoped that the general tone of and viewpoints regarding these anxieties have been communicated for with each technological innovation, moral and ethical controversies are seen to arise. Before closing the topic of issues arising from reproductive technologies, it may be instructive to direct our focus toward a more distant matter, the issue of cloning. The immediacy of solution here is not as pressing since the techniques for human cloning have not yet been worked out. Also, there is considerable hesitancy as to whether research dealing with human cloning ought to proceed. Since cloning is not yet a *fait accompli*, it may be useful to study this issue as an exercise in futuristic planning; although the technology in this case has not been perfected, its attainment is conceivable within the reasonably near future. Hence, society has the luxury of deciding in advance whether or not the good will be served by this innovation. In this regard, a consideration of the topic can be informative.

James Watson testified before the House Subcommittee on Science and Technology in 1971 that "if the matter proceeds in its current nondirected fashion, a human being—born of clonal reproduction—most likely will appear on the earth within 20 to 25 years and conceivably sooner if some nation actively promotes the venture." Using Watson's calculations, this would put the date for the achievement in the last decade of this century, the 1990s.

There can be many personal and clinical reasons for cloning (see p. 77). Robert Sinsheimer, a molecular biologist (while still an advocate of this kind of research), remarked that cloning will "permit the preservation and perpetuation of the finest genotypes that arise in our species—just as the invention of writing has enabled us to preserve the fruits of their work."[1] Professor Joshua Lederberg, Nobel Laureate in Biology, has written, "if a superior individual—and, presumably, genotype—is identified, why not copy it directly, rather than suffer all the risks, including that of sex determination, involved in the disruptions of recombination."[2] A contrasting view is presented by Leon Kass: "Among sensible men, the ability to clone a man would not be a sufficient reason for doing so. Indeed, among sensible men there would be no human cloning."[3]

The moral questions

Paul Ramsey poses the "first moral question" associated with initial attempts to clone humans. He asks, "in case of a monstrosity—a subhuman or parahuman individual results—shall the experiment simply be stopped and this artfully created human life be killed?"[4] It is worth noting that a significant number of grossly deformed creatures have resulted from frog cloning experiments, and there is no reason to be more optimistic about the first attempts in human cloning (note Fig. 5.1). According to Ramsey, the twin issues of the production and disposal of defectives provide sufficient moral grounds for precluding any attempts at cloning humans. When there are large risks associated with any experiment involving human subjects then that experiment ought not to be done. In an earlier discussion, this qualifier was expressed: "if the results of an important scientific experiment cannot be evaluated, then that experiment should not be done" (see p. 124). Could this be extended to include evaluation of experimentation with cloning, too? Presumably Ramsey would.

The scientific problem involved here is one that relates directly to the ethics of experimentation with human material (see Chapter 7). Although the techniques for manipulating human fertilized eggs are quite elegant, a percentage of these fertilized eggs do fail to progress normally through the early stages of embryonic development and degenerate. When introduced into the female uterus, some fail to implant into the endometrial lining; others undergo faulty or transient implantation. In many cases, the failure may be due to genetic and developmental abnormalities in the embryo. And while it is true that nature often aborts those embryos with serious

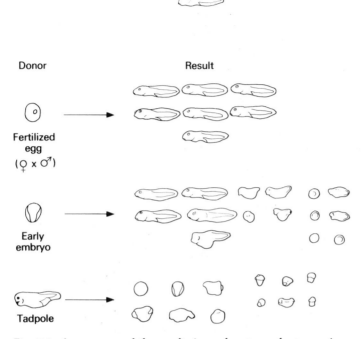

Fig. 5.1 *A summary of the results in nuclear transplant experi-*
ments using frogs. It is observed that the older the donor nucleus,
the greater the deviation from normal.

defects, she does not always do so. There is at present no way of finding out whether
or not the experimental procedures of *in vitro* fertilization, the transfer of human
embryos from donor to host, or any other exotic reproductive technique will result
in congenital anomalies, sterility, or mental or physical retardation in any of the
progeny. A suggestion has been made that it may be wise to postpone experiments
on cloning until gestation can be monitored closely enough to be sure that the fetus,
at least, meets expectations of normalcy.

And then there is the question of unused embryos. Dr. Gould, editor of *The
New Scientist*, has asked: "What happens to the embryos which are discarded at the
end of the day—washed down the sink? There would necessarily be many. Would
this amount to abortion—or to murder?" Or is it simply an expediency of the experiment with no ethical or moral connotations whatsoever? But, one might ask, isn't
that really a trivial question? For certainly, the present practice of abortion and certain kinds of chemical contraception (e.g., prostaglandins) also results in widespread
elimination of unwanted embryos. But does the present practice of abortion and
contraception excuse moral responsibility for new life if it is experimentally called
into being? Kass says no. He differentiates embryo disposal from elective abortion.
The two do not belong in the same category at all. In the case of experimentation, an
embryo is wanted and only those left over are deliberately destroyed. In elective
abortion, on the other hand, the embryo-fetus is unwanted right from the start, the

usual reason being a conflict of rights between the mother and the fetus. In cases of conflict like this, the mother's rights take primacy. In embryo disposal, there is no conflict of rights, hence, the moral circumstances are quite dissimilar. A human embryo flushed away in the laboratory because it is surplus constitutes willful manslaughter—an act, if it can be substantiated, of no small consequence.

Still another related issue concerns the experimental use of human embryos in which there is never any intention of carrying them to full term. This situation could arise if embryos are used for genetic experimentation. Human embryos would provide ideal experimental material since conducting good genetics experiments with adult humans is difficult at best, impossible usually. Long generation time, the number of progeny resulting from a single genetic mating, as well as moral compunctions against manipulating humans for experimental genetic purposes, preclude effective genetic experimentation. A partial way around this may be to have the matings done in a test tube, grown to the blastocyst stage, studied, and then discarded. These embryos may never be implanted into a human ovary nor would there ever be any intention to proceed with the experiments beyond some preestablished termination point. The unresolved ethical question is, Are these artificial matings alive, and if alive, are they human life? The response to this question will in no small measure determine the ethical validity of these experiments as well as cast light on cloning experimentation.

In the matter of cloning, the theologian Paul Ramsey warns that society is being led down the "primrose path" by the marvels of science. Each small step seems to contribute some tiny bit of new knowledge, usually judged to be desirable; each new biomedical technology in and by itself promises a little better existence. With each tiny increment we are further mesmerized by the achievement, accepting each in turn, without first working through its fundamental moral implications. But "the road to hell is often paved with good intentions," a wise man once said. Technology has a momentum of its own that once started is difficult to stop. The slow, almost unnoticed additions finally add up to something big but by the time this is realized, it may be too late to act (or react)! Moral quicksand has a hold on us and we are left with no other choice but to accept in toto what we have previously accepted in part. To prevent this from happening in the case of cloning, Ramsey's hope is that the first experiments with cloning result in monsters and that these get wide publicity. The shock value of publication could force a public assessment of the work, hopefully leading to a complete abandonment of it.[5] It seems that he would accept one moral transgression if it would prevent greater future evils.

But, the alarm bell may have already been rung even without the production of a monster. In early 1978, David Rorvik reported the first cloning of a man in a book entitled *In His Image* (Lippincott, 1978). The birth reportedly took place in December, 1976. Mr. Rorvik, an experienced science writer, is noted for his careful and meticulous reporting of scientific fact. Among his other works are *Your Baby's Sex: Now You Can Choose*, coauthored with gynecologist Dr. Landrum B. Shettles (Dodd, Mead, 1970), and *Brave New Baby* (Doubleday, 1971). Although almost no scientist took the report seriously since there are at present significant obstacles to human cloning (see p. 75), a number of people, including several scientists,* filed

---

* Jonathan Beckwith of Harvard University, Ethan Signer of MIT, and the Peoples Business Commission, a Washington, D.C. based lobby.

suit in federal court to gain access to information about grants involving cloning awarded by government agencies (e.g., NIH, NSF, CIA, and DOD). It is interesting to note that the suit-filers were also prominent in the opposition to recombinant DNA research. They insisted that the filing of their suit was not de facto acceptance of Rorvik's claim but rather that it was time to begin public debate on the issue since the real event may not be long in coming.

"We're worried that we're too close to cloning for comfort, even if the book is a hoax," said one member of the group. "All our values would be upset if we could xerox life."[6] Rorvik himself offers this caution: "It is my hope that this first successful cloning of a human being will alert the public to the far more promising and also far more perilous developments already occurring in the realm of genetic engineering."[7] What is being called for here is public discussion of a complex issue, socially sensitive and morally vexing; not an endorsement of cloning.

Leon Kass lists other questions which apply to cloning. Among these are the important issues of identity and individuality. Does each person have a right not to be deliberately denied a unique genotype? (Identical twins are exceptions since their formation is not intentional.) Is one inherently injured by having been made the copy of another human being, regardless of who that human being may be? Is individual dignity undermined by a lack of genetic distinctiveness? Kass states that membership in a clone with five to ten members (i.e., mass cloning) would doubtless threaten one's sense of self; but membership in a clone of two might do the same thing. This is probably so, since with the cloned individual the genotype with which it is saddled has *already* lived. Performance comparisons with progenitors will likely occur; personal potential will in all likelihood be stunted as he/she is forced into a mold that neither fits nor may even be wanted. Lederberg has written of this kind of cloning: "we would at least enjoy being able to observe the experiment of discovering whether a second Einstein could outdo the first." Would the cloned individual experience the same level of joy? To aspire to genius is laudable, to be the child of a genius can be dreadfully difficult, but to be expected to be a genius because you are a genetic twin to one is or could be crushing. Included in knowing your precursor's accomplishment is the anguish of knowing his ills as well—schizophrenia, heart attack at age 42, and the whole lot. Could one live a productive and happy life with such a burden?

A larger issue relates to the matter of power. As C. S. Lewis says in *The Abolition of Man*, "each new power won by man is a power over man as well. It is a well-documented fact of history that the number of powerful men grows smaller as power increases. Decisions then become concentrated into fewer and fewer hands. The problem of specific abuses grows proportionately." It is sufficient here to mention the prospects of involuntary breeding programs: the tyrant cloning himself; "gammas and deltas" bred for specialized purposes; five complete sets of spare organs stored until needed and the unused parts discarded; quintuplets for circuses; human clones raised for the single purpose of studying the relative contributions of nature and nurture; superstars who would be assured of winning gold medals in the Olympics; a cloning race between international powers. All sorts of scenarios with disastrous consequences can be readily conjectured.

But these science-fictionlike possibilities for the future, although not to be dismissed as mere idle speculation, are not the pressing problems which are more imminent. As Kass concludes, "we have great reason to be concerned about the private, well-intentioned voluntary use of the new technologies. The *major problem* to be feared is not tyranny but voluntary dehumanization!"[8] In the case of cloning, the total genetic blueprint of the cloned offspring is selected and determined by humans. What has been violated, even if only slightly, is the distinction between the natural and the artificial. In other words, laboratory reproduction of human beings is no longer *human* procreation. Humans themselves become simply another man-made thing. The depersonalization of the process of reproduction and its separation from human sexuality dehumanizes the activity that brings new life. The union of sex, love, and procreation is distinctly human, something that makes our species unique in the biological world. In all other species sexual reproduction is no different than a number of other bodily functions. In human society it has come to represent the highest form of sharing between two persons, conveying deep personal and social meaning. The loving feelings of physical and emotional well-being plus the sense of completion of self in one's offspring is done away with in clonal reproduction. People probably prefer to have children, their children, not specialized copies of someone else, even themselves. (Can you imagine the conflict between husband and wife in determining which partner should be cloned?)

Cloning adds an additional threat to our conception of humanness; the technique renders males obsolete. Human eggs, nuclei, and uteri are all it requires. All three can be supplied by women. Whatever value this might have can be countered with the humane and humanistic values growing out of a genuine sexual relationship.

On the other side of the issue, Robert Sinsheimer provides the rebuttal to some of the objections raised above:

> But here we are—at this juncture in our evolution. And we have really only two choices—to proceed with all the wisdom we can develop, or to stagnate in fear and in doubt. The choice seems to me to be: are we as a species to lead a furtive, timorous existence, in terror of our brute past—oppressed and confined by our finite vision and our unfinished state—or, using all that evolution has given us, do we seek to find the way to a higher state?[9]

These statements were uttered by him in the days when he was still enamored with genetic research (see p. 107); whether or not these remain his views is not important. The sentiments expressed here are still germane to those who would use technology without a consideration of the ethical or moral consequences.

It is appropriate to end this discussion by considering a less futuristic proposition. As is generally agreed, we live in an age of overpopulation. Zealous optimists are eager to engineer improvements in the human species when already a surplus of them exists. It has been said that the world suffers more from the morally and spiritually defective than from the genetically defective. In the absence of standards to guide and restrain our use of this new technology, we run the very real risk of dehumanizing ourselves much as other technologies have despoiled our planet. Fortunately, at least in the matter of cloning, there are no compelling reasons to proceed further with the research until we feel certain that the knowledge learned is worth the moral hazards. Perhaps our best efforts now should be directed to our survival, especially our survival as human beings.

VALUES PERTAINING TO HUMAN CLONING

1 Genetic cloning of human beings would make it possible to direct evolution along positive pathways and represents the next step in man's continuing journey from brute to saint, hence, it should be done.

2 The ultimate dehumanization of our species is the probable end-product of clonal reproduction; all attempts to achieve it must be stopped immediately.

3 In order to achieve the goal of successful human cloning, unethical or immoral experiments must be done. The end in this case cannot ethically validate the means.

4 Accepting in small increments the fruits of science and technology without thinking carefully about the moral consequences of each in advance could lead to the collapse in all that historically identifies humanhood.

5 Science is an ever-expanding frontier and although there are uncertainties about where it may lead, the quest for knowledge and the expected as well as the unanticipated benefits must beckon us on; cloning is only part of this greater mission.

REFERENCES

1 Robert L. Sinsheimer, "Ambush or opportunity?" *Hastings Center Report* 2, 4 (1972): 4.

2 Joshua Lederberg, "Experimental genetics and human evolution," *Bulletin of Atomic Scientists* 28, 8 (1966): 4–11.

3 Leon Kass, "New beginnings in life," in *The New Genetics and the Future of Man*, Michael Hamilton (ed.) (Grand Rapids: Erdmans, 1972), p. 44.

4 Paul Ramsey, "Shall we clone man?" in *Fabricated Man* (New Haven: Yale University Press, 1970), p. 78.

5 Paul Ramsey, "Genetic engineering," *Bulletin of Atomic Scientists* 28, 10 (1972): 14–17.

6 Barbara J. Culliton, "Scientists dispute book's claim that human clone has been born," *Science* 199 (1978): 1316.

7 David Rorvick (in Reference 6), p. 1316.

8 Leon Kass (in Reference 3), p. 61.

9 Robert L. Sinsheimer (in Reference 1), p. 6.

BIBLIOGRAPHY

Edwards, R. G., and Ruth E. Fowler, "Human embryos in the laboratory," *Scientific American* 223, 6 (1970): 44–54.

Galston, Arthur, "Here comes the clones," *Natural History* 84, 2 (1975): 72–75.

Gaylin, Willard, "We have the awful knowledge to make exact copies of human beings," *The New York Times Magazine* (March 5, 1972).

Grossman, Edward, "The obsolescent mother: a scenario," *Atlantic Monthly* (May 1971): 39–50.

6

EUTHANASIA

CONFUSION SURROUNDING DEATH

Birth control and death control go together, according to the ethicist Joseph Fletcher. To speak of living and dying encompasses the abortion issue along with the euthanasia issue. And just as genetics, molecular biology, fetology, and obstetrics have developed to a point where we have effective control over the start of human life, so the whole medical armamentarium for resuscitation and prolongation of life has enabled us to exert control over the terminal end as well.

To some, it seems an inconsistency in logic that, on the one hand, it is perfectly acceptable that therapeutic abortions be done for reasons of mercy and compassion, while on the other, it is unacceptable to take positive action to end a life where the prognosis is hopeless insofar as medical and social criteria can determine it to be. It would seem that life *in utero* and life *in extremis* are ethically inseparable, for the same questionnaire applies at both ends of the biological spectrum: What is human life? When does it become human? When does it cease to be human?[1]

The euthanasia issue, or the right to choose death, has become the "new think" question for several reasons, the primary one being the fear of a lingering death. The much discussed and highly publicized Karen Quinlan case turned public attention to the wisdom of prolonging some lives. There is little doubt that modern understanding of the human organism and the technology for sustaining it has changed the practice of medicine from an art to a science. The pronounced diminution in impact of many diseases which were once fatal has affected people's perceptions of the traditional views of death and dying. A new mysticism has grown up around man's achievements in medicine; it has become expected that whenever disease gains entrance into the body, the physician can almost ritually pull from his or her therapeutic bag of tricks a drug or an operation to reverse the course of the disease. One result of this has been a blurring of the line between life and death. People have come to believe that they can employ physicians to tell death to wait.

Today, degenerative diseases have replaced acute ones as the major killers as more and more people survive the early years of childhood and adolescence. Improvements in nutrition, living conditions, sanitation, and medicine have dramatically altered the age structure of the population in favor of the older categories. At the beginning of this century, 15 percent of the newborn died before their first birthday and 15 percent of the survivors were gone before adolescence. Today the mortality rate for the first year of life is less than 2 percent and about two-thirds of the population lives to reach age 70.[2] Accompanying this change in age distribution was a change in the shape of dying itself. "The old Victorian deathbed scene of final farewells at home is replaced: death comes in hospitals, from chronic rather than from acute diseases, (the former) . . . are more apt to be metabolic (rather) than infectious or contagious."[3] Medical therapies in responding to these ailments of old age are many times simply palliative or totally ineffectual. Care becomes emphasized over cure, not because the physician ordains it so but because medical science can do little about a human machine that is falling apart as a result of wear and tear. The care is costly and time-consuming, and rather than reversing the deterioration that naturally sets in, medical science merely slows down its progress. One important consequence of these technological advances is an ever-widening of the twilight that divides life and death. Even death itself defies simple definition since the transition from life to death can be protracted by artificial means. There are some who label it a "process"—a long drawn-out affair that commences when life itself begins and is not completed in any given organism until the last cell ceases to convert energy, sometimes well after vital functions cease.[4] Death, in this view, is a transition from the state of being alive to the state of being dead. On the other side are those who see death as an event, a distinct change in state: ". . . as long as you are, death is not; when death is, you are not. . . ."[5]

Physicians and lawyers who must deal with this sensitive question of death find little of practical value in these opposed views for they do not provide any assistance whatsoever in setting a line separating the living from the dead. Physicians desire some definition of death to protect themselves legally and to allow the performance of certain medical procedures like organ transplant operations; in general, they want to ease their conscience when dealing with death. Lawyers are wanting some definitive criteria for trying those kinds of cases where the "who," as in who caused a death, is uncertain.

WHEN IS DEATH?

The process of dying (as opposed to an event) can be likened to three concentric rings.* (See Fig. 6.1.) The outermost ring is one's social life, which is made up of one's behaviors and interpersonal relationships. Being outermost, it is most vulnerable and usually is the first to die. This has been called by Furlow, social death. After social death, the dying person retreats from the larger world to a narrowing ring of persons. The next circle symbolizes human intellectual life, that part of our constitution that sets us apart from the rest of the biological world. Consciousness and rational interaction deriving from that highest region of the brain, the cerebrum, characterize this level. Once dying has claimed this region, termed physical death, the innermost circle alone remains: biological life. Biological life, controlled

---

* Thomas W. Furlow, "Tyranny of Technology; A Physician Looks at Euthanasia," *The Humanist* **34**, 4 (1974): 6–8.

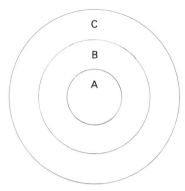

Fig. 6.1 *The three dimensions of life:* A - *Biological Life*
B - *Intellectual Life*
C - *Social Life*

largely by the brain stem, is not uniquely human because it shares features with non-humans. (For example, control of heartbeat, respiration, and other basic biological functions.) Loss of function in this brain region constitutes biological (or vegetative) death.

Traditionally, clinical and legal definitions of death have been founded on loss of biological life—the primary functions such as heartbeat, breathing, stereotyped reflexes, etc., are gone from the organism. The view is widely held that though the loss of these is indicative of death, the preservation of them is not tantamount to life, at least not human life. As our powers to sustain biological life have increased, dehumanization arising from a loss of those truly worthwhile aspects of human life has increased. Within this confusion, both physician and patient have fallen victims of technology. As a consequence, people are afraid and doctors are confused. It would seem that we had best be about the task of bringing a resolution to this conflict.

Most religious leaders have indicated a willingness to let doctors decide when death has occurred. Pope Pius XIII stated in 1957:

> Human life continues for as long as its vital functions, distinguished from the simple life (biological) of the organs, manifest themselves spontaneously without the help of artificial processes. The task of determining the exact instant of death is that of the physician.[6]

The legal profession, too, insists that the burden of definition and clarification rests with the physicians themselves. According to most interpretations of the law, the duty of the physician reflects the standard practice of the medical community.

> Doctors are in a position to fashion their own law to deal with cases of prolongation of life. By establishing customary standards, they may determine the expectations of their patients and thus regulate the understanding and the relationship between doctor and patient. And by regulating that relationship, they may control their legal obligations to render aid to doomed patients.[7]

The most prominent proposal put forward by the medical profession for determining "When is death?" has been offered in the Report of the Ad Hoc Committee of the Harvard Medical School to Examine the Definition of Brain Death; more often this is referred to as the "Harvard definition for death."[8] The following criteria were presented:

1. Unreceptivity and unresponsivity: total unawareness of externally applied stimuli and complete unresponsiveness to even the most intensely painful stimuli (no vocal or other response such as a groan, withdrawal of a limb, quickening of respiration).

2. Movements or breathing: no spontaneous muscular movements or response to any stimuli (pain, light, sound, touch), or spontaneous respiration; both of the above should not be observed covering a period of one hour. After patient is on a mechanical respirator, the total absence of spontaneous breathing is tested by turning off the respirator for three minutes and observing whether any effort to breathe spontaneously is made.

3. No reflexes: pupils fixed and dilated and do not respond to bright light; no ocular movements to head turning or following irrigation of eyes with ice water, and no blinking; no evidence of postural activity; corneal and pharyngeal reflexes absent; no swallowing, yawning, or vocalization reflexes; no motor reflexes whatsoever (biceps, triceps, pronator muscles, quadriceps, and gastrocnemius); all of the above indicative of irreversible coma.

4. Flat electroencephalogram: isoelectric or flat EEG (precise directions for the operation of the electroencephalograph are also included here); at least a full 10 minutes of recordings. This final test is confirmatory only, not diagnostic.

All of the above tests repeated 24 hours later should reveal no change. If the above procedures still reveal no activity, then the patient can be judged dead on the basis of irreversible cerebral damage. There are two exceptions to these criteria: The patient is suffering from hypothermia (internal body temperature is below 90°F) or from administration of central nervous system depressants (e.g., barbiturates).

The Harvard criteria are meant to be necessary for only a small percentage of cases where death is uncertain—where the traditional medical indicators of death are obscured because of the intervention of resuscitation machinery or where it is suspected that there is irreversible brain damage or permanent coma. The criteria are meant to complement, not to replace, the traditional signs which determine death. These are: the cessation of spontaneous respiration, no heartbeat, and complete lack of cephalic reflexes. Where the latter can be clearly ascertained, they are still used as the determinative criteria. As of January 1977, twelve states have enacted laws that define death as the end of total brain function even though a heartbeat may continue, either because of life-support equipment or the body's spontaneous electrical activity. Total brain function is meant to include both higher (i.e., cerebral) and lower (i.e., brainstem) brain function. It is seen then that both a medical and legal definition for death—at least in some states—is being formulated based on the loss of total brain activity.

Not everyone, however, agrees that the Harvard criteria go far enough. In some very few cases, spontaneous recovery was demonstrated by patients who could pass the Harvard test. The instance is reported of a 15-year-old Israeli boy who in 1969 sustained severe brain damage when he fell into a cave. By the Harvard definition, he was dead, but he was kept on drugs and artificial respiration. After two weeks, the EEG showed new activity in the brain and within two months of the accident, the boy was reported in good health, mentally and physically. Because of cases like these, one additional criterion has been suggested: the nonconsumption of oxygen by the brain and several methods may be used to determine this. In one procedure, nitrous oxide gas is injected into the carotid artery, the major artery to the brain, and the oxygen content is measured in blood which has passed through it. Another test injects a radioactive substance into the artery and subsequently seeks to locate it in the brain. If no oxygen has been used, then metabolism in the brain has stopped; the brain is irreversibly dead. It is well to remind yourself that in the vast majority of cases, the classical indicators of death—cessation of respiration, heartbeat, and reflexes—will continue to mark life's closing event. The Harvard criteria are applicable to those few instances where death cannot be easily determined.

The issue of when death is certain appears now in the twentieth century to be a very complex one. Not only is the matter of life's beginning difficult to establish; but as this discussion has shown, the matter of its closing is no easier to fix. And people are still uncomfortable about death, especially the thought of their own death.

A DENIAL OF DEATH

The blurring of the line between life and death is further confounded because our culture is a death-denying one as opposed to a death-affirming one. The nineteenth century produced physicians who began to shape the public's view of death. Over the years, death was transformed from "God's call," to a "natural event," to a "force of nature," to now when it is an "untimely event," the result of a disease certified by the physician and made official by the death certificate. Today medicine has advanced to a stage where the majority of deaths in America occur in hospitals. This phenomenon takes its origin from the desire to spare the dying person grief, but in recent times it has been transformed into protecting the healthy and minimizing the suffering of the survivors by removing the dying from their presence. This so-called covering up was especially accelerated between 1930 and 1950. When a person dies in a hospital, the body is quickly and quietly removed to the morgue before the evidence of death can upset anyone. We shelter our children from death and dying on the notion that we are protecting them from emotional harm. At least one authority, Elizabeth Kübler-Ross, sees this as a disservice to them by depriving them of the experience of death. She sees that by making dying and death a taboo subject and keeping children away from dead or dying people, we create a fear in them that need not be there.[9]

Even when dead, effort is made to make the body look natural by preparing it using sophisticated embalming techniques. Everything possible is done to help the survivors by being cheerful, turning the tasks of final preparation over to the professionals—undertakers or funeral directors—so that grief is minimized and rapidly disappears. It is not even acceptable to show your emotions upon the death of a loved one. Kübler-Ross believes this practice to be destructive as well. It is her opinion that survivors ought to participate in the events following the death of a loved one since such participation will help them in their grief and prepare them to accept their own death more easily.

Though it may be important to participate in thinking (and planning) their own death, the number of individuals who do are certainly a tiny fraction of the population. Dr. Robert S. Morison states, "the great majority prefer not to think about their own death in any way. Indeed, most people do not even leave a will directing what to do with their material possessions."[10]

Perhaps our society can learn how to better view death by examining the approach of other cultures. One death-affirming culture is the Trukese of Micronesia where once a Truke reaches 40 years, death begins first as a social event. At that time a Truke is judged mature enough to make decisions which guide his/her life and also prepare for death. Oriental people demonstrate this characteristic, too. The Japanese have two religions—Shintoism is the religion for the living and Buddhism is the religion for the dead. Death is viewed as a transition from one world to the next and the temples to each adjoin one another. The American Indians demonstrate a willingness about their death. They plan it and often have a certain amount of control over it. The Jewish culture provides laws which allow for a death with dignity and meaning. The dying person is to set his house in order, pass on any messages to his family, bless them, and make peace with God. This allows the dying person to take part in his/her death and continue to interact with the family until those final moments.[11]

This short detour on the death-denying characteristic of American culture perhaps provides some insights into our hesitation to approach the issue of euthanasia meaningfully, for as some have said, much of our past sex taboo has been transferred over to a death taboo. In our quest for happiness, we earnestly desire to avoid the sad, including what is perceived to be the greatest sadness of all—death. Perhaps the whole question of euthanasia can be viewed under greater light if we could begin again to view death as a natural process of life; that dying is part of living and we are still mortals subject to death. For example, in showing our care and love to those who are dying we not only make death more pleasant for them but we also help ourselves in preparing for our own death.

But some of this is beginning to change, at least in terms of limited euthanasia. The lingering and often painful death of the old and incurably ill has touched almost everyone's life. Most have had a relative or have known an acquaintance where the end did not come easily. People are speaking out more and expressing their views on this aspect of dying so that no longer is it only a moral dilemma for the medical profession, as it always has been, but it has become a dilemma for lawmakers and politicians, too.

FORMS OF EUTHANASIA

The very word euthanasia evokes a great deal of passion. For many persons euthanasia is but another way to spell murder. To others who see no point in merely prolonging the dying period, it is mercy killing. Marvin Kohl, an authority on the subject of euthanasia writing in *The Morality of Killing*, expressed the viciousness of the controversy this way:

When I first became interested in the problem of euthanasia, I was most impressed by the polarization of views and by the fact that few disputants believed that there was a middle ground for agreement. Almost all critics of euthanasia consider it to be morally outrageous, while advocates were the very opposite. According to the critics it is almost self-evident that euthanasia is morally wrong, and therefore unjustifiable homicide. To the advocates it seems to be equally obvious that a moral man is obligated to avoid, and help to reduce, needless misery, and that non-involuntary euthanasia ought to therefore be legalized. The disagreement is further aggravated by vicious name-calling. Opponents allegedly are cruel and heartless, advocates are heinous and barbaric murderers. Given this atmosphere, it is little wonder that underlying issues remain obscure and that disagreement is so rampant.[12]

In accepting the term euthanasia, one implicitly accepts an ethical judgment about it for it is by definition "good." The word is derived from the Greek *eu* meaning "well" or "good" and *thanatos* meaning "death"; thus "good death." However, the usage of the term in the literature is not consistent, and this adds to the confusion. It has even been suggested that the term itself be discarded because of many bad connotations associated with it and the phrase "modes of dying" be substituted.[13] Thus—

	Modes of Dying	
	Voluntary	**Involuntary**
Active	Suicide	Killing
Passive	Dying	Allowing to die

Applying these distinctions to euthanasia, the following forms can be identified:

1 Passive (or negative) euthanasia

This is the "letting the patient go" strategy, a practice which is already commonplace in many hospitals today. Code 90 designation on the patient's medical records signify the end has come and nothing is to be done to unduly prolong the life of that person other than trying to make him or her comfortable.

2 Active (or positive) euthanasia

a) Voluntary and direct; chosen and carried out by the patient (e.g., drug overdose left near at hand by the physician for the patient).

b) Voluntary but indirect; patient decides in advance that his or her life should be terminated under final conditions but gives to others the discretion to end it all (e.g., The Living Will).

c) Involuntary but direct; patient's life is ended without his or her present or past request (e.g., mercy killing).

Under traditional American law, the physician who withholds therapy that would probably prolong life can face prosecution for criminal negligence but he or she is almost never prosecuted. The hesitation here involves proving in court whether or not an affirmative act resulted in the death of the subject. An affirmative act may be one of commission or omission so that omission, too, is an offense when there is a duty to act—a legal duty, and not merely a moral obligation. Such an act of omission is considered murder if it is the immediate and direct cause of death. That line between treatment that is preserving life (i.e., ordinary means) or simply prolonging life (i.e., extraordinary means) has not been defined accurately by medical science, much less the law. Most prosecutions under the heading of omission depend on the whims of the local prosecutor (who may be motivated by the desire for higher office).

Active euthanasia or commission, on the other hand, is regarded in a different light. A physician who deliberately hastens the death of a patient comes under those laws prohibiting homicide. If it is a willful, premeditated act, it is normally considered first degree murder. Common and criminal law regard life as sacred and inalienable, and look upon any killing, especially premeditated killing, as homicide. Consent is never a defense to murder, nor are humanitarian motives. "He nonetheless acts with malice if he is able to comprehend that society prohibits his act regardless of his personal belief."[14]

All types of active euthanasia may also be considered a form of suicide. It is a crime in most states to "deliberately aid, advise, or encourage another to commit suicide." Even in those instances where an individual may take his own life, if another gives aid to the willing person, his actions would be considered criminal. Applied to euthanasia, any person (including physicians) who assists another in the taking of his or her own life in any way and regardless of the circumstances is open to criminal charges. Although the law in theory is very adamant on the issue of active euthanasia, in practice it is quite ambiguous. Conscientious searches of court records by legal scholars have yielded remarkably few cases involving the charge of euthanasia. Even when active euthanasia is alleged to have occurred, grand juries returned an indictment in only one U.S. case; the defendent was later acquitted.[15]

Some authors justify this disparity between law and punishment on the grounds that the law must remain since it is still a necessary deterrent for cases in which it is doubtful that euthanasia is the proper course of action. In other words, the law forces rational deliberation as to whether or not euthanasia is the best choice in a given case, rather than it being the easy or expedient thing to do. According to Yale Kamisar:

> If the circumstances are so compelling that the defendant ought to violate the law, then they are compelling enough for the jury to violate their oaths. The law does well to declare these homicides unlawful. It does equally well to put no more than the sanction of an oath in the way of an acquittal.[16]

As for cases in which the patient himself has refused life-saving treatment, courts have upheld the patient's right to refusal if withholding was based on religious scruples or on the treatment's limited probability of success. However, the courts have overridden this right, with the justification of state paternalism, where children, competent adults with dependents, or incompetent adults were involved.

The attitude of the medical profession toward the dying patient also presents a problematic situation, but in general it may be characterized as an emphasis on cure to the exclusion of care. This may be due in part to the constraints of the Hippocratic Oath: "On entering the medical profession the doctor pledges to prolong and protect life and also to relieve the suffering of his patient."[17] Perhaps a more important reason is the everincreasing number of malpractice suits being brought against physicians. It may be that in the absence of laws to the contrary, physicians feel they must do all they can to prolong the existence of even dying patients beyond any reasonable expectation of recovery in order to escape this threat. Such was reputed to be the case with Karen Quinlan; medical authorities, out of fear of a malpractice suit, decided against turning off the resuscitator, even though the Quinlans signed a form authorizing the attending physician to do so.[18] Medical technology has also contributed to the problem ". . . by failing to maintain the balance between the technological and the humane, . . . physicians have been seduced, if not actually betrayed, by their very competence."[19] The highly sophisticated life-sustaining therapies may blind the eyes of some medical specialists so that concern for the patient has been relegated to a secondary position behind the glamor of the machine. Finally, it is possible that the mechanization, so often a part of the care administered to the dying, reflects a defensiveness toward death common to most people. Within this context, physicians themselves may view death as an indicator of ultimate failure. The entire training and preoccupation of the doctor has emphasized the curative power of medicine, making the concept of "giving up" entirely foreign to this operational directive. If death is viewed as defeat, then strenuous effort must be exerted by whatever means is available to defeat that final event. Such an approach may be the means whereby health care personnel cope with and repress the anxieties that a terminally ill patient evokes in them.

There are some indications that the medical profession is beginning to grant greater importance to the issue of euthanasia and the care of the dying. In 1973, the American Medical Association House of Delegates condemned physicians agreeing to perform mercy killings but gave its approval to voluntary passive euthanasia for terminal patients:

> The cessation of the employment of extraordinary means to prolong the life of the body when there is irrefutable evidence that biological death is imminent is the decision of the patient and/or his immediate family. The advice and judgment of the physician should be freely available to the patient and/or his immediate family.[20]

Some medical schools are also placing more emphasis on the proper treatment of terminal patients, in no small measure due to the crusading efforts of Dr. Elizabeth Kübler-Ross.

The statement of the AMA quoted above is entirely appropriate, for it appears that a request for passive euthanasia by the terminal patient and/or his or her immediate family is not uncommon in the experience of most physicians. In a survey of over 400 doctors representing all major specialties, 38 percent reported hearing such a request from a terminal patient and 54 percent reported hearing such a request from the family of a terminal patient. A much smaller percentage (12 percent and 9 percent, respectively) of physicians indicated hearing requests for active euthanasia from terminal patients and their families.[21]

Doctors themselves generally favor passive euthanasia. In another survey, 59 percent of practicing physicians indicated they would practice negative euthanasia with a statement of authorization from the terminal patient. However, 90 percent of fourth-year medical students affirmed this view. Regarding active euthanasia, about one half of the medical students and one third of the practicing physicians surveyed favored permitting such a practice. Roughly half of the medical students indicated they would practice active euthanasia if legalized, but only about one fourth of the physicians indicated they would.[22] These discrepancies may be due to different value systems and/or the experience between the two groups. When it comes time to actually make the decision to terminate treatment, attitudes, particularly of medical students, may change. A 1977 AMA survey revealed that a still larger number of physicians respect the wishes of dying patients who do not want to be kept alive by extraordinary means. Only 5.5 percent of those responding said they do not favor this approach. Two thirds of the doctors indicated that legal constraint was the major factor that might prevent them from acceding to a patient's wish while others raised ethical reservations or personal religious convictions against carrying out the practice. Doctors under age 50 were more inclined to discuss imminent death with sentient terminal patients than were older doctors.[23]

Public awareness of the euthanasia issue is also on the rise, pushed on, no doubt, by the events of the Quinlan case in late 1975. In the few surveys that have been done, there is increasing support for permitting active euthanasia and almost overwhelming support for allowing passive euthanasia. In a 1950 Gallup poll, 36 percent of Americans said they approved of euthanasia (type unspecified). Contrast this with a 1973 survey in which 53 percent "expressed the view that physicians should be allowed by law to end the life of the incurably ill if the patient and family request it" (active euthanasia). As for passive euthanasia, an April 1972 *Life* magazine poll indicated that 90 percent of the 41,000 respondents believed that a terminally ill patient has the right to refuse artificial means of prolonging life.[24] When presented with the specific care of a hopelessly ill terminal patient and asked how they would respond, a majority of the public—two to one—opted in favor of passive euthanasia as opposed to making every effort to sustain life.

One might object that such surveys are of limited utility since they may not reflect the opinion of the group of people for whom the question of euthanasia is most important, namely, the elderly and those actually dying. Alex Comfort, the noted medical doctor and specialist in the area of aging, submits that the whole concern over euthanasia is a "red herring," the opinion of bleeding hearts but not that of the dying. Although the Gallup poll shows that the general public is becoming more accepting of the idea of euthanasia, there is one group strongly opposed and that is the patients themselves.[25] In one survey of the elderly in nursing homes, only 25 percent favored intervention to shorten life if it became hopeless. In another poll, half rejected euthanasia altogether, opting instead for "life at any cost." The wheel-chair-confined and deformed practicing psychologist, Saundre Diamond, who was born so severely brain damaged that doctors said she would never see, hear, speak, or walk and would be grossly mentally retarded, says, "those who ask to be killed or allowed to die often are listening to society's mandate that they die . . . I think they need careful, supportive counseling at these times so they can really see the options open to them of living, at what level, to enjoy the final stages of their lives."

On the other hand, a bill for passive euthanasia legislation in Florida elicited this commentary:

> The author of the statutory proposal reports few unfavorable responses among the hundreds he has received. The majority of responses are from those most likely to be immediately concerned—the aged.[26]

Much support for similar legislation in California came from the elderly. Over 2000 residents of Seal Beach Leisure World, a retirement community near Los Angeles, signed a petition urging the legislature to pass the bill and probably twice that many would sign a Living Will, the main provision of the legislation. In the words of one of them, "now there can be dignity in death—not to lay there with tubes and all sorts of apparatus trying to keep life when there's absolutely nothing." About all that can be concluded at this point is that there are some questions about the degree of public awareness and acceptance of euthanasia both among the elderly and the younger age categories.

THE ETHICAL ISSUES OF EUTHANASIA

The arguments for euthanasia focus upon two humane and significant concerns: compassion for those who are painfully and/or terminally ill, and concern for the human dignity associated with freedom of choice. The first argument is extended to include the patient's rights to choose how and when he or she will die. In the latter, the failure to permit a consideration of euthanasia demeans the dignity of persons in that the degree of dignity available and practiced by individuals is directly related to the ability to choose when, how, and why they are to live and to die.

A euthanasia ethic according to ethicist Arthur Dyck contains the following beliefs or propositions:[27]

1. an individual's life belongs to that individual to dispose of entirely as he or she wishes;

2. the dignity that attaches to personhood by reason of the freedom to make choices demands also the freedom to take one's own life;

3. there is such a thing as a life not worth living whether the cause be distress, illness, physical or mental handicaps, or even sheer despair for whatever reason;

4. what is supreme in value is the "human dignity" that resides in the human's rational capacity to choose and control life and death.

Essentially, this ethic operates from the premise that since wide latitude has been given in western societies to "live one's life at one's pleasure," the corollary of terminating one's life at one's pleasure should also be included if we are to be consistent.

On the other side, "Thou shalt not kill" is one of the clear and universal constraints upon human action observed in most societies—ancient and modern, primitive and advanced, religious and worldly. The injunction is part of a total effort to prevent the destruction of the human community (see Chapter 1, p. 39). According to critics of euthanasia, it is the nature of the constraint not to kill that is at stake in decisions regarding euthanasia. The absolutist position is, of course, to prohibit all forms of euthanasia. This view submits that life is intrinsically good, and that it is better to be living than not living, regardless of the potential for accomplishments or achievement of goals; or even if life itself has no meaning. Further, this view fears that a relaxation of the present strong prohibition against killing will weaken social resistance to violence. For example, euthanasia may be extended to those who some may see fit to eliminate: the defenseless, the senile, the nonproductive, the aged. The best way to protect life is to make protection exceptionless. That which cannot be used cannot be abused.

The prohibitionist position is buttressed by the religious conviction that humans do not own their lives but hold them in trust from God. If this be true then mere humans cannot destroy life, even their own since to do so is to destroy what essentially belongs to God. Numerous arguments opposing euthanasia arise from this religious position. Many Christian authors, basing their position on the sanctity-of-life principle, offer the Biblical verse, "The innocent and just man thou shalt not kill" (Exodus 23:7 or Daniel 13:53) in defense. Thus, the moral code of God forbids absolutely the killing of anyone except an unjust aggressor in self-defense.

A more moderate view contends that there are conditions when interventions to prolong life are no longer justifiable after a point has been reached. Unlike the ethic of those who opt for free and voluntary euthanasia, this ethic distinguishes between acts that *permit* death (acts of omission) and acts that *cause* death (acts of commission). Orthodox Judaism forbids active euthanasia of any kind but demonstrates a permissive attitude regarding passive euthanasia. Christian moralists, too, insist that the use of extraordinary means to prolong the life of the terminal patient is not required. As for what constitutes extraordinary means, Catholic ethicians define them as "all medicines, treatments and operations which do not offer a reasonable hope of benefit and which cannot be obtained and used without excessive expense, pain, or other inconvenience."[28] (It is in this regard that the orthodox Roman Catholic stand is more liberal than that of some Protestants.)

Nonetheless, mainstream Judeo-Christian thought clearly condemns active euthanasia, whether involuntary or voluntary. Jewish and Christian tradition as well as legal interpretation have maintained a clear distinction between the failure to use extraordinary measures (permitting death) and direct intervention to bring about death (causing death). In the first case, the physician does not assist in the act of killing by withholding treatment, hence, it is not morally wrong. Since he is not participating in a direct act, he is not abandoning the first principle of the medical practice, namely, to do no harm to one's patient. A moderate euthanasia ethic submits the following beliefs and values:[29]

1. An individual's life is not solely at the disposal of that person; every human life is part of the human community that bestows and protects the lives of its members; the existence of a community at all depends upon constraints against taking life.

2. The dignity that attaches to personhood by reason of the freedom to make moral choices includes the freedom of dying people to refuse noncurative, life-prolonging interventions but does not extend to taking one's life or causing death for someone who is dying.

3. Every life has some worth; there is no such thing as a life not worth living.

4. The supreme value is goodness itself, to which the dying and those who care for the dying are responsible; less than perfect human beings require constraints upon their decisions, including decisions regarding those who are dying; human beings or the human community cannot presume to know who deserves to live or to die.

This perspective does recognize that the conditions under which people die have greatly changed and submits a more humane proposal to dying. It recognizes the rights of patients to refuse medical care as well as advocating greater concern for the terminally ill. This position derives its moral justification by differentiating between absolute and relative good. Although most humans hold life to be good, few would hold it to be good in an absolute sense. To validate the latter claim it must be shown that mere physical life is *always* a good thing. This has not been done and there is a great deal of doubt that it can ever be done. Death, under some conditions, can be a friend. The presumed flaw in the prohibitionist view is not in its intention to protect life but in the effects it produces; for unless the position is more carefully qualified, pointless suffering must be experienced by some. As the previous discussion reveals, this view is probably that of the majority in our country as well as in the Western world.

Objections to euthanasia from a nonreligious perspective have also been submitted. Perhaps the most popular of these is the so-called wedge argument. The wedge argument submits that since killing is wrong, it should be restricted to as narrow a range of exceptions as possible, for if the number becomes large, wide latitude is given to legitimizing the taking of life and it becomes an easy policy for society to approve of. Thus, accepting passive euthanasia or worse yet, accepting voluntary active euthanasia will lead to involuntary active euthanasia. Those holding this opinion frequently support their views by citing the Nazi experience. Joseph Sullivan, for example, states that the Nazi government abused their euthanasia laws and put millions of innocent people to death. The murders were justified by reason of the compulsory euthanasia legislation which at the time of its enactment was thought to include only "incurable mental cases, monstrosities, and the incurables that were a burden to the state. . . . However, once the state held this power of life and death over innocent members of society, the lives of all citizens were in danger."[30] (See also Leo Alexander, "Medical Science Under Dictatorship," *The New England Journal of Medicine* 241 (1949): 39.)

While the wedge argument regarding the relationship between voluntary and involuntary euthanasia may be true, the use of the Nazi experience to validate it is incorrect, as Joseph Fletcher points out. In those instances where people thought it right to kill others judged to be inferior, their actions stemmed from almost unlimited political power, not from the seductiveness of killing. If their beliefs included cruelty (at the start), their actions also reflected this. As Fletcher says, "what they (the Nazis) did was merciless killing, either genocidal or for ruthless experimental purposes."[31] The Nazis' form was involuntary and its objective was to maximize benefit to the state. The political policy of liquidation had been determined far in advance and justification for it was sought later on medical grounds. It was not a case of the population being led down the proverbial primrose path. On the other hand, active euthanasia practiced within a medical context is voluntarily sought and is designed to maximize benefit to the recipient. Only the deepest kind of love and humane concern for the terminally living motivates the latter act and not the simple expediency of eliminating a life judged to be useless. Clearly, there is an ethico-moral-legal wall of separation between voluntary and involuntary euthanasia which has been ignored by those citing the Nazi example, according to Fletcher.

Another secular objection to euthanasia is that all rational beings are ends in themselves. Their lives may not be taken except, possibly, in self-defense. This position also assumes that life is intrinsically good. (Every rational being, as defined by Immanuel Kant, is deserving of respect and this right must not be violated. See Chapter 2.) Some opponents of euthanasia caution against the possibility of making a mistake in so grave a matter as hastening the death of another. The act of taking a life is a radical closure of options. The decision is irreversible. In euthanasia, the possibilities are ruled out that (1) the patient may spontaneously improve, (2) the patient may recover with continued medical treatment, and (3) an unknown or unanticipated discovery of a treatment for the particular illness may benefit the patient at some future time. Since human beings are fallible, they ought to choose that alternative that allows them the opportunity to change their minds. Killing a person closes this option. Still another presumption against taking a life states that in situations of imperfect knowledge, one should avoid the worst of all possible moral errors, i.e., killing. As implied in the three reasons given above, there always exists some uncertainty about the future of the life under question. There are few questions more complex than that of trying to put a value on someone else's life. In many cases, it must be admitted that error-prone human beings are hopelessly ignorant to pass judgment concerning whether another's life is worth living. When we are in a state of ignorance, the morally right behavior demands that the life not be taken. To do less involves one in the gravest of all moral abuses!

Some supporters of euthanasia, for instance Joseph Fletcher, counter that the fear of mistake is merely rule worship. Simply because there exists a universal commandment against killing to protect life, as indeed there must, does not mean that life is an absolute good. Life may reach a point where it is no longer worth living. This does not imply that the human being has no worth but rather that the worth of the person's life is beyond that point where it is no longer worth rescuing. A person whose life involves only intense pain, who can no longer enter into personal relationships, no intellectual activity, who may not experience even a fleeting moment of joy—then the merciful and moral thing to do is rescue such a life from further agony or dehumanization. Rule worship itself is morally degrading in the judgment of Fletcher. "To reject control and responsibility, to deny human beings the role of decision maker . . . is to deny human beings their status. We become puppets, cease to be people."[32]

Certain proponents of euthanasia present the interesting proposition that if a person is no longer human, it cannot be murder to kill the person. Indeed, the act could not be called euthanasia at all and "the issue would leave the realm of the moral and devolve into a question of pure pragmatics".[33] The obvious problem here lies in deciding upon the necessary criteria of personhood (see Chapter 5d, p. 168). It seems that any such system is subject to the objection that it is arbitrary and open-ended.

The argument that one is not murdering if the being in question is not a person is clearly not a majority opinion. However, a variation on this theme, that it is not murder if the being in question is already dead, has wider support. What is referred to here is the Harvard definition of death—complete cessation of all reflexes and no spontaneous brain activity (flat EEG). If one accepts this definition as the indicator of death, then the termination of artificial means of life support for patients with a flat EEG is a pragmatic and not a moral decision. As stated earlier, this position has already been adopted by some states as a legal definition for death; numerous hospitals use it, too.

Clearly, the issues involved in euthanasia are difficult and discussion is needed at all levels if disentanglement of the many positions as divergent as these is to be worked out. The insight of Joseph Fletcher provides a handle for approaching the problem. He poses the issue in the form of four questions.[34]

1. Which do we prefer, quantity or quality of life? Do we prefer personal or human life or do we favor biological life at any cost to personality and humanity?

2. Can death sometimes be a friend, not always an enemy? Life and death are fundamental aspects of the same creative process; this means that death is part of the natural order of things. A recent best-seller recounts the experiences of people who had "crossed-over" only to return to life (e.g., heart stoppage, no EEG, etc.)[35] Many people report that an intense calm was experienced unlike anything encountered before, a release from the physical world (the ultimate trip).

3. May we humans assume any *initiative* in dying? We have implemented a stewardship of life; we exert control over disease and injury interfering with natural processes; we prevent conception or birth. Can human intervention in hastening or contriving death fit the same rationale?

4. Is there any difference between killing a person and letting him die by omitting a remedy, so long as his death is intended in both cases? (If passive euthanasia is practiced, then why not active euthanasia?) Euthanasia of either kind is right or wrong depending on the situation; neither is intrinsically good or evil. Both are forms of hastening death.

Fletcher's position arguing on consequentialist grounds is essentially this: In a medical context, it may be moral or legal to accelerate the death process by taking direct action; therefore the use of extraordinary means is morally optional.

Consequentialist arguments are not favored by proponents of euthanasia for they require that assumptions be made about what is necessary to promote the common good. Are not patience, perseverence, and the respect for life of moral value to a society? "The argument(s) from the common good . . . is guilty of a fundamental confusion between good and good and therefore remains a non sequitur."[36]

The key question remains: Can an act of euthanasia ever be right or morally justified and if so under what conditions? Marvin Kohl, in *The Morality of Killing*, submits that active euthanasia is morally good when the dominant motive is the desire to help the intended recipient.[37] The act must involve the inducement of as painless and quick a death as possible and it must result in beneficial treatment for the recipient. Further, the act must be preceded by the fully informed consent of the recipient, or, if the recipient is not free to choose for physical and/or mental reasons, then consent by a proper legal guardian; or, if this is inappropriate, then society through its representatives should determine the course of action (in that order). If there is reasonable doubt that the purported act is not kind or the kindest alternative possible, one should always refrain from so acting. The principle here is that euthanasia must be avoided if the evidence concerning the best interest of the patient in any way is ambiguous.

The argument of active euthanasia under these specifications is twofold: (1) Since it is kind treatment, and society has an obligation to treat its members kindly, this form of action is a prima facie obligation—that is, under certain circumstances, we have a moral obligation to induce death; and furthermore, it is not only virtuous, it is a duty. (2) Justice requires society, where possible, to give to each according to his basic needs; since human beings have a basic need to live *and die with dignity*, it is only just that we treat them accordingly. In practice, this means the right to live, the right to die, and the right to die with dignity. Kohl says, as long as the exercise of the right to choose death does no harm to anyone else or to society, it would seem that society has no right to deny it.

A contrary opinion to the above rationale would say that a kindly and intrinsically just act is not necessarily moral. Consequences do not make an act moral. The rule against killing the innocent must be universally binding for two reasons:

1 History tells us that killing the innocent under permissible conditions is conducive to killing the innocent under nonpermissible circumstances.

2 Although active euthanasia may have good consequences, still the rule must be kept, for even one breach of it would weaken the authority of that rule.

We have already discussed that there is probably no evidence that killing per se is necessarily contagious.

Regarding the second objection, proponents of euthanasia would argue, why dogmatically adhere to a single principle that on the one hand protects innocent life but at the same time creates needless suffering in other innocent lives? As Professor J. J. Smart observes, "to refuse to break a generally beneficial rule in those cases in which it is not most beneficial to obey it seems irrational and to be a case of rule worship."[38] If rule worship is wrong, why not formulate a better rule? We will return to this question shortly.

Ethicist Sissela Bok cautions "going slow" in the practice of active euthanasia.[39] First, she claims that the proviso that a patient is dying is not without ambiguity. Where does one draw the line and determine that the patient is definitely dying? In his article "Choosing the Good Death," Wayne Sage cites several examples of dramatic recovery, or spontaneous remissions, even after a terminal diagnosis had been made (recall the earlier cited case of the Jewish boy). Even in more benign circumstances, errors in diagnosis do occur. Second, there are no clear lines of demarcation to distinguish between acts of omission and acts of commission. There are borderline cases where the distinction is nearly impossible to make; for example, is there any difference between pulling out the plug of an oxygen machine and simply not replacing the tank of oxygen when it has run out? The distinction between passive and active euthanasia is artificial. If one can support passive euthanasia, then active euthanasia can be supported for the same reasons. As Joseph Fletcher claims, the end—the death of the patient—is the same in both cases, hence, the two forms are morally indistinguishable. Third, Bok argues that the matter of informed consent raises serious questions:

Is there a distinction between requesting something and consenting to something?

Might someone ask to die out of concern for his or her family?

Could the consent be a temporary response to depression or confusion induced by medication?

Could the desire to die be based on an unrealistic view of a situation resulting from insufficient information or inability to understand?

In view of these and other uncertainties, Bok advocates the prohibition of active euthanasia plus greater efforts to make dying easier, for example, by humane care and concern, recognition of patient's rights to refuse medical care, etc.

SOME FURTHER CONFOUNDING ISSUES

A great deal of intense argumentation has been elicited on the issue of distinguishing active from passive euthanasia. As Richard B. Brandt suggests, once a decision for death has been made, "hesitation to use more positive procedures is surely nothing but squeamishness."[40] However, not all agree that the two forms of euthanasia are so easily lumped. If there is a general reluctance to actively cause death, it is a reflection of a common-sense perception that there is a significant moral difference between killing and allowing to die. Killing does involve a "definite and in its implications momentous change of policy. . . . the distinction between 'killing' and 'allowing to die' may serve to indicate the important difference between an agent who wants someone dead and another agent who does not."[41] Although the easing of pain is an important goal and taking of a life may be the only way to achieve it, this awesome judgment carries with it heavy responsibility; errors may happen! The argument "supposes that the fact of suffering (of the dying patient), not the way it is removed, is morally decisive."[42] While this line of reasoning seeks to maximize mercy for the dying, opponents to active euthanasia argue that it is still not at all clear that killing the suffering terminal patient is the humane way to end that suffering.

The second issue that dominates the euthanasia debate is the procedural question, who should make decisions for death? The issue of consent is the major theme of a highly recommended volume by Robert Veatch, *Death, Dying and the Biological Revolution: Our Last Quest for Responsibility* (New Haven: Yale University Press, 1976). His primary commitment is to individual liberty and he opposes any person or policy that limits it. In his view, something has gone wrong when "authority over the life and death of one individual is . . . placed in the hands of another."[43] He proposes legislating policy that asserts the competent patient's right to refuse treatment, gives proxy decision-making powers for the incompetent to a chosen agent (family or court-appointed guardian but not the physician), requires the honoring of written judgments made by the patient (e.g., the Living Will), and protects the rights of medical personnel to nonparticipation for reasons of conscience.

SOLUTIONS IN THE LAW

It is clear from these discussions that current practices are much confused in this matter of shortening another's life—moralists disagree, religious viewpoints vary, and medical practice is inconsistent. Even in legal matters, law as it is written and law as it is practiced are vastly different. This in its turn encourages disrespect for the law and is a situation that should be remedied. According to Ruth Russell the "best solution is to enact a comprehensive euthanasia law—one that would provide for active and passive euthanasia and that would meet a broad spectrum of needs and provide adequate safeguards for every case."[44] We are not entirely without precedent here for other countries have enacted this type of legislation. Most European countries do not classify passive euthanasia as homicide, and Switzerland even allows a physician to make poison available to a fatally ill patient provided the physician does not administer the poison himself. Several countries recognize "homicide upon request," which carries a more lenient punishment than would normally be exacted for murder. Thus far, only Uruguay has legalized active euthanasia performed at the request of the terminal patient.[45]

Russell lists these as partial solutions to the euthanasia issue in the United States:

1. Amend the Constitution to recognize the right of an individual to life, liberty, and happiness which includes the right to death when one is suffering from an irremedial condition and happiness is no longer possible.

2. Amend the suicide laws to make assisted suicide legal in certain circumstances and in accord with legal safeguards permitting doctors to practice life-shortening tactics.

3. Amend the criminal code to distinguish euthanasia from murder (the Swiss Code identifies a murderer as a dangerous person or one with a depraved mind).

4. Make "brain death" a legal criterion of death (this would solve only a minor part of the problem).

5. Legalize the Living Will (see Fig. 6.2—The Living Will).

6. Enact euthanasia laws pertaining to passive euthanasia to provide legal and professional immunity to physicians who discontinue life-prolonging treatments (Death with Dignity Acts).

7. Enact active euthanasia laws which recognize the right of a patient to choose death and have the assistance of a qualified person to bring it about (Voluntary Euthanasia Acts).

Russell submits, however, that any of these by itself is only a half-step or partial solution; what is needed is a comprehensive euthanasia law that would combine the best features of the above proposals as well as some additional provisions. The three parts of such an act should include:

1. provisions for passive euthanasia, voluntary and nonvoluntary;

2. provision for active euthanasia at the request of the patient, including the proviso for deciding, with an advance declaration stating his or her wishes, when an irremediable condition occurs (Living Will);

3. provision for positive euthanasia at the request of the next of kin or legal guardian when the individual is unable to speak for him/herself.

She further suggests that the following safeguards be included:

1. Legislation would be permissive only, not compulsory.

TO MY FAMILY, MY PHYSICIAN, MY LAWYER, MY CLERGYMAN
TO ANY MEDICAL FACILITY IN WHOSE CARE I HAPPEN TO BE
TO ANY INDIVIDUAL WHO MAY BECOME RESPONSIBLE FOR MY
HEALTH, WELFARE OR AFFAIRS

Death is as much a reality as birth, growth, maturity and old age—it is the one certainty of life. If the time comes when I, _____ can no longer take part in decisions for my own future, let this statement stand as an expression of my wishes, while I am still of sound mind.

If the situation should arise in which there is no reasonable expectation of my recovery from physical or mental disability, I request that I be allowed to die and not be kept alive by artificial means or "heroic measures". I do not fear death itself as much as the indignities of deterioration, dependence and hopeless pain. I, therefore, ask that medication be mercifully administered to me to alleviate suffering even though this may hasten the moment of death.

This request is made after careful consideration. I hope you who care for me will feel morally bound to follow its mandate. I recognize that this appears to place a heavy responsibility upon you, but it is with the intention of relieving you of such responsibility and of placing it upon myself in accordance with my strong convictions, that this statement is made.

Signed _____

Date _____

Witness _____

Witness _____

Copies of this request have been given to _____

_____

_____

_____

Figure 6.2 *The Living Will as developed by the Euthanasia Education Council (250 West 57th St., New York, N.Y., 10019. Reprinted with permission.)*

2. No secret action should be permitted for either active or passive euthanasia; the decision and proceedings should be part of the public record.

3. A written, witnessed, and notarized request for euthanasia would be required from either the patient or the next of kin or guardian. It could be made in advance while in good health but could be revoked at any time by the person making it. If made in advance it would have to be reaffirmed before euthanasia could be administered.

4. Two or more physicians would verify that the patient's condition is irremedial and that the request is a bona fide one executed without duress from others.

5. In cases where it is possible, application for euthanasia should be preceded by consultation with others—clergyman, hospital chaplain, psychologist, social worker, members of the family, etc.).

6. The formal application should be filed at the County Court House or other legally constituted authority where, after review, a permit may or may not be issued (application is authentic and properly completed, there is no evidence of coercion or foul play, etc.).

7. A waiting period would ordinarily be required to ensure that emotional distress did not prompt the application (e.g., 15- to 30-day wait period).

8. The administration of euthanasia would be the responsibility of the patient's physician or other medical person designated to carry out the physician's instructions and the patient's wishes.

9. The death certificate would indicate the action taken.

10. No physician or other medical personnel would be required to administer euthanasia if it is contrary to his/her conscience, judgment, religious beliefs, etc.).

11. No medical person or other specialist who performs an authorized act of euthanasia would be guilty of any offense.

12. No insurance policy in force would be vitiated.

13. Each person who has reached the age of maturity should be encouraged to lodge with the appropriate office his or her desires pertaining to euthanasia. Such persons would be issued cards to carry indicating these wishes.

The legislation Russell proposes should not be overly rigid but it should define the rights, roles, and responsibilities in the relationship between the doctor and the terminally (or critically) ill patient.

Dr. Robert Veatch, from the Institute of Society, Ethics, and the Life Sciences, suggests that these inclusions be part of effective legislation:[46] (1) provision be made to ensure that the wishes of the person, expressed while competent and never disavowed, remain valid even though that person may be unable to reiterate them during terminal illness; (2) penalty clauses for failure to follow instructions or foregoing a document should be inserted; (3) the rights of medical personnel to withdraw from a case for reasons of conscience, with the provision that adequate medical care be provided; (4) that deaths resulting from withdrawal of treatment are not suicide (for legal and insurance purposes) and that medical attendants are not guilty of homicide for following directions.

It is inevitable, given our system of jurisprudence and constitutional law, that legislation lags behind public opinion, but a number of legal proposals for both passive and active euthanasia have been presented. A number of state legislatures have considered such laws. Perhaps the most popular is a call for the legalization of the so-called Living Will. This document is a statement declaring a person's wishes regarding treatment if that person should become terminally ill. It is to be signed by the person while still of sound mind and would serve as an expression of his/her wishes in the event that he/she would be unable to communicate them. The most commonly referenced form of the Living Will was developed by the Euthanasia Education Council, a nonprofit organization in New York City. (See Fig. 6.2.) This will asks that no artificial means or heroic measures be used to keep the patient alive if there is no real chance of recovery, and requests only the alleviation of suffering. Less popular are proposals for comprehensive legislation permitting both passive and active euthanasia.

California was the first state to enact a euthanasia law, the Natural Death Act, which went into effect on January 1, 1977. The introduction to the act states:

> The Legislature finds that adult persons have the fundamental right to control the decisions relating to the rendering of their own medical care, including the decision to have life-sustaining procedures withheld or withdrawn in instances of a terminal condition.
>
> The Legislation further finds that modern medical technology has made possible the artificial prolongation of human life beyond natural limits.
>
> The Legislature further finds that, in the interest of protecting individual autonomy, such prolongation of life for persons with a terminal condition may cause loss of patient dignity and unnecessary pain and suffering, while providing nothing medically necessary or beneficial to the patient.
>
> The Legislature further finds that there exists considerable uncertainty in the medical and legal professions as to the legality of terminating the use or application of life-sustaining procedures where the patient has voluntarily and in sound mind evidenced a desire that such procedures be withheld or withdrawn.
>
> In recognition of the dignity and privacy which patients have a right to expect, the Legislature hereby declares that the laws of the State of California shall recognize the right of an adult person to make a written directive instructing his physician to withhold or withdraw life-sustaining procedures in the event of a terminal condition.

The law allows a doctor to discontinue life-support equipment from a dying patient who has authorized it in advance. It can be acted on only after two doctors certify a patient hopelessly ill, with death imminent no matter what treatment is used. Under the law, a physician cannot be sued or prosecuted for implementing a Living Will. The document must be renewed every five years to remain valid.

The bill had a wide base of support on the way to its passage and signing including religious, professional, and senior citizens' organizations. However, fifteen months after its enactment (March 1978) doctors reported only a few of their patients had directed them to cut off life-sustaining procedures when death was imminent. Indeed, one of the main objections to it is its narrowness. For example, the directive is legally binding only if a patient has been certified as terminally ill at least fourteen days before the directive is signed. Moreover, the law contains a strict witness requirement and, coupled with the five-year renewal provision, diminishes the operational effectiveness of the law. According to one elderly citizen, "they've made it too difficult." Another voiced the objection that "people don't trust this act." It is feared that physicians would become insensitive to the needs and requests of terminal patients who did not have the proper documentation or whose case did not fit the narrow specifications of the Natural Death Act. (For example, Karen Ann Quinlan would not have qualified even though she might have signed a directive.) However, the bill's authors had deliberately constructed a limited bill anticipating subsequent legislation to clear up some of its vagueness. They felt it was important to get legislation on the books dealing with the easier cases first. This is exactly what is feared by the antieuthanasia position. Dr. Philip Dreisbach, of Concerned Physicians and Attorneys Against Euthanasia, represents the views of several pro-life groups that fought its enactment. He said, "The governor has made a tragic mistake for the future of helpless patients and his own political future. This is the Act that euthanasia groups in the United States and Europe have been waiting for. Governor Brown will be known as the first American governor to point us toward legalized medical homicide and suicide."[47]

According to opponents, legislation like this is making it all too plain that an antilife philosophy is being adopted by the American medical and legal professions. The abortion of live babies, fetal experimentation, neonatal euthanasia, and now legally mandated euthanasia—the "death brigade" is claiming an even wider circle of victims, with no apparent end in sight.

In spite of some fundamental opposition, the movement to legislate death with dignity has gained momentum. In 1977 alone, forty states had considered legislation and eight have enacted legislation of some kind (Arkansas, California, Florida, Idaho, Nevada, New Mexico, North Carolina, and Virginia). Most of these assert the rights of competent persons to execute documents indicating that certain kinds of intervention should not be used when they become terminally ill (e.g., California Natural Death Act). Others sought to clarify who could make a decision for cessation of treatment for the incompetent, terminally ill patient. For example, the Florida Act transfers the Living Will authority to the next of kin, then to physicians.

It remains to be seen whether the California Natural Death Act or any of the other death-with-dignity legislation does in fact let the genie out of the bottle. Whatever their outcome, these do represent landmark efforts at legislation; an important step has been taken in trying to clarify some of the issues encompassed by euthanasia. The recognition is growing that care for the dying does have limits. By accepting passive euthanasia, a legal differentiation is made between ordinary and extraordinary means of treatment for terminal patients; some treatments are medically indicated and expected to be helpful while others are not. Passive euthanasia does not mean that the health care professional has given up on the terminal patient. The question does not seem to be whether to treat or not to treat but rather *how* to treat. "Decisions to cease curative attempts are not abandonment of a patient but (now are) a part of good medicine."[48] Here we are in the midst of something new in medical therapy—*no* treatment may also be good for the patient!

AN ALTERNATIVE TO EUTHANASIA

An alternative to enthanasia designed to accommodate the needs of the dying patient is the hospice movement. The objective here is to ameliorate one of the greatest fears of the dying person, namely, the feeling of being alone, of having to face the unknown without any of the familiar surroundings that may support him/her during the final days. The preoccupation of most health services (i.e., hospitals) with their emphasis on equipment, routines, impersonality of therapies, and the insistence on regulation of body functions all tend to exaggerate the depersonalization of the patient. Surrounded by busy nurses, orderlies, residents, and lab technicians who manipulate sophisticated scientific equipment and administer a variety of concoctions, "he (the patient) slowly but surely is beginning to be treated like a thing. He is no longer a person . . . he becomes an object of great concern and great financial investment."[49] Since present day hospitals are unable (or unwilling) to facilitate the dying, the reasoning goes, why not create another kind of institution which has an atmosphere designed to comfort and accommodate the needs of the terminally ill? The hospice provides that possible solution.

The word hospice has been used since medieval times to designate a place of rest. Originally designed for travelers on long journeys, its meaning has been expanded to include this new kind of traveler on a different kind of journey. The best known hospice, St. Christopher's Hospice, was founded by Dr. Cicely Saunders in London in July 1967. Personalized care and the virtual elimination of all types of suffering are the hallmarks of Dr. Saunder's philosophy and practice of medicine. Pain control, one of the major advances here, is accomplished with oral doses of the "Brompton Cocktail"—a mixture of diamorphine (heroin), cocaine, gin, sugar, syrup, and chloropromazine. The cocktail is administered generously and yet not given to the degree where the body becomes addicted. The other major feature of the hospice is the unique atmosphere in which the staff's constant attention and care help ease the dying patient. Often families stay all day visiting and eating with their loved ones. The dying person is encouraged to take home visits when his/her condition allows and to stay at home as long as possible.

There is none of the usual hospital atmosphere. The rooms are cheerful and flowers are prevalent. Doctors do not make rounds in white coats ordering this and that; rather, they do a lot of hand-holding, touching, listening, explaining, and making occasional changes in pain medication. The emphasis is on communication and honesty with the dying person as well as with the person's family. In this manner, everyone concerned is better able to face the situation of the death of a loved one realistically and to accept it "with dignity."[50]

There are about thirty hospices in England and only recently have hospices come to the United States. The first was founded in New Haven, Connecticut; others are at St. Luke's Hospital in New York, at Harrisburg Hospital, and at the Vince Lombardi Cancer Center at Georgetown University in Washington. Groups throughout the country are seriously evaluating the hospice idea with the view of establishing them in local communities. There are now more than eighty located in thirty states.* The hospice concept, where it has been put into practice, has been a tremendously effective means for providing terminal care. In these specialized hospitals, "there is a surprisingly cheerful atmosphere of faith and hope." Dr. Saunders declares that "in such hospitals . . . none of the patients would accept voluntary active euthanasia."[51] Perhaps this is part of what Sissela Bok has in mind when she suggests that we ought to "reduce the suffering of patients through a much greater concern for humane care of the dying."

Certainly, this discussion has not exhausted the topic of euthanasia. The problems pertaining to it are another demonstration of inadequate public awareness coupled with the need for clarification. It seems inevitable that laws will be passed which will provide this clarification. It is a challenge to every citizen to participate in their formulation.

---

*   For more information write: Director of Information, Hospice, Inc., 765 Prospect St., New Haven, Conn. 06511.

Issues related to euthanasia

There are still a number of issues related to this whole matter of dying. For example,

The work of Elizabeth Kübler-Ross on death and dying and its implications for developing a euthanasia policy.

The physician's duty to preserve life.

The right to suicide.

The Karen Quinlan case and the right to die.

Space does not permit a discussion of these; the included bibliography may provide resources to those who desire to study these or related issues further.

VALUES PERTAINING TO EUTHANASIA

1 To assist in any way to bring about another's death is homicide.

2 The sanctity-of-life ethic requires that all life be treated with respect.

3 The quality of life must take precedence over mere physical survival.

4 The primary obligation of the medical profession is to preserve life.

5 Death with dignity is to be preferred over life which defaces one's humanity.

6 Society has a right to intervention in order to protect individuals from themselves even if the intervention is against their will.

7 What we owe the sick is not help to die but help in dying.

8 Each person is considered to be master of his/her own body, and he/she may, if in sound mind, expressly prohibit the performance of life-saving medical treatment.

9 The universalizing of the Living Will, although in itself an acceptable document, is to be resisted nonetheless because it is the first step leading up to a legalization of active euthanasia.

10 Ordinary means must always be used by the physician in administering to his patients; heroic or extraordinary measures may or may not be used depending upon the circumstances.

11 We are all morally obligated to reduce pain and suffering in the world.

12 There is no moral difference between allowing to die or accelerating death.

13 There is a limit to the amount of pain a person should be allowed to bear.

14 A sound mind is difficult to maintain if the body is not healthy, therefore, competency in the case of the terminally ill is questionable at best.

15 The prolongation of life should not in itself constitute the exclusive aim of medical practice.

16 Decisions to stop life-sustaining treatments properly belong to the physician.

17 The rights of the patient are to be respected at all times (the right to information, to participate in decisions concerning his/her own treatment, to refuse treatment, etc.).

18 The patient has the right to refuse treatment to the extent permitted by law, and to be informed of the medical consequences of his action (from "The Patients' Bill of Rights").

19 Passive euthanasia is a morally acceptable act; active euthanasia can never be tolerated.

20 The consciences of medical personnel must be respected to the extent that they not be required to participate in those procedures they find morally repugnant.

21 Direct killing is always wrong, only protective killing is permissible.

22 A person could change his/her mind between the time of signing of a living will and the time he/she is faced with death.

23 The problems of erroneous prognosis and health professional error as well as the possibility of spontaneous remission make the practice of active euthanasia morally risky.

24 Proxy decision-making power for the incompetent should be in the hands of the family or a court-appointed guardian, not the physician.

25 Only God has the right to terminate life since He is the author of it.

REFERENCES

1 Joseph Fletcher, "The 'right' to live and the 'right' to die," *The Humanist* 34,4 (1974): 15.
2 Robert S. Morison, "Dying," *Scientific American* 229, 3 (1973): 55–62.
3 Joseph Fletcher (in Reference 1), p. 13.
4 Robert S. Morison, "Death: process or event?" *Science* 173 (1971): 694.
5 Paul Ramsey, "The indignity of death with dignity," *Hastings Center Studies* 2, 2 (1974): 49.
6 Vincent J. Collins, "Considerations in prolonging life—a dying and recovery score," *Illinois Medical Journal* (June, 1975): 46.
7 George P. Fletcher, "Legal aspects of the decision not to prolong life," *Journal American Medical Association* 203 (1968): 119–122.
8 "A definition of irreversible coma," *Journal American Medical Association* 205, 6 (1968): 337–340.
9 Elizabeth Kübler-Ross, *Death, The Final Stage of Growth* (Englewood Cliffs, N.J.: Prentice-Hall, 1975), pp. 5–6.
10 Robert Morison (in Reference 2), p. 62.
11 Elizabeth Kübler-Ross (in Reference 9), pp. 28–43.
12 Marvin Kohl, "Understanding the case for beneficent euthanasia," in *The Morality of Killing* (New York: Humanities Press, 1974), pp. 92–110.
13 Roy Branson, "Allowing to die is not killing," *Liberty* 70 (Nov/Dec, 1975): 5–6.
14 W. H. Baughman, J. C. Bruha, and F. J. Gould, "Euthanasia: criminal, tort, constitutional and legislative considerations," *Notre Dame Lawyer* 48 (1973): 1202–1260.
15 O. Ruth Russell, "Moral and legal aspects of euthanasia," *The Humanist* 34, 4 (1974): 22–27.
16 Yale Kamisar, "Euthanasia legislation: some non-religious objections," in *Euthanasia and the Right to Die*, A.B. Downing, (ed). (London: Peter Owen, Ltd, 1969), pp. 85–133.

17   Howard W. Brill, "Death with dignity: a recommendation for statutory change," *University of Florida Law Review* **22** (1970): 368–383.

18   Tabitha M. Powledge and Peter Steinfels, "Following the news on Karen Quinlan," *Hastings Center Reports* **5**, 6 (1975): 5–6; 28.

19   Robert Morison, (in Reference 2), p. 61.

20   Roy Branson and Kenneth Casebeer, "Obscuring the role of the physician," *Hastings Center Report* **6**, 1 (1976): 8–11.

21   N. K. Brown, "The preservation of life," *Journal American Medical Association* **211** (1970): 76–82.

22   E. H. Laws, "Views on euthanasia," *Journal of Medical Education* **46** (1971): 540–542.

23   "Poll: doctors respect dying patient's wish," *Champaign-Urbana News Gazette*, (Jan. 24, 1977).

24   Eric Cameron, "Euthanasia: mercy or murder?" *Liberty* **70** (Nov/Dec, 1975): 2–5.

25   Wayne Sage, "Choosing the good death," *Human Behavior* (June 1974): 18–22.

26   Howard W. Brill (in Reference 17), p. 374.

27   Arthur Dyck, "An alternative to the ethic of euthanasia," in *To Live and To Die: When, Why and How.* Robert H. Williams (ed.), (New York: Springer-Verlag, 1974), pp. 98–112.

28   John F. Dedek, "Euthanasia," in *Human Life* (New York: Sheed and Ward, 1972), pp. 119–141.

29   Arthur Dyck (in Reference 27), p. 112.

30   Joseph V. Sullivan, "The immorality of euthanasia," in *Beneficent Euthanasia*, Marvin Kohl (ed.), (Buffalo: Prometheus, 1975), pp. 12–33.

31   Joseph Fletcher, "Ethics and euthanasia," in *To Live and To Die, When, Why, and How?* Robert H. Williams (ed.), (New York: Springer-Verlag, 1974).

32   Joseph Fletcher (in Reference 1), p. 14.

33   Eike-Henner Kluge, *The Practice of Death* (New Haven: Yale University Press, 1975), pp. 131–181.

34   Joseph Fletcher (in Reference 1), pp. 13–14.

35   Raymond A. Moody, *Life After Life* (New York: Bantam, 1975).

36   Eike-Henner Kluge, (in Reference 33), p. 146.

37   Marvin Kohl, "Beneficent euthanasia," *The Humanist* **34**, 4 (1974): 9–11.

38   J. J. Smart quoted in Marvin Kohl (in Reference 37), p. 11.

39   Sissela Bok, "Euthanasia and the care of the dying," *Bioscience* **23**, 8 (1973): 461–466.

40   Richard B. Brandt, quoted in "Fatal choices: recent discussions of dying," by David H. Smith, *Hastings Center Report* **7**, 2 (1977): 8.

41   Joseph V. Sullivan (in Reference 30), p. 14.

42   Joseph V. Sullivan (in Reference 30), p. 14.

43   Robert Veatch (in Reference 40), p. 8.

44   O. Ruth Russell (in Reference 15), p. 22.

45   Howard W. Brill (in Reference 17), p. 374.

46   Robert M. Veatch, "Death and dying: the legislative options," *Hastings Center Report* **7**, 5 (1977): 5–8.

47   Bob Egelko, " 'Living Wills' cranked out in California," *Champaign-Urbana News-Gazette* (Nov. 22, 1976).

48   Richard A. McCormick, S. J., "Notes on moral theology," *Theological Studies* **37**: (1976): 87–107.

49   Elizabeth Kübler-Ross, *On Death and Dying* (New York: Macmillan, 1969).

50   Cicely Saunders, "Living with dying," *Man and Medicine* 1 (1976): 227–242.
51   Raanan Gillon, "Suicide and voluntary euthanasia: historical perspectives," in *Euthanasia and the Right to Die,* A. B. Downing (ed.), (London: Peter Owen, 1969).

BIBLIOGRAPHY

Alexander, Leo, "Medical science under dictatorship," *The New England Journal of Medicine* **241** (1949): 39–47.

Glasser, Ronald J., *Ward 402* (New York: Pocket Books, 1973).

Heifetz, Milton D., *The Right to Die* (New York: Berkeley, 1975).

O'Rourke, Rev. Kevin D., "Christian affirmation of life," *Hospital Progress,* (July, 1974).

Veatch, Robert M., *Death, Dying and the Biological Revolution: Our Last Quest for Responsibility* (New Haven: Yale University Press, 1976).

SUICIDE

Binstock, Jeanne, "Choosing to die: the decline of aggression and the rise of suicide," *The Futurist* **8** (1974).

Gibbs, Jack P., (ed.), *Suicide* (New York: Harper & Row, 1968).

Pretzel, P. W., "Philosophical and ethical considerations of suicide prevention," *Bulletin of Suicidology* (July, 1968): pp. 30–38.

Szasz, Thomas S. "The ethics of suicide," *The Antioch Review* **31** (Spring, 1971): 7–17.

Tonne, Herbert, "The right to suicide," *The Humanist* **34**, 6 (1974); 33–34.

7

HUMAN
EXPERIMENTATION

PUBLIC CONCERN OVER HUMAN EXPERIMENTATION

In February of 1975, the National Academy of Sciences convened a two-day forum: "Experiments and Research with Humans: Values in Conflict." The ambitious forum objectives were, among others, to explore thoroughly: "the triumphs and failures of human research; the conflict between individual rights and benefits to society; the ethical and legal aspects of free and informed consent; the equitable distribution of risk among different segments of the population; and the implications of proposed legislation and its impact on the future of research."[1] More than 500 natural and social scientists, physicians, lawyers, philosophers, government officials, and public interest advocates participated.

The conference objectives summarize in a nutshell the issues involved in human experimentation, an area where controversy and emotionalism have run rampant. Highly publicized abuses in experiments on humans (e.g., prisoners in research, the mentally retarded as research subjects, and the like) have had the effect of putting scientists and physicians on the defensive, and public demands for a system of regulations to curb or preclude altogether potential dangers to humans who are participants in experimentation. Scientists counter with the warning that the advancement of biomedical knowledge and efforts to save lives will be seriously retarded, if overly cautious constraints are placed on experimentation. One of the tasks of the aforementioned National Commission for the Protection of Human Subjects (see p. 178) was to investigate and prescribe guidelines for dealing with the complex problems of obtaining informed consent from children, prisoners, and the mentally ill when they participate in experiments. It is fair to say that among all the questions raised by an increasingly concerned public about science, technology, and medicine, an especially sensitive one deals with biomedical experimentation on humans.

Historically, societal regard with matters related to human experimentation are of recent origin. Concern was generated from events of World War II that convulsed the world not only physically but morally as well. World War II marked the first time in the history of warfare that large civilian populations were exposed to the enormous destructiveness of both property and human life resulting from war. One need only mention such new phenomena as the detonation of the nuclear bomb on civilian populations of Japan with its hundreds of thousands of casualties, the fire-bombing of Dresden with the same devastating results, the horrifying and dehumanizing events made public by the war crimes trials following the war, the charges of genocide as entire populations of people were exterminated, and the individual as well as the public conscience experiences disgust and nausea at the gross inhumanity that was commonplace. Following the war, an organized effort was made at reassessing the world moral order and codifying standards of ethical behavior. Thus, the United Nations Organization was born with such phrases as "the protection of human rights" and the "brotherhood of the human community" motivating its birth. These were to serve as anchor points in nations dealing with one another. Another example illustrative of this movement was the infamous Nuremberg war crimes trials that brought before a world judicial tribunal, for the first time, those accused of perpetrating the morally revulsive events of World War II. Defendent after defendent pleaded innocence, arguing that they were merely implementing the law of the land, that is, they were simply carrying out orders. They reasoned that they were in the untenable position of obeying others higher than they in authority, and that not to do so seriously threatened their own personal safety. By only doing what they were told, and by not initiating any independent action, they could not therefore be judged guilty. However, the prosecution countered that there were basic human rights, self-evident and inviolable, that all persons owed allegiance to. There are primary values or basic inclinations of human nature that need no validation, and one is obligated to conform his/her behavior to these (e.g., protection of the innocent). These sovereign principles must take precedence over any other considerations; to do less would serve to undermine the moral basis on which society's very being rests. In short, society could not afford to sacrifice some of its members beyond defined duty without risking the foundations on which its existence depended. To be certain, society has struggled for centuries over the conflict between human morality as a universal absolute applicable in all times and in all places and a relative system where the conditions of the day determine its definition. World War II, however, pointed out the inescapable necessity of clarifying and, if possible, codifying forms of ethical behavior.

THE NUREMBERG CODE

One of the more shameful episodes brought out by the Nuremberg trials concerned the matter of human experimentation where large numbers of concentration camp prisoners were used for purposes of medical experimentation.[2] A great many of those confined were non-Germans whose incarceration was often tantamount to death. Certainly it can be assumed that few, if any, volunteered themselves as experimental subjects. Some of the physicians and scientists conducting these researches were persons of high standing within the profession, enjoying both national and international reputations. The standard arguments made in their defense were first, that they too were simply carrying out orders given them, and second, that the prisoners were going to die anyway. If the latter be the case, why not extract some benefit for humankind from the evil of their hastened death—an inevitable event in any case and one over which the scientists had no control. But more sinister and threatening to the concept of basic human rights was a third argument in defense of their deeds, namely, that the acquisition of knowledge and the advancement of social ends must override the individual. In other words, the welfare of society must take precedence over the welfare of any single person. Scientific knowledge that is socially beneficial must be sought at whatever cost. This is another overt manifestation of science itself becoming prostituted in the cause of knowledge, a case where any means justifies some desired end. The inherent dangers of such an approach are so great that most sane people would recoil in shock and horror, as did those trying the war crimes cases. They asserted that there is a more fundamental morality at stake, one that must be protected from abuse if society is to avert disaster. (For a description of some of the grisly details of human experimentation conducted by Nazi researchers see Ivy and/or Alexander referenced in the Bibliography.)

After the Nuremberg trials, the judicial tribunal with the help of expert physicians drafted a code of conduct, the Nuremberg Code, a landmark document in human experimentation specifying the relationship between experimenter and experimental subject. It is a lengthy document containing some ten propositions. In the main, these can be summarized as follows:[3]

1. The voluntary consent of the human subject is absolutely essential.

2. The experiment should yield fruitful results for the good of society unprocurable by other methods or means of study.

3. The experiment should be designed and based on the results of previously conducted animal experimentation.

4. The experiment should be designed to avoid all unnecessary physical and mental suffering and injury.

5. No experiment should be conducted where there is an *a priori* reason to believe that death or disabling injury will occur.

6. The degree of risk should never exceed the determined humanitarian importance of the problem under investigation.

7. Adequate preparation should be made to protect the experimental subject against even remote possibilities of injury, death, or disability.

8. The experiment should be conducted only by scientifically qualified persons.

9. During the course of an experiment, human subjects should be at liberty to bring the experiment to an end.

10. During the course of an experiment, the scientist in charge must be prepared to terminate the experiment at any stage if in his judgment continuation of the experiment is likely to result in injury, disability, or death to the experimental subjects.

The ethical values of human freedom and the inviolability of the human person are the root of this code. Throughout these propositions, emphasis is placed on full disclosure of all experimental details and voluntary informed consent of the human subject. In effect, the Nuremberg Code reaffirmed the great traditional safeguard so long practiced between the physician and his patient: "first of all do not do injury." Just as the welfare of the individual patient must be of basic importance in the physician/patient relationship, so the first responsibility of the researcher is the safety of the human experimental subject, objectives of the planned research notwithstanding.

The Nuremberg Code was followed by several others, among them the Principles of Those in Research and Experimentation (World Medical Association, 1954), the Declaration of Helsinki (WMA, 1964), and the AMA's Principles of Medical Ethics (AMA, 1971), and the DHEW Guidelines of 1974 concerning the Protection of Human Subjects. Each of these reiterated the principles of the Nuremberg Code, in some cases extending them to cover aspects of human experimentation not directly covered in the Nuremberg document. Throughout, the *sine qua non* of the medical practitioner is reiterated: "the health of my patient will be my first consideration." The inviolable moral principle implied in these statements asserts that every human being has the right to be treated with decency and that right belongs to each and every individual and should supersede every consideration of what may benefit humankind, what may contribute to the public welfare, or what may advance medical science. No doctor or experimenter is justified in placing science or public welfare before his or her obligation to the patient or the human experimental subject. An end, no matter how worthy, cannot justify unworthy means! To this day, this pronouncement of the Nuremberg Code remains the fundamental consideration guiding all human experimentation.

THE INTENSIFIED SEARCH FOR KNOWLEDGE

A second source of concern relative to human experimentation originates from the intensified search for medical knowledge following World War II. There are a number of reasons why this push for new knowledge exacerbated the general problem. Of primary importance is the enormous and continuing availability of research funds, as shown by the comparison below:[4]

Money available for research each year		
Year	Massachusetts General Hospital	NIH
1945	$500,000	$701,800
1955	2,228,816	36,063,200
1965	8,384,342	436,600,000

As is shown, since World War II, the (NIH) budget for medical research increased a whopping 624-fold. The availability of research funds is further added to by individual or foundation-supported research programs; for example, Jerry Lewis and Muscular Dystrophy, March of Dimes and research on birth defects, and War on Cancer programs. The obvious corollary follows: As great sums of money are devoted to medical research, the dangers of ethical error will also increase as larger numbers of experiments are conducted on human subjects by larger numbers of scientists.

But the problem is not only one of absolute numbers. Medical schools and university hospitals are dominated by medical investigators. Every young scientist knows that his/her professional future in a major institution is determined by his/her ability as investigator, and publication is still the measure. Coupling the two factors—the ready availability of money for conducting research and pressure to publish—one can see how great the chances become of committing ethical error on human subjects.

There is a third practical point contributing to the concern over the use of human subjects. The newer sophisticated technologies represent innovative approaches to the treatment of disease. But greater power for good also carries with it greater potential for harm. For instance, the whole new issue of side-effects has become painfully evident. Who would have made the connection back in 1943 between DDT and environmental health hazards? Or, who would have dreamt that advances in antibiotic and chemotherapy would create a whole new antibiotic-resistant pathology? Or that certain chemicals used in therapy have the potential to increase some forms of cancer? The new medical technologies—remedies, operations, and investigative procedures—have multiplied the possibilities of injury to experimental human subjects. As the many facets of a new technique are refined, ethical dilemmas not previously experienced are raised; for example, the distinction between what is clearly experimental and what is clearly therapeutic becomes blurred. Almost every medical procedure involves some degree of uncertainty and so results cannot be predicted with certitude; they are, at least in part, experimental. The newer techniques complicate the problem still further—to clarify results in advance simply is not possible. It is apparent that the drive for new knowledge has placed modern medicine in a position it has not been in before; new therapeutic weapons produce much good but also new dangers to individuals and to communities as a whole.

Finally, the whole matter is exacerbated by the general awakening of an increasingly concerned general public whose sources of information are an active public communication system. Newspapers are quick to play up presumed abuses, engendering thereby controversy and emotionalism. The highly publicized Tuskeegee syphilis study or the intentional feeding of pesticides to humans are instances where public resentment over this form of science can be brought very quickly to the flaming point. No longer is it likely that human experimentation will escape the critical scrutiny of the public eye.

THE ETHICAL ISSUE—HUMAN INVIOLABILITY

When science takes up humans as its experimental subject, the conflict immediately rises between two basic values in Western society: freedom of scientific inquiry on the one hand and individual inviolability on the other. Especially in human experimentation, the clear division between these two spheres is lost. Scientists point with justifiable pride to the enormous past successes made possible by a free science. The unrestricted exercise of scientific experimentation is asserted to be a First-Amendment right where the freedom of inquiry includes the freedom to generate new ideas. Ethicists submit the equality of worth of every human being and the right of everyone to be treated with dignity and decency. What is wrong with making a person an experimental subject is that he/she becomes a thing—a passive non-being merely to be acted on. At least ethically, some justification is needed if an infringement of the primary inviolability of the human person is to be allowed, and the justification must be by values and needs of a dignity commensurate with those sacrificed.[5] In other words, what values are being gained to compensate for those being surrendered? Thus the questions arise: When, if ever, may society expose some of its members to harm in order to seek benefits both for the individual and society as a whole? Who is to be martyred? In the service of what cause and by whose choice?[6]

Although it is nearly axiomatic, the observation bears emphasizing that even though much testing is carried out with laboratory animals, the ultimate tests must be made on humans. In fact, federal regulations require that these tests be done. There is no way one can extrapolate with certainty from animal experiments to human response. In the end, humans themselves must provide information about themselves. Furthermore, there are many instances where animal experimentation is simply not suitable, for animal models do not exist (e.g., in species-specific infection). The only tests possible are on human subjects and there the question of conscience arises for where results cannot be perfectly prophesied, then hazards of injury are courted. As expressed by researcher Dr. Walsh McDermott, "it is impossible to do clinical investigation without putting people to some risk."[7] Thus, a variety of experiments requiring large numbers of human subjects will continue, heightening concern and elevating the clamor for regulation.

However, not everyone agrees that ethical violations are serious enough to warrant the concern aroused. Some feel that regulations pose needless constraints on continued and necessary experimentation. They add that the widely publicized horror stories convey a totally false impression of the real situation for these represent only an infinitesimal percentage of the total experimentation now being conducted. The arguments on this side of the question go like this:

1 Most subjects in most experiments do volunteer.

2 Details in some studies cannot be told in advance (e.g., placebo research).

3 Nobody intends to harm human subjects, and besides, almost nobody ever does.

4 Benefits for humanity make the rare accidents bearable.

Thus, although nearly everyone agrees that ethical violations do occur, the practical question is, How often? Those who have specifically studied this question conclude that the problem is widespread. Henry K. Beecher of the Harvard Medical School describes a large number of studies where questionable ethical practices were involved.[8] One Hastings Center report of cases in their files where humans were the experimental subject showed that in less than 25 percent of them was consent obtained from the participants; not one paper documented the nature of information given subjects.[9] Another study evaluated 100 reported human experiments from reputable scientific journals in one year and judged 12 unethical. Less than 25 percent of all scientific papers provide adequate information on the ethical procedures followed. The English physician Dr. M. H. Pappworth, a researcher long concerned with the ethical problems of human experimentation, documents in his book *Human Guinea Pigs*[10] over 500 cases where questionable or unethical procedures were used. In a most recent report, it was indicated that EPA (Federal Environmental Protection Agency) planned to test a potential carcinogen on humans by feeding it to hospital patients (in Mexico City) at levels 1000 times the normal daily exposure. The planned project was rejected when it came to the attention of an agency attorney.[11] Sociologist Bernard Barber, in reporting the results of his survey of scientists conducting human experimentation, concluded that "research with human subjects has produced . . . some instances of ethical abuses. Studies of the attitudes and practices of investigators suggest that better controls are required."[12] It would thus seem from these and many other observations unreported here that unethical or questionable ethical procedures are not so uncommon as to be readily excused.

Experimentation with humans takes place in several settings: (1) with self-experimentation; (2) with patient volunteers where the objective is to benefit the patient (experimental therapies); (3) with patients where the objective is not their benefit but that of other patients in general; and (4) with normal subjects.[13] It is in the latter two categories that the majority of concern has been expressed, and this discussion will be limited to these.

The controlled medical experiment designed to gain information rather than to try out new therapeutic techniques is a relatively modern one. It has only been within recent times that medical experimentation has been able to involve more than attempting benefits to the ill patient. This requires a new ethical perspective for patient benefit is no longer the sole consideration. Answers to three major questions must be sought by those serious about the issue of human experimentation:[14]

1   What limits, if any, should be placed on scientific inquiry and what are their implications?

2   Who should have the authority to formulate these limits?

3   By what means should they be imposed?

Regarding the first question, all participants in human experimentation have a unique set of value preferences and motivations whereby they chart their courses: the investigator who initiates and conducts the experiment, the human being who is its subject, and the state which supports or restricts the research. Frequently the respective values are in conflict. In this study we will investigate but one of them, the matter of informed consent.

THE ISSUE OF CONSENT

Since Nuremberg no aspect of human experimentation has received greater attention than the issue of consent. It is the first commandment held in common by all codes dealing with this form of research and it is the single issue over which the most heated debates have been held. Ethically, it can be argued that a moral claim on another cannot be made without consent of the donor. To this day this proposition continues to ignite much controversy. The ethical question demanding satisfaction is this one: How can the rights of individuals as subjects be protected? Specifically, how does one obtain meaningful and informed consent? The immediate and naive response is that it is readily available for the asking. However, as the subsequent discussion will show, this is not as easily done as might be first thought. And in fact, some have argued that any fully informed consent may never be obtainable; the whole issue of full and informed consent is an abstract and theoretical one only. To get fully informed consent, the argument goes, would require the transmission of not only endless technical details but also a lifetime's scientific education. Moreover, it is impossible to fully inform the subject since the researcher himself does not know all the answers or he would not be doing the research in the first place.[15] However difficult it may be to obtain, informed consent remains the criterion of highest persuasion.

The Department of Health, Education, and Welfare's regulations on the protection of human subjects (1974) calls for six basic elements of information to be transmitted for consent to be reasonably informed:[16]

1. A fair explanation of the procedures to be followed and their purposes, including identification of any procedures that are experimental.

2. A description of the attendant discomforts and risks reasonably to be expected.

3. A description of the benefits reasonably to be expected.

4. A disclosure of appropriate alternative procedures that might be advantageous for the subject.

5. An offer to answer any inquiries concerning the procedures.

6. An instruction that the person is free to withdraw his/her consent and to discontinue participation in the project or activity at any time without prejudice to the subjects.

It is apparent that these guidelines recognize the near-impossibility of full and informed consent; rather they seem to be satisfied with *reasonably* informed consent. Perhaps this is the best that can be hoped for anyway.

THE PATIENT AS RESEARCH SUBJECT

Let's examine several instances where obtaining reasonably informed consent may be questionable. In the first case, the patient is the subject; the experimentation, though, may benefit him/her directly by alleviating an illness, or the research is used to gain knowledge which may benefit others but not the person being experimented on.

All such requests are filtered through the illness setting; patients generally do not complain or question the physician's judgment. The patients have placed themselves under the care of a physician for the purpose of getting well so that if suitably approached, they will accede, on the basis of trust, to almost any request the physician may make. Certainly, so it is thought, the physician would not prescribe anything known to be harmful. Furthermore, if the physician's request is refused, there is the danger that no treatment or only minimal treatment will be given. In this case, the risk of losing treatment outweighs an informed objective choice. Also, the rejection of a proposed therapy can be interpreted as a denial of the physician's wisdom. Our society still clothes the physician with the mystic of wisdom; therefore, to even entertain the thought that the doctor would suggest a therapy that would purposely harm the patient is not only contrary to every ethical guideline in the book but is inconceivable as well. Another problem in obtaining informed consent is that many times the patient, unaware of either the real nature of his illness or the proposed therapy, tends to equate research with treatment. This is a particular difficulty with the poor, uneducated, or functionally illiterate (e.g., those who do not understand English, are senile, etc.), and it is this group that comprises over eighty percent of the human subjects used in this aspect of human experimentation. The connection between university and public hospitals and a large fraction of the patients being medically indigent accounts for the disproportionate representation. At the same time, this group is the least likely of all groups in society to be able to give voluntary and informed consent.[17] Finally, one more factor that complicates this picture is that the experiment is usually free, of cost engendering the very common response, "what have I got to lose?" It seems to be part of the human psyche that monetary cost is somehow equated with value, and although the experimental subject may entertain some risks, the gamble is favorable since there is no money given for the service. Under any of these conditions, it can be seriously questioned whether any genuine and informed consent can be procured. If these be the circumstances, although no coercion is intended, one might question whether there is any real difference between implied pressure and coercion. The philosopher Hans Jonas has insisted that if patients should be experimented on at all, it should be in reference to their own disease only! It is totally indefensible to conscript an unfortunate sick person who by reason of his/her illness is readily available into an experiment where he or she cannot in any way benefit. Then Jonas contends, the patient is made "into a thing—a passive thing merely to be acted on . . . his being is reduced to that of a mere token or 'sample'.[18] This distinction firmly establishes that there is a fundamental difference between the permissible and impermissible in matters pertaining to patients as research subjects.

THE HEALTHY PERSON AS RESEARCH SUBJECT

A second instance where obtaining reasonably informed consent may be difficult involves the subject who is not ill. Healthy human subjects are especially necessary for testing the toxicological effects of drugs and other chemicals. For these experiments the Federal Food and Drug Administration (FDA) guidelines stipulate several distinct requirements:[19] Extensive studies on animals must be carried out before human tests are permissible; the scientific credentials of the investigator must be compatible with the proposed human experimentation; and the design of the experiment must be well thought out and specified in advance. After these requirements have been satisfied, three distinct phases of testing are compulsory:

> *Phase 1 testing:* The first time a new drug is introduced represents the riskiest stage of testing. The objectives are to determine such things as toxicity, metabolism, absorption, elimination, other pharmaceutical actions, the preferred route of administration, safe dosage range, prominent side effects, etc. Phase 1 testing is not done to determine therapeutic value but is rather a test of safety in human administration. This phase of testing is best done with large samples of normal, healthy individuals under controlled conditions of diet, exercise, rest, etc. Two major populations, the military and prisoners, satisfied these requirements, with prisoners providing the largest number of research subjects. (Military volunteers were formerly obtained from the ranks of conscientious objectors or those doing alternative service. With the all-volunteer military, this source of recruitment is shut off. The present stringencies regulating prison research has curtailed the use of prisoners. See p. 255.)

Phase 2 testing: After satisfactorily passing the first phase, the new drug is tried out on a limited number of patients suffering from the disease the drug is intended to cure.

Phase 3 testing: This is the clinical trials stage; a large number of patients suffering from the disease are given the experimental drug to assess still further its safety and effectiveness as well as to determine optimal dosage schedules.

Furthermore, FDA guidelines insist that the experiments be scientifically valid, human subjects be protected by institutional review committees, and participants be informed of the nature of the experiment. Written consent must be obtained for Phases 1 and 2; Phase 3 requires oral consent only.

A particular difficulty arises when it is essential to the success of the experiment that the participant, sometimes even the researcher, be uninformed about certain aspects of the experiment, for example, the control-group-placebo experiment or the "double blind" experiment. There is no way to do such experiments and still get completely informed consent from the subjects. Some have seriously challenged the ethics of these protocols, especially in cases where the subject volunteers in anticipation of some useful outcome, for example, the administration of an inert substance instead of a birth control chemical. Philosopher Jonas feels that especially in the case of a sick patient, the subject is definitely wronged even when not physically harmed for the giving of placebos betrays the trust of the patient who believes that he/she is receiving treatment. Even apart from ethics, the practice of deception holds the danger of undermining the faith in legitimate treatment, the very basis of the doctor-patient contract. Clearly the prescription of placebos is intentionally deceptive and makes informed consent impossible. Even benevolent deception is not allowable because it makes a mockery of human individual freedom and dignity. Some argue, however, the prohibition against the use of placebos should not be absolute. In these instances, great care should be exerted in balancing benefits over costs.[20] Ethicist Sissela Bok suggests the following principles in trying to decide the difficult cases:[21]

1. Placebos should be used only after careful diagnosis.

2. No active placebos should be employed, merely inert ones.

3. No outright lie should be told and questions should be answered honestly.

4. Placebos should never be given to patients who have asked not to receive them.

5. Placebos should never be used when other treatment is clearly called for or all possible alternatives have not been weighed.

The whole matter of deception is especially sensitive in social or psychological experimentation. Experimentation without consent, deceit, and even compulsory participation of psychology students were commonplace before the new insistence on openness. One of the concerns here is that although no one is physically at risk, psychological damage may be done. Sociological research involving interviews and questionnaires must now meet the same review procedures as medical research. Informed consent is seen to be more important than any scientific considerations. Secret observers, researcher role-playing, and other unobstructive techniques are being seriously questioned. The main ethical criticism is the violation of the subject's privacy.[22 and 23]

It is apparent that silence sometimes is necessary in certain experiments and so is deception; but they are never desirable if they can be done without. Psychologist Perry London suggests these three questions to be answered by researchers before using deception or purposely withholding information:[24]

1. Is there any way to get the information without such a practice?

2. Is the sought-for information so valuable that it is worth misleading, debriefing, and apologizing to subjects?

3. Is there significant risk of damaging the subject's psyche so that even an explanation of the truth following the experiment will not correct the psychological harm or reduce the sense of humiliation of having been duped?

London concludes that there is far too much deceptive research going on in the psychological and social sciences.

PRISONERS AS RESEARCH SUBJECTS

The use of prisoners as research subjects has raised some of the hottest confrontations over the ethics of human experimentation. While prisoners normally do not lack the capacity to offer a reasonably informed consent, their capacity to do so voluntarily is problematical. Consequently, most states have taken steps to either completely abandon or more stringently control those activities within their boundaries. Some are calling for an outright ban on all prison research. In 1975, the Federal Bureau of Prisons issued an indefinite moratorium on all forms of nontherapeutic research in any federal prison. Essentially, the issue returns again to that most singular anxiety, the necessity of insuring voluntary participation and obtaining informed consent. A second matter of ethics concerns the use of penitentiaries as the experimental setting; openness and public inspection are not as easily maintained under conditions which are intrinsically secretive.

In recent times prisoners formed the largest pool of potential subjects, especially for drug testing, and most drug companies had working agreements with prisons. Although the extent and nature of experimentation with prisoners cannot be determined, at least 3600 prisoners in the United States were used for drug testing during 1975 alone, according to the National Commission for the Protection of Human Subjects. Besides these tests, performed primarily by drug companies, the commission also determined that the federal government funded a number of other studies in which prisoners were used: within the Public Health Service, 124 biomedical studies and 19 behavioral projects between 1970 and 1975; the Department of Defense sponsored numerous studies for research on infectious diseases; and the former Atomic Energy Commission had supported research involving radiation of male prisoners' genitals.[25]

During the year 1975, eight states and six county and municipal prisons were used. One of the largest and most elaborate research facilities is located at the State Prison of Southern Michigan at Jackson. This is a maximum-security prison, one of the biggest penitentiaries in the United States. Of its 5000 inmates, 800 prisoners form an available pool for research in special facilities built within the walls of the prison by two of the country's largest pharmaceutical manufacturers, Parke-Davis and Upjohn. Between 1964 and 1968, over 100,000 tests on human subjects were performed here. Approximately eighty to ninety percent of all Phase I testing by drug companies has been done in prisons.

By contrast, in no country surveyed by the National Commission other than the United States were prisoners used as volunteer subjects for medical experimentation. And in fact, virtually no country except the United States conducts any clinical pharmocological studies on healthy subjects in or out of prisons. Also, unlike the United States, other countries will accept data generated from studies made in other countries. (The countries surveyed were Belgium, France, Germany, Italy, the Netherlands, Spain, Sweden, Australia, Canada, New Zealand, South Africa, the United Kingdom, Brazil, Colombia, Mexico, Peru, and Japan.)

Prison abuses of all kinds have been widely publicized. Jessica Mitford's book *Kind and Usual Punishment* on prison conditions points out that some experimentation conducted in prisons is dangerous and has little scientific value. At the Iowa State Prison, for example, the experimental induction of scurvy in eleven prisoners led to acute episodes of swollen and bleeding gums, joint swelling and pain, hemorrhaging, etc. In some, the effects proved to be irreversible (two of the prisoners later escaped). All this was done even though the cause and cure of scurvy are well known. Another example of questionable research is the infamous Tuskeegee syphilis study, where 400 black men with syphilis were not treated so the course of the disease could be followed. Here again, the etiology and cure of this affliction are well known. The list could be added to from medical literature as well as popular reporting.

However, the personal welfare of the prisoners is not the only ethical consideration. The issue of whether any nontherapeutic research should be allowed in prisons arises from several factors:

1. The subjects involved are captives of the state and are made available by the permission of the state. Does this put the state in the position to decide who is to be martyred and in the service of what cause? Society first creates the conditions of loss of freedom and then exploits it. Prisoners, as a group, are generally held in low esteem by society and, in fact, are considered inferior by most. There can be no informed consent, according to Jay Katz (psychiatrist), when one of the parties is not free. It is far too easy to strike a bargain between unequals. If the ultimate concern with human experimentation involves personal dignity and individual inviolability, then the setting for conflict becomes real when the long and the short range interests of society, science, and progress are set up against the rights of the individual.[26]

2. The prisoner participants' position of confinement renders their consent to participate questionable; prisoners are not free agents and true consent without overt or implied coercion is impossible in prisons. In a study (McGuire, personal communication) 1200 prisoners at the Cook County Jail (Ill.) were evaluated relative to their ability to give consent. It was found that over 95 percent of them could not render adequate and informed consent. The largest share of them were pretrial detainees, hence ineligible for any state assistance or rehabilitation programs. Even basic necessities such as soap and toothpaste had to be personally furnished. Unable to come up with bond, unable to hire lawyers, and convinced they would not be

defended well, they would do anything to get out or to improve their situations. At the California Medical Facility at Vacaville, research on "aversive conditioning" using the drug anectine (it creates a muscle paralysis and a sensation of suffocation) with 64 extreme-acting criminal offenders determined that 5 signed up against their will and 18 involuntarily signed because of implied pressure.

3. Research in prisons is carried on in an environment which lacks the kind of peer review or openness found in other research settings. Because such research is not in the public eye, there is the possibility of abuse even if it is unintended. Such abuse can be easily covered up if negative publicity may result.

4. The special problem of informed consent implies or even requires that information be given and that it be understood by the candidate for participation. The intellectual capacity of most prisoners disqualifies them on these grounds. Thus, unconscious motivations, psychopathologies, states of deprivation, wretched conditions and the like, all mitigate against giving free and informed consent.

It is especially this issue of voluntary informed consent that raises the greatest ethical question. Prisons, as total institutions, by their very purpose and character, make it highly questionable whether free consent to research is possible. As Patricia King, one of the commission's most adamant opponents of prisoner experimentations, expressed it: "I, personally, do not believe that theoretically one can ever remove enough of the constraints from a prison to afford self-determination because by the time you removed them all you would not have a prison."[27]

The National Prison Project of the American Civil Liberties Union filed a complaint in the U.S. District Court on behalf of seven prisoners who were involved in viral diarrhea, malaria, shigella, and typhoid experiments. The complaint asked that the court declare that "the use of prisoners in nontherapeutic biomedical experimentation of this type is unconstitutional per se because of the impossibility of truly voluntary consent.[28] Eight states have prohibited the use of state prisons for these purposes: six by departmental policy, one by moratorium, and one by legislation (Oregon). The Board of Directors of the American Correctional Association adopted this statement:

> The American Correctional Association has long viewed with concern the use of prisoners as subjects of medical pharmacological experimentation . . . It now urges that efforts to eliminate such practices be undertaken by responsible bodies at the Federal, State, and local levels . . . The authority which authorizes or permits prisoners to become subjects of human experimentation ignores his historic obligation as a custodian to protect and safely keep those for whom he assumes legal responsibility.[29]

The use of prisoners has been stoutly defended by some. Dr. Albert Sabin (of oral polio vaccine fame) noted at the National Academy of Sciences Conference on human experimentation that basic studies on his own polio vaccine were done on prisoners. If research using prisoners was stopped, he says, "it would greatly impede medical research."[30] Dr. William N. Hubbard, Jr., president of Upjohn Company, at the same meeting stressed that meticulous care has been taken over the past 15 years at the Michigan facility to safeguard inmate welfare and rights and to ensure that the participants are true volunteers giving their informed consent. Dr. C. Joseph Stetler, president of the Pharmaceutical Manufacturers Association (representing 131 member firms), testified before a congressional subcommittee that (1) prisoners are the best subjects for Phase I testing since within that population there are the least number of variables; (2) prisoners volunteer readily to achieve financial rewards, to relieve boredom, or, in some cases, to make amends to society; and (3) all major drug research would be severely curtailed or stopped if the use of prisoners was prohibited.

The Pharmaceutical Manufacturers' Association has established the following guidelines for drug studies carried out with prisoners:

1. There must be complete freedom from coercion.

2. Adequate medical protection must be given to all research subjects.

3. Full information about the nature of the testing must be made available.

4. There should be suitable monetary compensation for participation.

5. The prisoner-subject has the right to withdraw from the experiment at any time.

6. Refusal to participate or withdrawal from an experiment should have no effect on parole eligibility.

The effectiveness of the PMA guidelines was perhaps demonstrated by this testimony before the commission where it was stated that "to the best of our knowledge, not a single prisoner has died or been permanently injured as a result of drug-firm–sponsored (Phase I) testing."[31]

Since it is universally asserted by those who defend the practice of using prisoners that the rights of the individual are being protected and that informed consent is obtained, one might inquire as to the validity of this claim. In an extensive study prepared for the commission by the University of Michigan, interviews with 181 prisoners in four prisons found 87 percent very willing to participate in research projects.[32] Commission members personally interviewed prison research participants at Jackson and were startled to find that subjects were among the best educated and intelligent at the prison (56 percent had completed twelve grades or more). They were very indignant that they might lose the opportunity to participate for several reasons: (1) they are housed in a decent environment (not in jail); (2) they get real money—up to $200 per research project as opposed to 50¢ per day with an $8 maximum per month for routine prison work; and (3) they receive good medical care.

Money, it turns out, is no less important in prisons than in the free world. A person in prison gets only the bare necessities; any extras, such as toiletries, books, magazines, snacks, art supplies, and cigarettes, must be purchased with personal funds. Money is also an important contact with the outside world. Prisoners send money home to their families; others continue to pay union dues so they have a better opportunity to work once released; and money saved can help them get started again when they get out. In addition, money is an effective "cooling" agent in prisons. Where money is freely available, there is less prison violence since the need to fight for simple ammenities (e.g., cigarettes) is minimized.[33]

On the con side of the issue, in the case where prison volunteers are offered money payments, the position of pretrial detainees is extremely tenuous. In the time before sentencing, the state has no obligation to supply anything. A study in Philadelphia revealed that only fifteen percent of the prison population were employed; the rest were ineligible for any aid. Under these circumstances one could seriously question the reality of free consent. If the payments of money are large, whether they be to those awaiting trial and sentence or to those already sentenced, the undue influence of money may obscure an appreciation of risk and weaken the will for self-preservation (e.g., Evel Knievel phenomenon—"anyone would try to jump the Snake Canyon for $6 million"). As John Freund warns, one ought not to be put in the business of buying lives.[34] Of prisoners who volunteer for research, seventy percent said it was to get money, a reason given three times more often than any other. If, on the other hand, the payments are small, the charge of exploitation can be made. (In all of these cases it is well to remember that the prisoner is *not* a free agent; he/she has very few options open to him, hence the parallel between this group and those not confined—e.g., college students—is invalid.) Alternatively, if no payment is offered, then is consent to be included as part of a prisoner's record? Will it have some bearing on parole or commutation of sentence? The fear of parole refusal or the denial of special privileges for those who do not participate can be as effective in hiding the real situation as are threats of harm or other forms of coercion.

CHILDREN AS RESEARCH SUBJECTS

The problem of full capacity to render informed consent presents another urgent case when children are the experimental subjects. Present FDA regulations require that drugs be tested on all age groups for whom the drug is intended. This includes tests for safety on normal subjects before the drug can be released for use on patients. In research involving children, the ethical considerations are quite different from the two groups previously discussed; it requires a distinction between therapeutic and nontherapeutic research. The law states that parents may consent for the child if the treatment is for the child's welfare or benefit, that is, for therapeutic purposes. Proxy consent is permissible here because parents have the obligation to care for and protect the welfare of their children. Parents are frequently called upon to make decisions for their children and this right is highly praised (e.g., the school attended). However, parents are not morally (or legally) permitted to make decisions for their children that carry with them high risks; only those decisions that will not infringe on the child's physical or mental welfare may be made. This position has legal support on its side; "parents may consent for the child if the invasion of the child's body is for the child's welfare or benefit."[35] One of the difficulties, though, is how broadly to interpret welfare or benefit. This has generated an important controversy, particularly as it applies to nontherapeutic research on children.

If an experiment is for nontherapeutic purposes, the generally followed guideline stipulates that the child be at least fourteen years of age and intelligent and mature enough to understand the nature of the procedure, including potential hazards, and that no coercion be applied or guilt feelings engendered. With these conditions satisfied, child consent coupled with parental or guardian permission completes the requirement of this guideline. In some extreme cases such as organ donation, the age minimum may be lowered to six years if the recipient is a sibling and/or the child understands the procedure, including risks and loss.

Protestant theologian Paul Ramsey argues strenuously that in no circumstances can proxy consent be given for children when the experiments are nonbeneficial to them.[36] The covenant of loyalty between parents and children demands that children be protected. There is a sacred obligation to defend the child's interests; therefore, parents have no right to force children to undertake nonobligatory behavior. When the latter happens, the child is treated as a mere means rather than an end, a thing, not a person. (Ramsey does allow the one exception when an epidemic threatens. Then proxy consent is acceptable for subjecting the child to research on a disease not suffered by that child since the aim of the research is the protection of the child's future health and welfare since he/she runs the high risk of contracting the contagion at some time later.)

Medical researcher Henry Beecher has a slightly different view. He submits that nontherapeutic research is permissible if the studies have no discernible risk, if they are approved by a high-level review committee, if the child is not taken advantage of, and if the studies are "necessary and valuable for human progress."[37]

Catholic theologian Richard McCormick proposes a novel interpretation of proxy consent. Consent for children to participate in experimentation even if it does not benefit them directly is "morally valid precisely insofar as it is a reasonable *presumption* of the child's wishes, a construction of what the child would wish could he consent for himself."[38] The reason the child would wish this is because "he *ought* to do so." McCormick argues that since a certain level of involvement in nontherapeutic research is good for the child, he/she ought to choose it. He further contends that such participation is morally obligatory since it enhances moral sensitivity or a disposition toward the good. Of course, he is talking about "no risk" clinical research.

Dr. William G. Bartholome of the Department of Pediatrics, University of Texas, presented the following guidelines to the National Commission for carrying out nontherapeutic research on children ages 5–14 years:[39]

1. The experimental protocol must be subjected to careful institutional peer review.

2. The experiment would provide significant and essential new knowledge.

3. The knowledge to be gained by the experiment can be obtained only by experimentation involving children.

4. The experiment must involve no greater risk or discomfort than would be encountered by the child in his/her family life.

5. Where possible, the same or similar experiment must have been performed on adult subjects and been found to be without risk.

6. Informed parental consent is mandatory.

7. The consent of the child subject must be obtained by a member of the research team and by an independent subject-representative.

8. The research must be reviewed by an ethical review board and reviewed and supervised by an institutional protection committee.

He justifies the use of children for nontherapeutic research on the grounds that such involvement can contribute to moral development of that child. He differs from McCormick in that participation requires the child's willingness and consent.

NONPENAL-INSTITUTIONALIZED PERSONS AS RESEARCH SUBJECTS

Lastly, there is the special problem of subjects who are not possessed with full capacity to consent and who are inmates at state nonpenal institutions (e.g., mental hospitals, children's homes, etc.) In terms of legal standing, the state has assumed the obligation of ward or guardian. These populations are composed primarily of individuals with mental retardation or physical defects or both, with the largest number being in the first group. According to lawyer John Halperin, these institutions represent conditions of total deprivation where individuals surrender all control of their lives. Inmates are completely dominated by staff discretion. The mentally retarded, especially, are frequently treated as subhumans: The design of the institutions is to shorten the lives of those committed and to keep inmates out of sight of the public (personal statement, American Association for the Advancement of Science, Annual Meeting, New York, 1975). The issue is obvious: Is there any way at all for these persons to give informed consent or is the matter for the state to decide? The clearest example of questionable ethical procedures is the controversial Willowbrook experiments on hepatitis where institutionalized, mentally retarded children were intentionally given hepatitis to study the course of the disease and to develop a potentially useful vaccine for the disease. According to one source, permission for participation in the experiment was a contingency for admittance to the hospital (personal communication). The experiments were defended on the grounds that the children would contract hepatitis normally and that getting it under controlled conditions was more likely to result in a less severe case and would result in lifetime immunization to the disease. Experiments like this have led to a permanent prohibition against using institutionally confined persons except for purposes of therapeutic research where they themselves may benefit from the research. This recommendation was contained in the final report of the National Commission for the Protection of Human Subjects rendered in March, 1978.

PROTECTION OF HUMAN SUBJECTS

Much more discussion could be devoted to the problem of human experimentation; the literature attacking and defending it is voluminous. However, the point has been made. The central ethical issue is this: The welfare of the individual must be of basic importance when he or she is placed in the experimental environment. Can adequate protection of the human subjects be effected? Various suggestions have been put forth that could ameliorate risks and minimize future abuses. At the one extreme Alexander Capron (law professor), after his studies of abuses of prisoner-subjects, concluded that a prompt and complete moratorium should be placed on all prison research until procedures involved with its practice are thoroughly examined and proper controls are initiated.[40] A stronger opinion insists that all research using prisoners, other than therapeutic research, be absolutely forbidden. On the other hand, the Pharmaceutical Manufacturers Association rejects all regulation, asserting that the industry can and does regulate itself in these matters. The more moderate view supports continued human experimentation but with more federal regulations and built-in enforcement procedures.

DHEW guidelines, covering only those experiments supported by federal grants, place the basic responsibilities for safeguarding subjects' rights on the person(s) receiving the grant.[41] The guidelines stipulate that:

1. No grant or contract for human experimentation will be made unless the application has been first reviewed and approved by an appropriate institutional committee.

2. This committee should determine that the rights and welfare of subjects involved are adequately protected; that benefits to be derived from the experiment outweigh risks either to the individual or to the knowledge gained; and that informed consent be obtained by methods adequate or appropriate (see earlier discussion, p. 244, for directions on providing information).

3. The local committee is responsible for continuing review of the experiment.

Some criticisms of these guidelines have been leveled particularly because of their vagueness; they do not specify what is minimal and acceptable risk. Further, they left too much in the hands of local review committees, groups frequently unable to make effective ethical decisions. The special problems with in-house review committees are well-known: They include the lack of training by members of these committees to deal effectively with ethical problems—many are staffed by professional scientists, not ethicists, or others similarly trained; the time required to do a good job. On the one hand it is desirable to have people who are knowledgeable in the area under consideration; on the other, these same persons are actively engaged in their own research and activities; the unwillingness to censure colleagues especially if they are well-known; the pressure for publication associated with institutional fame (see Reference 42 for a discussion of review committees). Some of these loopholes were covered in amendments to the guidelines by providing greater protection to children, prisoners, and the mentally ill. The National Commission, in the fall of 1978, recommended that federal procedures for regulating and accrediting Institutional Review Boards (IRB) be adopted to be sure that the rights of human subjects are protected. Among these new procedures are measures to ensure that HEW be the sole agency for accrediting IRBs and that compliance with federal regulations be followed by on-site inspection and federal licensing of each of the 500 IRBs in the nation.

However, the HEW rules apply only to federally supported research. Critics claim that the greatest abuses occur with experimentation carried out under the aegis of private support (e.g., drug companies, local hospitals, etc.) Further, as history has shown, it is difficult for an agency to police itself; conflict of interests inevitably arise (a historic example of the unworkable nature of conflict of interest is demonstrated by the Atomic Energy Commission experience). In the more general case, it is argued that the medical profession is not qualified to regulate itself since, by training, its area of expertise is not ethics but science. Professional researchers do not have the capabilities to properly weigh ethical costs against benefits. Critics insist that federal legislation is required, and they defend their position on the grounds that the federal government, by reason of its delegated responsibility of safeguarding society, is the appropriate institution to insure the protection of human subjects.

Again, the U.S. is not without precedent in this matter; several countries have already enacted legislation to regulate human experimentation. The British Law of 1963, suggested by some as model legislation, declared it illegal to use prisoners in medical research. A number of other western European countries have done likewise. In the United States, largely through the efforts of Senator Edward Kennedy (D-Mass.), the previously mentioned National Research Act was signed into law

July 12, 1974. Among its several provisions, it created a federal commission on ethics, officially named the National Commission for the Protection of Human Subjects of Biomedical and Behavioral Research. The commission was given the charge to report on three general types of topics:

1 Propose guidelines for regulation of research on certain populations.
   a) human fetuses
   b) prisoners
   c) institutionalized psychiatric patients
   d) children below the age of understanding
   e) other "captive groups" (the comatose and the terminally ill patients)
   f) the use of psychosurgery—its extent in the U.S. and circumstances, if any, when it should be permitted.

2 Survey existing arrangements for an ethical review of research projects involving human subjects, funded by the federal government, and submit revisions and modifications if necessary.

3 Submit to Congress a general report on the legal, social, ethical, and public policy implications of novel biomedical and behavioral technologies.

The commission's first task dealt with deciding what to do about fetal research and it reported its recommendations to the Secretary of HEW on May 1, 1975 (see p. 181).

The study and recommendations on the uses of psychosurgery were completed and submitted in August 1976, and will be dealt with in Chapter 8. The commission concluded its investigation of the prisoner research question and tendered the following recommendations in October 1976:[43]

Recommendation 1

Studies of the possible causes, effects, and processes of incarceration and studies of prisons as institutional structures or of prisoners as incarcerated persons may be conducted or supported, provided that (a) they present minimal or no risk and no more than mere inconvenience to the subjects, and (b) the requirements under recommendation (4) are fulfilled.

Recommendation 2

Research on practices, both innovative and accepted, which have the intent and reasonable probability of improving the health or well-being of the individual prisoner may be conducted or supported, provided the requirements under recommendation (4) are fulfilled.

Recommendation 3

Except as provided in recommendations (1) and (2), research involving prisoners should not be conducted or supported, and reports of such research should not be accepted by the Secretary, DHEW, in fulfillment of regulatory requirements, unless the requirements under recommendation (4) are fulfilled and the head of the responsible federal department or agency has certified, after consultation with a national ethical review body, that the following three requirements are satisfied:

   a) The type of research fulfills an important social and scientific need, and the reasons for involving prisoners in the type of research are compelling.
   b) The involvement of prisoners in the type of research satisfies conditions of equity; and

c) A high degree of voluntariness on the part of the prospective participants and of openness on the part of the institution(s) to be involved would characterize the conduct of the research; minimum requirements for such voluntariness and openness include adequate living conditions, provisions for effective redress of grievances, separation of research participation from parole considerations, and public scrutiny.

Recommendation 4

a) The head of the responsible federal department or agency should determine that the competence of the investigators and the adequacy of the research facilities involved are sufficient. . . .

b) All research involving prisoners should be reviewed by at least one human subjects review committee or institutional review board comprised of men and women of diverse racial and cultural backgrounds that includes among its members prisoners or prisoner advocates and such other persons as community representatives, clergy, behavioral scientists and medical personnel not associated with the . . . research or institution. . . .

Recommendation 5

In the absence of certification that the requirements under recommendation (3) are satisfied, research projects covered by that recommendation that are subject to regulation by the Secretary, DHEW, and are currently in progress should be permitted to continue not longer than one year from the date of publication of these recommendations in the Federal Register (January 14, 1977) or until completed, whichever is earlier.

In essence, the commission said no to human experimentation with prisoners is permitted unless there are compelling reasons for carrying on the research, unless voluntary participation is meticulously carried out, and unless the principle of equity is satisfied, that is, specific ethnic or racial groups are not disproportionately represented in the experimental population. The burden of proof is placed on the researcher to demonstrate compelling reasons for using prisoners for research purposes. Fairness requires more equitable distribution of the research burden; however, the commission does not specify how this should be done.

Although the objective of the report was not to declare an outright ban on prison research, critics of the recommendations argue that they would probably result in a moratorium on most medical research conducted in prisons in the United States. And, indeed, HEW ruled that prisoners cannot be used at all in nontherapeutic research if it involves more than minimal risk (January, 1978).

Returning to the general question of nontherapeutic research, a number of writers have suggested various ways to strengthen protection of human subjects. Some of these are the following:

1 Examination of possible methods of compensation for subjects, who, in spite of all precautions, are harmed by the research activities; this would require a form of indemnification or insurance for subjects to cover all consequences of their participation arising unforeseeably and without negligence.[44] This policy would force a greater concern on the part of the experimenter as well as providing compensation to the participant in the event something goes awry. Fewer but more carefully run experiments may result. There are some ethical as well as practical questions here: Is consent a waiver of damage or harm? How much

harm is compensable? Are economics of overall greater concern than ethical or moral issues? Are dollars to be equated with humanness or humanitarian goals?

2 Research proposed should be more carefully evaluated in advance of the actual experimentation. Perhaps limits do exist in our search for knowledge and ends do not always justify the means. The principle here could well be that an experiment is ethical or not ethical at its inception and is not determined by some later measure of success. Consider the following example: Liver biopsy is a very dangerous and potentially lethal procedure; the first several pioneer attempts resulted in death; the experimental subjects, however, were moribund patients where death was imminent. Were these experiments ethically acceptable? Does every human being have the right to be treated with decency regardless of his/her state of health? Also, there is much duplication of research in a number of laboratories. Is this necessary and could it be controlled? Should data gotten from other countries be used in the United States (see p. 248)?

3 Evaluation of the review process: Peer review is still held up as a mystical force which ensures quality in science; however, in ethical matters at least, it is no safeguard, as an earlier discussion showed (see p. 254). A way around the peer review problem is to expand local committees to include other professional and lay input (e.g., ethicists, social scientists, citizen representatives, etc.) Greater visibility could be generated by making the review process open, thus precluding dubious or clandestine procedures. There exists a need to know more about what is going on in research. A suggestion to accommodate this is to initiate a communication system among review committees out of which could evolve some common law or limits of permissibility. Furthermore, by turning to other cases of a similar kind, local committees needn't begin anew on experiments presented to them for review.

4 Information and consent: A system is needed to ensure that someone knowledgeable clearly and accurately conveys all needed information, including all hazards, to subject-participants. Many investigators leave this to subordinates, some of whom are nonmedical personnel. To protect the interests of the subject during the experiment, an intermediary person or ombudsman should be available who has free access to all information on both sides and has no vested interests in the experiment; such an individual would function to enhance the freedom of the subject, e.g., to change the terms of the agreement, to withdraw from the experiment, etc.

5 Publication of experimental results: Reporting of an experiment in a scientific journal should make unmistakeably clear that ethical proprieties have been observed; data obtained unethically should never be accepted for publication.

FUTURE SOURCES OF RESEARCH SUBJECTS

As one studies the immensities of the problems surrounding the single issue of human experimentation, there looms the uncertainty of how to contain and accommodate the rising public pressures to regulate clinical research while at the same time preserving vital research activities. Sorting out this value conflict cannot be left to scientists alone. More stringent guidelines on using human subjects must and will have their effects on society. Already, one of the spin-offs over denying the use of prisoners has been the forcing of much of Phase I testing outside of the country. The poorer areas of Central South America and Africa are some locations where stringencies are few and experimenters are welcomed. Who is to regulate in this area? In our own country, where will experimental subjects come from who can meet the same controlled conditions as those found in prisons? Some have suggested a national lottery from which names would be selected at random and to which everyone is subject, not just the poor or the captive, or certain ethnic groups. The justification here is a simple one: If all members of society benefit from medical research, then the risk should be distributed equitably among all members. Here again, the principle of fairness validates this proposal. Another opinion submits that if medical care is a right—and more and more it is being considered so (see Chapter 9 on Health Care in America)—then volunteering oneself for experimental purposes is an obligation incumbent on every citizen. A third possibility considers the development of a semiprofessional class of people whose job it is to participate in human experimentation. There is a reasonably large segment of our population which has disowned the work ethic. These people are not psychotic or otherwise unhealthy, and their physical needs are minimal. Such persons are usually quite knowledgeable, especially in matters concerning their own self-interests. Members of this group include the ski-bums, coffee-house transients, and others living the free life.

A modification of this plan is to establish a clearing house administered by some agency and/or commercial enterprise. Healthy individuals might be enlisted to participate on a part-time basis for payment: the unemployed between jobs, housewives who desire to supplement family incomes, college students working their way through school, and the like. This register would list the names of those who would participate in human research for a fee. The person would be free to accept or reject those experiments he/she does or does not wish to be involved in. Such a clearing house would not be without its own unique ethical problems. (For example, how forceful are the compunctions motivating participation? Again, could the desire for a cash reward occlude a clear realization of the risk involved in some kinds of experiments?) Finally, a last opinion proposes that progress in terms of new medical knowledge is an optional goal, not an absolute one. We have not made a binding commitment to the future to develop new medical therapies for the generation yet unborn. Why, after all, must we search for a cure to every disease? Individual mortality is an event none can escape. If this be so, then it is not unethical or immoral to impose restraints and even to stop certain kinds of testing if the stakes are simply too high.

In raising these questions about human experimentation, it is no one's intention to indict science for malfeasance or even to stifle research. The real need is for greater conscious awareness of the issues—the pursuit of knowledge to better relieve the sufferings of humankind versus the need to protect the experimental subject. We need to minimize harm and preserve personal dignity, and we need to guarantee individual autonomy and promote justice as fundamental human principles. In addressing this task contributions can and must be made by many if democracy is to operate at its most efficient level.

VALUES PERTAINING TO HUMAN EXPERIMENTATION

1   An experiment utilizing human subjects is ethical at its inception and is not to be judged ethically valid or invalid on the basis of its results.

2 Respect for persons as human beings in the experimental setting includes the protection of their autonomy and the insistence that justice prevails.

3 The voluntary consent of the human subject is the sine qua non of human experimentation.

4 It is impossible to obtain full and informed consent; rather, the best that can be hoped for is reasonably informed consent.

5 The risks that an experimental subject takes must be outweighed by the benefits to the subject and/or the importance of the knowledge to be gained.

6 Among the experiments that can be tried on humans, only those that can harm are forbidden.

7 Every adult human being of sound mind and body has a right to determine what shall be done with his/her own body.

8 Where it is impossible to obtain the free and informed consent of individuals, proxy consent is permissible if the subject benefits by the experimentation.

9 No experimentation that does not directly benefit the patient should be performed on patients who are ill.

10 The mentally incompetent should never be used as research subjects unless the objective of the research is to directly help them.

11 Persons are free to volunteer themselves for any kind of research whether the motives are altruistic or self-serving.

12 Researchers cannot always have the subject's best interest in mind.

13 It is an excessive extension of paternalism to prevent a person from participation in research he/she has judged to be personally acceptable.

14 The subject of an experiment is entitled to full and frank disclosure of all the facts, probabilities, and opinions which a reasonable person might be expected to consider before giving his/her consent.

15 Compensation to volunteers in human experimentation should never be so much as to constitute an undue inducement.

16 It is morally wrong to put patients at risk in an unnecessary experiment or one improperly designed.

17 Human experimental subjects should never be treated as means but always as ends.

18 In situations where the giving of informed consent is questionable, it is best not to proceed.

19 Scientists have a moral obligation to carry out those experiments that may do good.

20 The principle of equity requires that the selection of subjects be nondiscriminatory against the sick, certain ethnic classes, prisoners, and the less fortunate.

21 Any proposal for undertaking human research which fails to consider all reasonable possibilities of harm is morally irresponsible.

22 No persons should be compelled to be research subjects, either by force or coercion or subversion.

23 An experiment involving humans which is poorly or improperly designed in that it could not yield significant scientific facts relevant to the question under study is by definition unethical.

24 It is incumbent on the researcher to prove that a proposed experiment is ethical in all of its aspects.

25 The willingness to provide equitable compensation in case of injury should be regarded as one of the necessary conditions for an ethically acceptable human experiment.

REFERENCES

1   Richard J. Seltzer, "NAS forum debates human experimentation," *Chemical and Engineering News* 20 (March 3, 1975): 25.

2   Andrew C. Ivy, "Nazi war crimes of a medical nature," *Federation Bulletin* 33 (1947): 133–146.

3   "The Nuremberg Code," *Readings* (Hastings-on-Hudson, N.Y.: Institute of Society, Ethics and the Life Sciences.)

4   Henry K. Beecher, "Ethics and clinical research," *New England Journal of Medicine* 274 (1966): 1354–1360.

5   Hans Jonas, "Philosophical reflections on experimenting with human subjects," in *Readings on Ethical and Social Issues in Biomedicine*, Richard Wertz (ed.), (Englewood Cliffs: Prentice-Hall, 1973).

6   Hans Jonas (in Reference 5), p. 19.

7   Walsh McDermott (in Reference 1), p. 20.

8   Henry K. Beecher (in Reference 4), p. 1355.

9   Robert M. Veatch and Sharmon Sollitto, "Human experimentation—the ethical questions persist," *Hastings Center Report* 3, 3 (1973): 1–3.

10 M. H. Pappworth, *Human Guinea Pigs* (Boston: Beacon Press, 1968).

11 "Science and technology concentrates," *Chemical and Engineering News* (May 16, 1977): 27.

12 Bernard Barber, "The ethics of experimentation with human subjects," *Scientific American* 234 (1976): 25–31.

13 Henry K. Beecher (in Reference 4), p. 1354.

14 Jay Katz, Alexander Capron, and Eleanor Swift Glass, "Some basic questions about human research," *Hastings Center Reports* 2, 6 (1972): 1–3.

15 Robert M. Veatch, "Ethical principles in medical experimentation," in *Ethical and Legal Issues in Social Experimentation*, Alice M. Rivlin and P. Michael Timpane (eds.), (Washington, D.C.: Brookings Institution, 1975), p. 31.

16 Robert M. Veatch (in Reference 15), p. 32.

17 Joseph Fletcher, "Patient consent to medical research," *Hastings Center Studies* 1, 1 (1973): 39–49.

18 Hans Jonas (in Reference 5), p. 25.

19 Janice Crossland, "Human experimentation," *Environment* 16, 4 (1974): 18–20; 25–27.

20 Hans Jonas (in Reference 5), p. 32.

21 Sissela Bok, "The ethics of giving placebos," *Scientific American* 231, 5 (1974): 17–23.

22 Robert M. Veatch (in Reference 15), p. 49.

23 Donald Warwick, "Social scientists ought to stop lying," *Psychology Today* (February, 1975): 38–40; 105–106.

24 Perry London, "Experiments on humans: where to draw the line?" *Psychology Today* (November 1977): 20, 23.

25 Roy Branson, "Prison research: National Commission says 'No, unless' . . . ," *Hastings Center Report* **7**, 1 (1977): 15–21.
26 Alexander M. Capron, "Medical research in prisons," *Hastings Center Report* **3**, 3 (1973): 4–6.
27 Patricia King (quoted in Reference 23), p. 17.
28 American Civil Liberties Union (quoted in Reference 23), p. 16.
29 American Correctional Association (quoted in Reference 23), p. 16.
30 Albert Sabin (quoted in Reference 1), p. 25.
31 Pharmaceutical Manufacturers Association (quoted in Reference 23), p. 16.
32 University of Michigan (quoted in Reference 23), p. 16.
33 Frank Hatfield, "Prison research: the view from inside," *Hastings Center Report* **7**, 1 (1977): 11–12.
34 Paul A. Freund, "Ethical problems in human experimentation," *New England Journal of Medicine* **273** (1965): 687–692.
35 Paul A. Freund (in Reference 34), p. 691.
36 Paul Ramsey, "The enforcement of morals: nontherapeutic research on children," *Hastings Center Report* **6**, 4 (1976): 21–30.
37 Henry Beecher, (quoted in Reference 15), p. 43.
38 Richard McCormick, "Proxy consent in the experimentation situation," *Perspectives in Biology and Medicine* **18**, 11 (1974): 2–20.
39 William G. Bartholome, "Parents, children and the moral benefits of research," *Hastings Center Report* **6** (1976): 44–45.
40 Alexander M. Capron (in Reference 26), p. 5.
41 Robert Q. Marston, "Medical science, the clinical trial and society," *Hastings Center Report* **3**, 2 (1973): 4–7.
42 Robert M. Veatch, "Human experimentation committees: professional or representative?" *Hastings Center Report* **5**, 5 (1975): 31–40.
43 Roy Branson, (in Reference 25), p. 19.
44 Clark C. Havighurst, "Compensating persons injured in human experimentation," *Science* **169** (1970): 153–157; also "Compensating injured research subjects: I. The moral argument," by James. F. Childress and "II. The law," by John A. Robertson, *Hastings Center Report* **6**, 6 (1976): 21–31.

BIBLIOGRAPHY

Beecher, Henry K., *Research and the Individual: Human Studies* (Boston: Little, Brown, 1970).
Goldiamond, Israel, "Protection of human subjects and patients: a social contingency analysis of distinctions between research and practice, and its implications," *Behaviorism* **4** (1976): 1–41.
Ivy, Andrew C., "Nazi war crimes of a medical nature," *Federation Bulletin* **33** (1947): 133–146.
Ivy, Andrew C., and Leo Alexander, "Medical science under dictatorship," *The New England Journal of Medicine* **241** (1949): 39–47.
Rivlin, Alice M., and Michael P. Timpane (eds.), *Ethical and Legal Issues of Social Experimentation* (Washington, D.C.: The Brookings Institute, (1975).
White, Robert R. (ed.), *Experiments and Research with Humans: Values in Conflict* (Washington, D.C.: National Academy of Sciences, 1975).

8

THE CONTROL
OF BEHAVIOR

FACT AND FANTASY OF BEHAVIOR CONTROL

It has been said that the age of psychotechnology has arrived. The physical and chemical control of the mind, behavior prediction and modification have all been made possible by our new understandings of the brain and its function. It does not require much imagination to see that the power to regulate minds would raise unique ethical and moral problems about such matters as the surrender of constitutional freedoms and human dignity. The power has the potential to change our whole system of life—politics, economics, war, and more—if it is ever misused. It is a frequent occurrence to read in the daily newspapers, popular magazines, and paperbacks and see pictured in the movies the nature and force of behavioral control technology. In Ken Kesey's *One Flew Over the Cuckoo's Nest*, a lobotomy puts a permanent halt to Randle Patrick Murphy's heroic struggle against Big Nurse. In Michael Crichton's *Terminal Man*, Harry Benson learns to stop worrying and instead learns to love the electrical charge he gets from forty electrodes planted in his brain. David Rorvick's *Esquire* article "Someone to Watch over You" portrays a society governed by ESB (electro-stimulation of the brain), as does Karen Waggoner's piece in the *Yale Alumni Magazine*, "Psycho-civilization or Electroliarchy: Dr. Delgado's Amazing World of ESB." These and other plays, articles, and books convey the impression that psychotechnology has a wide range of applications to medical and social problems now or in the near future. Even Dr. Kenneth Clark, in his presidential address to the American Psychological Association in 1971, proclaimed that society was on the threshold of a new era. Biochemical intervention was called for to stabilize the moral and ethical propensities of man. No longer could world leaders be trusted to subordinate or eliminate their negative and primitive behavioral tendencies.

The particular impression conveyed in these writings is that mass behavior control is imminent; the world will soon face the far-reaching applications and the social consequences of this awesome new power exemplified in Orwell's *1984* or Huxley's *Brave New World*. It goes without saying that control means power and behavior control means power over people. And so we might begin this discussion with the questions: How valid are these claims? Can mass control over minds lead to a world of human robots? Eating, drinking, sleeping, sex—can these all be managed on demand much like puppets on strings?

Although there has been and continues to be a large number of these predictions for the future, Dr. Eliot Valenstein, professor of psychology and neuroscience at the University of Michigan, labels such claims modern "myths." Here again, as in the case of genetic intervention (see Chapter 3, p. 98), the popular reporting is usually distorted and oversimplified, exaggerating the degree of control possible. It is quite true that animal studies have demonstrated that brain stimulation can initiate eating, drinking, and aggression, or intensify sexual behavior and many other responses that are characteristic of a particular species. And some of these demonstrations are very dramatic. However, first impressions can be misleading, as can be the extrapolations from these to human behavior.

One of the main reasons why a mere listing of all the behaviors ever evoked by stimulation can be very deceptive is that it creates the impression that a greater amount of control and predictability exists than actually is possible. One can easily be impressed with the observation that electrodes implanted in specific brain regions of monkey brains always elicit a particular behavior—flexing a leg, opening the mouth, or change in facial expression; they can cause unlimited sexual gratification in rats if a lever is pressed or a continuation of eating even after complete satiation. However, those who have participated in the research know that electrodes placed in a given part of the brain do not always invoke a particular behavior. In a large percentage of the cases, animals do not display any specific behavior in response to stimulation even though great care and precision may have been exerted in placing the electrodes. Even in rats, where behavior is much more stereotyped than in monkeys or humans, stimulation of the same brain region produces variable results. For example, one rat may eat, another may drink, another may initiate sexual behavior, while still others will actively explore the environment searching for a reward. All of these behaviors may be evoked when the same region is stimulated in different animals. In another experiment, rats ate food pellets when a certain brain region was stimulated. However, if the food offered was first ground up, the same rats would not eat the food in this new form; instead they would drink. Non-stimulated rats would eat the food in either form.

Thus a great amount of uncontrolled variability in behavior triggered by electrostimulation of the brain has been observed in a variety of species. Such factors as the composition of the group, social rank, role of the individual in the group, its sex, and physical environment were important determiners of behavior (see Valenstein, Reference 1, for a detailed discussion of these experiments).

Experimental data clearly indicate that electrodes that seem to be in the same brain locus in different animals often evoke different behavior, and electrodes located at different brain-sites in the same animal may evoke the same behaviors. Even the often referenced work of Dr. Jose Delgado—the dramatic taming of aggression in fighting bulls—is an exaggerated claim of presumed control. What is thought to occur in this case is not pacification of the aggression center of the brain but a general motor effect. In the original experiment, electrodes were implanted in that region of the brain, the amygdala and the caudate nucleus, presumed to be the aggression-inhibition region. A charging bull was brought to a sudden stop when this region was electronically stimulated. Newer studies, however, suggest that the stimulated region of the brain controlled neck muscle movements and the animal lost motor control of his head, leading to confusion and frustration. Under these conditions, the animal simply could not launch an effective attack. It hardly seems necessary to point out that the same stimulation will very likely disrupt almost any behavior that happened to be going on at the time, even if it was only a peaceful pleasantry occurring in a pasture.

Another set of observations which were thought to be indicative of direct brain correlates and behavior was Dr. Wilder Penfield's dramatic work at the Montreal Neurological Institute. He demonstrated that stimulation of the temporal lobes elicited auditory and visual memory. Presumably what was described by the patient was a real past event. As one patient described it: "I see my mother coming toward me; she is wearing a blue dress; she is calling my name." The patient's mother had been dead for over thirty years. From observations of this kind came the general theory of memory which suggested that every conscious experience is stored in a specific location in the brain. Stimulation of that locus would elicit recall much like opening a book to a specific page and locating a certain line. What is not generally reported in these experiments is that in many instances the patient's responses are very sketchy and abbreviated, and much of the time there is no response at all. Others who tried to duplicate Dr. Penfield's results report total failure. Even in those instances when a vivid memory is reported, it is very difficult to verify if the patient is actually reliving the past. Also, it has been determined that some of the images reported were not derived from memories of real experiences at all. Subjectivity of the patient influences response and this may change from hour to hour. A more reasonable interpretation has been put on these phenomena, namely, that these images are nothing more than evoked hallucinations; when neurons are stimulated they do something, from recalling some particular past event to manufacturing experiences which may *seem* very real.

There is little convincing evidence that electrostimulation of the human brain can elicit specific and predictable behavior, not even the simple responses of hunger and thirst. What is more likely to occur is an effect on the general emotional state of the subject—feelings of relaxation, euphoria, well-being, confusion, anger, or rage. Stimulating the same region in the brains of human subjects at various times in the day may trigger completely different responses; stimulating the same region in different patients also produces varying results. Even the environment or those present in the room may determine the behavior demonstrated. It would seem that the physiological-psychological state of the total individual is of utmost importance in effecting the final response. Valenstein lists a number of other instances where, in general, the same kind of indeterminacy is shown. The point here is that behavior cannot be predicted accurately on the basis of brain anatomy alone even with precise placement of electrodes.

And these observations are exactly what one would expect in the light of what is being learned about brain function. In the first place, individual brains differ as much as individual fingerprints. Both macro- and micro-architecture of the brain have been shown to be another facet of human uniqueness. The three brains pictured (see Fig. 8.1) demonstrate a considerable amount of cytological variation. An inspection shows that brains A, B, and C resemble each other in the certain areas

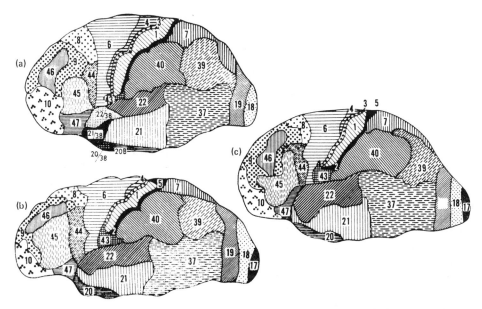

Fig. 8.1 *The architecture of brains. Note the differences in the size and placement of the numbered regions. (From "Heredity, human understanding, and civilization," by Roger J. Williams in* American Scientist, Summer, 1969. Used with permission.)

shown but differ from each other in the size, shapes, and placement of these areas. Since no two brains are alike, either in terms of their gross physical dimensions or in the details of their wiring patterns, electrodes cannot be positioned so that they will elicit the same response in different subjects.

It is also thought that neuronal networks overlap one another extensively. Neurons may be part of many circuits; which circuit will be fired depends on a number of factors. Hence, implanted electrodes may trigger a variety of behaviors, depending on a number of inputs, not just that of the stimulating electrode. The behavior elicited depends on which pathway is being accorded priority at the time of the stimulation and this can be conditioned by a number of other stimuli not related to the experimental one. Many experiments have suggested that stimulation seldom produces specific goal-directed behavior; rather, it produces a more general motivational state which itself is influenced by one's own personality and previous history. Many responses are dependent on the situation; such things as who is present, what has just happened, where the subject is located, the physiological state of the subject, and other such factors can all affect the response even though the same region is being stimulated. Lastly, response may change over time as individuals acquire new association networks from the state previously induced (in other words, the subject, or more correctly, the subject's brain, "learned" from the experimental stimulation).

Most everyone in the field of neurophysiology agrees that electricity is a very crude stimulus that has its effect by grossly disrupting neural circuits rather than by causing them to subtly reveal normal function. Electrical stimulation can be compared to a bull in a china shop, crashing here and there, disrupting neural circuits in chaotic fashion rather than directing fine control of function.

If electrical intrusions are crude, can chemical control provide a higher degree of specificity and finesse? It is thought that chemical stimulation may not violate the normal physiology of the brain to the same extent as electricity. However, the problem of diffusion of the introduced chemical over a wide neural area can occur as the chemical mixes with intercellular fluids. Diffusion can be reduced by using a chemitrode or a double-barrelled cannula. (See Fig. 8.2.) Such an arrangement makes it possible to apply extremely minute quantities of a drug to specific neural sites without many of the undesirable side effects. The strategy in chemical stimulation of the brain is to either mimic or antagonize the action of the brain's own chemical transmission system. To gain an appreciation of the difficulties inherent in interpreting results from these experiments, consider that there are only six major known neurotransmitters—acetylcholine, norepinephrine, dopamine, serotonin, glutamic acid, and GABA (gamma amino butyric acid); but with these few chemicals an infinitely large number of behaviors is possible. It is apparent that the relationship between brain chemistry and behavior cannot be simple.

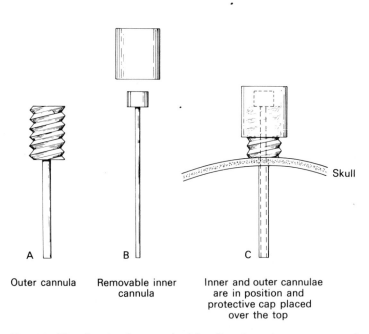

A — Outer cannula

B — Removable inner cannula

C — Inner and outer cannulae are in position and protective cap placed over the top

Skull

Fig. 8.2 *The chemitrode, a method for directing minute amounts of chemical to specific brain regions. (Source: "A double-barrel cannula system" from Eliot S. Valenstein,* Brain Control, *John Wiley, New York, 1973. Used with permission.)*

Without going into detail, much the same story can be observed here as was seen with electrical control. For example, although physical aggression can be reduced by pharmacological treatment (e.g., through injecting biogenic amines such as norepinephrine or dopamine), the effects are not restricted to aggressive behavior alone. Subjects given such agents are less responsive in general and have been described as being neurologically numb. Also, the effect of any drug can vary enormously in different individuals. One need only think of alcohol and its effects on people—some fight, some sleep, others become the life of the party, while still others wax philosophical. Another factor affecting response to drugs is the internal state of the body as directed by internal rhythms; a whole new biology—chronobiology, or the study of the function of biological clocks—informs us of these varying effects. Dr. Jonathan Cole of the National Institute of Health put the whole situation this way:

> Even if one were only attempting to control the mind of a homogeneous group of psychiatric patients with a drug with which one had considerable experience, the desired effect would not be produced in all patients and one would not be able to plan specifically that any particular effect would be produced in a particular patient. A drug designed to speed up mental processes could lead to increased activity and productivity in one person while producing an increase in frustration and aggression in another and an exacerbation of anxiety in a third.[2]

The picture of brain function that is emerging from these researches then is this: There are few areas of the brain that are concerned with the regulation of one and only one behavior and there is no single area in the brain that has complete control over any single behavior. The brain is not organized into spatially discrete units that conform to categories of behavior, as specified by the older localization theory of brain function. More recent interpretation holds that no part of the brain by itself contains a bit of information or particular memory. The functional brain, it turns out, does not fit our labels. Even those neatly drawn diagrams of brain maps one sees in biology books are not that definitive in relating behavior to brain structure; much overlap and interdependence exist.

The one-region, one-function idea has been replaced by what neurobiologist E. Roy John has called the statistical configuration model. He proposes that many brain functions are distributed throughout most brain regions. For example, vast areas of the brain are involved in every thought process. Some regions may contribute more than others to certain functions. Thus, the auditory regions of the brain play the major role in hearing, motor areas have the biggest roles in muscular movement, and the like. When something is learned, according to John, small groups of cells do not form new connections. Rather, cells distributed in many parts of the brain learn new firing patterns corresponding to the learning. If this be true, then what is learned cannot be found in any specific brain region. Brain function, in this model, is not just a matter of the physical parts or the connections between them. The brain rhythms are at least as important as the way the brain is put together.[3] The relationship of a light bulb to an electrical circuit might describe the association between the brain parts and behavior. Just as the essence of the light bulb is not the light switch so the discrete brain regions do not control single behaviors.

The strength of the evidence linking specific brain regions to behavioral functions depends to a great extent on the sophistication of the methods used to gather data and on the completeness of the theory employed in analyzing it. Simple, rather naive, overly mechanistic theories of brain function lead to strong conclusions linking discrete areas of the brain to specific behavioral responses. Such views often include the logical fallacy that given a presumed relationship, stimulation of that region will result in a definite behavior, anything from lifting a finger to robot-like aggressive actions.

More complex (and newer) theories of brain function view this magnificent organ as an interacting complex of relationships. We are beginning to think in terms of brain circuits rather than brain centers. Each specific area participates simultaneously in a number of behavioral response circuits. Subtle functional relationships exist between structure and function which cannot be directly or easily controlled by experimental stimuli.

For all of these reasons it is considered unlikely that in the foreseeable future at least we will acquire the capacity to control specific behavior, to administer a drug, or to implant an electrode that can modify neural activity so that discrete, fine behavior can be elicited. The external stimulation of the brain using either electrical or chemical means does, though, produce less specific responses—changes in motivation, attention, or sensory sensitivity. Valenstein contends that effective education can go far in dispelling the myth of directed behavior control. But this is not to deny there are significant ethical concerns in the matter of behavior control. Rather, they are of a different sort than some of the popular literature may lead us to believe.

REFERENCES

1. Elliot S. Valenstein, *Brain Control* (New York: John Wiley, 1973).
2. Elliot S. Valenstein (in Reference 1), p. 130.
3. E. Roy Jones, "How the Brain Works—A New Theory," *Psychology Today* (May 1976), pp. 48, 51–52.

PHYSICAL INTERVENTION INTO THE BRAIN

Electroshock

There are at least three methods for physical intervention into the brain. These are (1) electroshock, (2) electrostimulation of the brain, and (3) psychosurgery. They are listed in the order of severity relative to their physical intrusion into the brain, as well as the ethical issues each raises; from least to most. Each of these has as its target the alteration of some function of the subjective experience—the "mind." This assumes that subjective experiences are somehow related to specific processes taking place in the brain. It further presumes that predictable and therapeutically useful changes in mind function can be obtained through alterations of activity in the brain either through direct physical (surgical) or physiological (electrical or chemical) manipulation. On the basis of the previous discussion, these presumed relationships are open to argument on many theoretical and empirical grounds.

Perhaps one of the least understood is electroshock, also known as electroconvulsive treatment (ECT) or shock treatments. There is no general agreement on how electroshock works although it has been known for almost four decades that the induction of convulsive seizures is an effective treatment for the relief of acute psychoses. According to one theory, electrical stress to the nervous system triggers a therapeutically useful reaction—for example, it may escalate the interaction of ACTH (adrenodorticotrophic hormone) and epinephrine, elevating the production or utilization of certain neurotransmitters which regulate mood-biogenic amines such as norepinephine. The treatment can have beneficial effects on some patients, especially the severely depressed, and is considered safe if muscle relaxants are used first. (It is known that some forms of psychotic depression may result from a deficiency in norepinephrine.) ECT is not administered as a single treatment but in a series. The typical ECT series for depression is 6 to 12 separate shocks given at two- to three-day intervals. A schizophrenia series may involve 18 to 25 shocks depending on severity (and administering physician). The electricity may be applied in one of two ways: bilaterally, where the electrodes are placed on both temples resulting in both sides of the brain being shocked; or unilaterally, in which case the electrodes are placed one on the forehead and the other on the rear of the scalp. In unilateral ECT, only one hemisphere is exposed to the shock, usually the less dominant hemisphere (as determined by right or left handedness).

A single shock consists of an electrical current of between 500 and 900 milliamperes which is approximately the energy needed to light a 100-watt light bulb. The amount of current that actually passes through the brain is about one-tenth of that; most of it travels between electrodes on the skin surface. Seventy to 150 volts powers this current. The duration of the charge varies from 0.2 to one full second. The objective is to produce the grand mal convulsions of the type demonstrated in epileptic episodes.

Patients are lightly anesthetized so that no pain is felt. They are administered succinylcholine or anectine to produce a placid paralysis; these chemicals function by detaching the motor endplates of nerves from muscles so that violent muscular contractions cannot occur that might fracture the long bones (e.g., arms and legs) of the body. Ventilation of the lungs with 100 percent oxygen is supplied during the procedure since the muscles controlling breathing are also paralyzed. The whole procedure, from start to recovery, requires a total time of three to five minutes.

Although no firm records are kept as to the number of these procedures performed, estimates range from 50,000 to 200,000 a year.[1] For what it is worth, two-thirds of all shock recipients are females. ECT enjoys almost total acceptance in the medical community and electroshock units are found in almost every psychiatric hospital or ward.

Not everyone within the profession, however, agrees that ECT is a desirable therapy; and, in fact, some are calling for its complete ban in this country. The most serious side effect is memory loss. That is not surprising since the electrodes are discharged directly over the temporal lobes, where the most recent memory is thought to be encoded. Retroactive amnesia inevitably follows treatment and in some cases, the memory loss can be long-term, even permanent. The effect of this loss can be devastating—particularly for those who require their memory in their professions. Pathological brain damage has also been observed in autopsy when long-time treatments have been employed (50 to 100 separate shocks). (The author Ernest Hemingway committed suicide in 1971 following an ECT series. Prior to his self-annihilation, he complained of memory loss. This, of course, does not prove cause-effect.)

Whether or not ECT is a valid therapy has been argued strenuously within the medical community. The number supportive of this treatment is still larger than those opposed. It remains the therapy of choice for certain mental conditions and for certain patients. The use of antidepressant and tranquilizer drugs has narrowed its use somewhat. It is considered to be a very crude form of therapy, much like an electronic shotgun, but to its advantage, the effects of ECT are very quickly evidenced in patients.

Electrostimulation

Electrostimulation of the brain (ESB) employs electrode implantation to specific regions of the brain. This is the method championed by Dr. Jose Delgado.[2] Using suitable cerebral maps, electrodes can be accurately placed within any desired brain structure. Guided by micromanipulators, assemblies of very fine wire are introduced through small openings in the skull. The terminal contacts remain outside the skin and can be stimulated electrically or recordings can be made from them. Electrodes may remain implanted for months or even years. Multichanneled transdermal stimulators consisting of microminiature integrated circuits enclosed in biologically inert silicon are implanted subcutaneously. Energy and signals are transferred through the intact skin by radio induction. The subject may be thus wired up for life. According to Delgado, the use of electrodes represents a more conservative approach than psychosurgery, in which portions of the brain are destroyed.

There are several medical reasons for implanting electrodes in humans.[3] They are especially effective as inhibitors where they can prevent responses by disrupting neural circuitry or by activating inhibitory circuits (Delgado's specialty), e.g., overcome chronic insomnia, block epileptic convulsions, suppress aggressiveness, etc. In pain relief, electrostimulation applied directly either to regions of the brain or to the spinal cord probably closes the so-called gating mechanism of pain. In the gate control theory of pain, there are two types of neural fibers: A fibers that are of large diameter, have low thresholds of firing, and elicit somatic sensations like touch; C fibers that are small diametered, have high thresholds, and respond to noxious stimuli. In locations where nerves enter the spinal cord, a gating mechanism is theorized to be present. A can inhibit C; thus any stimulation that increases the firing of A over C closes the "gate" and the noxious (or pain) sensation is blocked. Diminution of pain can be effected by such things as clenching the fist, biting the bullet, listening to music, etc., since any of these stimuli change the proportion of firing between A and C. Electrical stimulation of A fibers closes the gate; this is the principle of electrical analgesia. However, direct stimulation of the spinal cord has a high risk of inducing permanent damage.

The area of the brain most generally stimulated for therapeutic reasons is the septal region. After stimulation, the mood of some schizophrenic patients, for instance, seems to improve for as long as several days. ESB also relieves psychological pain caused by anxiety, or depression, by evoking a feeling of pleasure; this is potentially its most useful aspect.

The method is much misunderstood by the general public. It can trigger or modify only what is already in the brain. It cannot insert new experiences into the brain. It cannot teach mathematics; nor can it create new skills. ESB may activate or suppress physiological mechanisms but it cannot create them. One personality cannot be substituted for another by electrical stimulation nor can it implant ideas. It is only in science fiction that students will learn calculus through positioned electrodes. Further, ESB is not a way to achieve spontaneous orgasms or an electronic "high." The most it can do is influence emotional reactivity—individuals can become more aggressive or amorous but always the response is related to the patient's past experiences.

Although its usefulness as a therapeutic tool is limited, not because of any intrinsic limitations but because there are easier ways to achieve the same results, the method does have its critics. The danger here again lies in the abuse of the technology. For example, it could be used to teach, by either rewarding or punishing certain behaviors. The scenario might go like this: After the electrodes are implanted, the subject can be requested to perform a desired behavior on the threat that if he didn't comply, a bad headache would be his reward. Alternatively, a light feeling of euphoria may be induced if he cooperated.

Another projected misuse goes like this: A condition for parole from prison requires that two electrodes be inserted into the parolee, one to stimulate pain, the other to monitor his location. Using remote sensing methods hooked into a computer, his exact position within the community could be monitored. If the computer detects that he is spending too much time in unsavory locations, the pain stimulator is turned automatically on and the parolee is electronically reminded to change his behavior. If he decides to stay low or leave town, the computer would no longer detect his presence and an all-points bulletin could be put out for his pick-up (made easier by the fact that he has a monitoring device in his scalp). All of this could be done with present technology and not a single human being would be involved in his supervision (think of the economics here!). It is this potential for misuse that frightens some. It is the general opinion of neurosurgeons that there is little evidence that direct stimulation of the brain via electrodes has made significant contributions to the alleviation of psychiatric problems. ESB may be able to affect mood, but the consequences of prolonged stimulation are unknown. However, a major advantage of ESB over more drastic interventions such as psychosurgery is its reversibility.

Psychosurgery

And this is the third direct intervention into the brain, brain surgery or psychosurgery, where part of the brain is surgically removed or destroyed. Of all the behavior control techniques, psychosurgery has roused the most divisive controversy, probably because it is the most drastic in the public mind. Psychosurgery is the physical destruction of brain cells for the primary purpose of altering behavior or emotions. The cells destroyed may or may not be pathologic. In the relatively long history of psychosurgery, different areas of the brain have been tinkered with in attempts to modify a long list of behaviors: emotional stress, hallucinations, hyperkinesis, anxiety, obsessive-compulsive acts, phobias, impulsive aggressive behavior, depression, drug addiction, alcoholism, sex perversion, homosexuality, and pain.

Other categories of psychological disorders attacked by surgical techniques are schizophrenia and paranoid psychoses as well as the more traditional medical problems, including epilepsy and movement disorders (e.g., Parkinsonism).

The first published account of the use of psychosurgery in mental patients was given by Dr. Gottlieb Burckhardt in Switzerland in 1891.[4] He removed parts of the cerebral cortex to quiet patients suffering from hallucinations. In spite of the fact that all patients remained psychotic and that he was strenuously opposed by his colleagues, he was encouraged by the small gains in peacefulness shown by some of the patients as compared to the others in near hopeless condition in the mental hospital.

Not much was heard about psychosurgery again until the middle 1930s when a Portuguese psychiatrist, Egas Moniz, attempted to transfer the results of animal experimentation to clinical practice in humans. Experimental ablation of the frontal lobes in chimps effected a dramatic calming of previously demonstrated emotional disturbances without interfering with performance ability of learned tasks. Lesioning of the frontal lobe tracts using a surgical knife called a leucotome was carried out on a limited number of seriously disturbed patients. Here too, calming effects were observed following the surgery. In 1936, Drs. Walter Freeman and James Watts introduced a modified precision-lobotomy technique into the United States. It has been estimated that anywhere from 40,000 to 70,000 frontal lobotomies were performed in the United States alone up to 1955.[5]

The behavioral side effects produced in animal subjects following the destruction of the frontal lobes were overlooked by these scientists; they recognized only the calming effects and the release from obsessive compulsions. In humans, the operation often resulted in a general intellectual decline which showed up as reduced ability to plan for the future. Personality changes also were sometimes reported. These included inappropriate behavior such as a lowering of moral standards and a general lack of emotional responsiveness. The latter, when especially pronounced, gave rise to the vegetative existence of some patients who had undergone this procedure and in general, caused frontal lobotomies to be tainted in the eyes of the public. In an effort to reduce the untoward side effects and to maximize benefits, psychosurgical procedures have undergone a continuous evolution in refinement. The original leucotome of Egas Moniz was a hollow shaft with a cutting wire loop which was extended through a longitudinal slit near the tip of the instrument once it was in place. The leucotome, with the cutting wire retracted, was inserted through a burr hole in the top of the skull, eased into the white fiber tracts filling the frontal lobes, and rotated. The extruded cutting wire removed a roughly spherical core of the white material. The wire loop was then retracted, the leucotome withdrawn and reinserted at a different angle and another cut was made. This sequence was repeated until a total of six lesions, three in each hemisphere, had been produced. Freeman and Watts developed the precision leucotome, a narrow-bladed, dull-edged, and blunt-pointed knife with depth gradations marked along its length. This was inserted to the desired depth through a hole in the side of the skull and with a single sweeping motion of the blade, the fiber tracts within the frontal lobes were severed. Depending on how far the leucotome was inserted, the procedure was referred to as moderate, standard, or radical frontal lobotomy. Later Freeman, over the vehement opposition of Watts, introduced the infamous transorbital lobotomy (or ice-pick surgery) into the United States. In this technique, a surgical instrument much like an ice-pick was inserted through the soft tissues above either eye and hammered (using a mallet) upward through the thin bones above the eye sockets (orbits) and with a side-to-side sweep of the handle, the fibers at the lower depths of the frontal lobes were severed. (See Fig. 8.3.) This procedure had several advantages: A hospital stay was not necessary; it could be (and was) done in a doctor's office; it was fast and easy to perform even by unskilled hands; and no cosmetic disfigurement of the patient resulted. The only immediate effect was two black eyes. It was because of these advantages that this technique made possible the greatest number of abuses and literally thousands of these operations were done by nonspecialists in their own offices across the country in the 1940s and early 1950s.

The procedures mentioned so far are considered *closed* because the tissue being sectioned is not directly visible. Such operations were criticized on the technical grounds that they could result in potentially lethal hemorrhages which could not be detected and the exact extent of the lesion could not be accurately controlled. In response, an *open* approach to the brain was developed in the late 1940s. In this technique, a relatively large opening is made in the skull and the brain is gently spread to expose the desired site. This technique allows direct visualization of the area to be lesioned, resulting in less damage to tissues. Several procedures have been developed to effect the lesioning. Skill in locating exactly the area for surgery has been refined, using stereotaxic instrumentation. A 3-D picture of the brain is made, using anatomical landmarks and x-ray. The stereotaxic instrument has made it possible to produce small and precisely located lesions deep within the brain, utilizing electrocautery, thermocoagulation, cyrogenic cooling, radio-frequency energy, and ionizing radiation emitted by implanted granules of radioactive yttrium.

An almost endless variety of techniques have been applied at one time or another to most areas of the brain in attempts to alleviate this or that symptom, but in the final analysis, the technique employed makes little difference in terms of the *correction* effected. It is not necessary to make different lesions in different areas of the brain for various mental illnesses since there is little specificity between region and behavior. The benefit derived is determined largely by the quantity of brain tissue removed or destroyed. Also, the success of the procedure is largely determined by selection of the patients suffering from specific categories of mental illness. For example, for frontal lobotomy to be helpful in schizophrenia, the disorder must be the pseudoneurotic variety with obsessive thinking and hysteria, and must be of long duration with the patient exhibiting suffering (psychopaths never benefit from lobotomy); also the patient must be genuinely desirous of assistance. Patients suffering from severe neuroses of the anxiety-tension type, or of the obsessive compulsive type with repetitive phobic or ritualistic thoughts, are considered good candidates for lobotomy since these disorders are generally intractable to all other sorts of therapy and ECT may exacerbate the symptoms.[6]

Brain surgery has also been used to control pathological aggression or uncontrollable, destructive, and violent behavior (most such individuals are also mentally retarded). The model is the dramatic taming of aggressive animals following amygdalectomy. India and Japan lead the world on the number of amygdalectomies done, especially on children. The danger associated with this procedure is that many brain areas influence multiple behaviors, not just one; thus the destruction of one region can affect other unintended behaviors. Especially is this true with the region of the

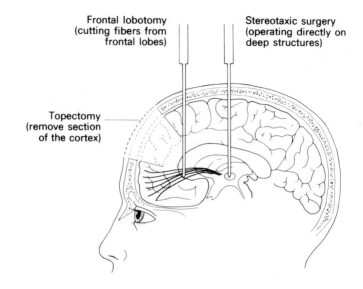

Frontal lobotomy
(cutting fibers from
frontal lobes)

Stereotaxic surgery
(operating directly on
deep structures)

Topectomy
(remove section
of the cortex)

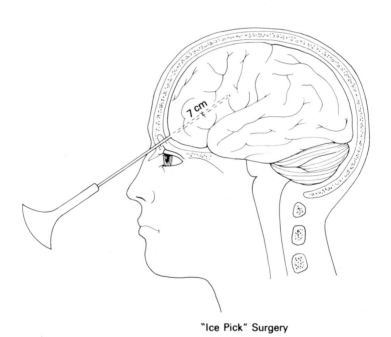

7 cm

"Ice Pick" Surgery

Fig. 8.3 *Types of psychosurgery.*

amygdala for this structure is involved in the regulation of a number of functions (e.g., in monkeys the region controls the "4 F's": feeding, fighting, fleeing, and sexual activity, as well as visceral and endocrine functions). It may require a long time before the secondary effects show up so they often go undetected. Also, follow-up studies on long-term effects are very difficult since baseline behavior prior to surgery is very difficult to determine as the patient is violent and uncontrollable before surgery; after surgery he/she is manageable. But the condition of the other behaviors was not (and could not) be determined because of the emotional problems. In such cases, qualitative data are lacking; hence, there is virtually no evidence that intellectual or emotional changes do occur.

With any of the procedures described there is no way at present of exactly predicting the consequences, either short or long term; consequences range all the way from complete relief, to some or little alleviation, to no effect on the symptoms, but devastating side effects, such as obliteration of personality, have been observed. Furthermore, it is a difficult problem to decide the point at which the patient's mental state cannot be improved by some as yet untried treatment that is less drastic than irreversible surgery. Psychosurgery performed on children presents a special problem. One psychosurgical team recently reported results of limbic system lesions made in 115 children, including 39 who were under age eleven. O. J. Andy, a well-known psychosurgeon at the University of Mississippi, has reported operations on a number of children six to nineteen years of age. The majority of these were institutionalized, demonstrating violent and uncontrollable behavior. Following the surgery, they became manageable. Yet, who can predict what the long term effects of this or that lesion will be? The temporal and frontal lobes and the limbic region are structures involved in a wide range of behavioral activities. The so-called Kluves-Bucy Syndrome, in which the subject loses grip of reality, directs sexual activity at a variety of objects, is deranged, bites objects, carries things in its mouth, etc., has been produced experimentally in monkeys after lesioning of these systems, and has been identified in humans. Is this too high a price to pay? Is it morally unacceptable to invade this ultimate perimeter of personhood or might it be better to operate and risk sacrificing some potential that may never be fulfilled anyway? Many medical practitioners involved in these procedures defend the latter view and emphasize that surgery does not always have devastating effects as many believe; particularly is this so with the new, more restrictive kinds of surgery. For example, in one study of 200 cases, 90 percent were generally improved, 25 percent showed marked improvement, 5 percent were completely freed of previous symptoms, 42 percent returned to full-time jobs, and 60 percent of the others held part-time jobs. It would thus seem that frontal lobes are not necessary for a good day-to-day adjustment to society or a good performance on IQ tests. What lobotomies seem to do is to separate emotional involvement from a given task. Thus, to cross a street, a lobotomized person must think himself or herself through the potential dangers to which he/she is exposed; the emotional element of danger or the potential for physical hurt is lacking.

Space here is not sufficient to evaluate the efficacy of psychosurgery nor to weigh the benefits gained against losses, instead the reader's attention is directed toward Valenstein's review in his excellent book *Brain Control* (Reference 1, p. 268).

The proponent view represented by neurosurgeons Mark and Scoville, Delgado, and others is that the values of psychosurgery have been established.[7]

Modern operative procedures are safe and produce few, if any, side effects, and the philosophical objections of the critics relative to intrusions into the mind are spurious because they are based on incorrect conceptions of it. In the words of Delgado, "the inviolability of the brain is only a social construct, like nudity."[8]

The opponent view, represented by psychiatrist Peter Breggin,[9] is that the efficacy and safety of psychosurgery has not been determined and furthermore, it represents a direct attack on the psyche, mind, or soul. Also, the danger of abuse for effecting political oppression is far too real to allow the practice to continue. Breggin, as well as a number of others, is calling therefore for a complete moratorium on any further brain operations to control behavior. Some ethicists submit that there may be substance to this fear.

Opponents of psychosurgery point to the following as an example of what could happen if brain lesioning, behavior control, and political power are all lumped together. Several years ago, the National Institute of Mental Health awarded large grants to several institutions to test procedures for screening habitually violent prison inmates with the possibility of performing brain surgery on them. These proposals drew some sympathetic listeners, especially from some public office-holders and administrators, for the reason that the cost to incarcerate one violent criminal for twenty years is about $100,000 while for a $6000 medical treatment the person is made socially acceptable. The other side on this issue asserts that there is little evidence to support the view that abnormal brain function is the major cause for the majority of violent crimes. The surgery, if performed in these cases, is a flagrant abuse of medical technology. It is generally agreed that no human behavior, normal or abnormal, comes from the brain alone without the environment. Since psychosurgery destroys not just the symptom being focused upon (e.g., violence), but the brain's overall capacity to respond emotionally, the entire human being is subdued (not cured). The person is psychically disarmed!

A moderate view makes no global judgment of psychosurgery. Rather, it takes each operative procedure, and the theory behind it, and evaluates it on its own merits, including any possible threats to personal freedom presented by the psychosurgery. The moderate view seeks to establish a proper balance between the interests of society and the interests of the patient, not by attacking the psychosurgical procedure, but by providing safeguards against the abuses of power.

This is precisely the position of the National Commission. The National Commission for the Protection of Human Subjects of Behavioral and Biomedical Research was charged by Congress to review the question of psychosurgery along with a number of other issues (e.g., fetal research, human experimentation, see p. 255). The commission's final report on the subject of psychosurgery was issued on March 14, 1977. Some of its provisions did not please either the promoters of psychosurgery or those favoring its complete ban.

Briefly, the commission found that psychosurgery is an experimental procedure, that in certain cases it could have beneficial therapeutic effects, that a potential patient's status should *not* prohibit him/her from undergoing psychosurgery. (Those under legal confinement as well as free persons are eligible. This is contrary to a court ruling that prohibits any form of psychosurgery on persons detained against their will.) The commission also stipulated that safeguards should be set up to ensure that psychosurgery be performed only when it is medically indicated and the subject has given informed consent.

The commission's primary recommendation is this:

> Until the safety and efficacy of any psychosurgical procedure have been demonstrated, such procedure should be performed only at an institution with an institutional review board (IRB) approved by DHEW specifically for reviewing proposed psychosurgery, and only after such IRB has determined that: (a) the surgeon has the competence to perform the procedure; (b) it is appropriate, based upon sufficient assessment of the patient, to perform the procedure on that patient; (c) adequate pre- and post-operative evaluations will be performed; and (d) the patient has given informed consent . . .[10]

If the last provision is at all questionable, more elaborate safeguards are required, such as a court hearing for prisoners, the involuntarily committed mental patients, and children.

Several objections to the report have been raised. The first considers the potential for future abuses. The commission's mandate for present caution is contained in the first sentence, "until the safety and efficacy . . . have been demonstrated." The question arises, What happens after that? Could the procedure then be performed without the safeguards listed? The second criticism is that no method is specified for determining "safety and efficacy." As already pointed out in this discussion, the problem is a difficult one, and in fact, there is at present no consistent theory that explains how psychosurgery even works.[11] Some critics assert that there is absolutely no evidence of psychosurgery ever being beneficial for children.[12]

The commission's recommendations represent a reasonable attempt to establish safeguards for the application of this potentially useful but controversial method of behavior modification. An outright ban would probably be unsatisfactory since it would deny some patients relief from their illnesses even when practiced under appropriate conditions.

With the introduction of psychopharmacologic agents (see the next section) and public awareness of the many abuses in the practice of psychosurgery, the procedure as a method of choice is not used that frequently, with only about 400 to 500 operations per year performed by about 140 surgeons. In comparison, about 250 million people in the United States have taken neuroleptic drugs since 1950; tens of thousands take them regularly. It should be pointed out, however, that prolonged use of these drugs can lead to serious complications such as Parkinsons-like symptoms, fatal decrease in white blood cell count, and tardive dyskinesis (slow rhythmical movements around the mouth, smacking of the lips, blowing out of the cheeks, side to side movement of the chin, and other bizarre muscular activities; it can be dangerous if it impairs breathing; there is no known treatment.)

The following principles governing the use of psychosurgery are generally adhered to by neurosurgeons: Psychosurgery is justified only[13]

1 as a last resort when drug or other forms of therapy have proved ineffective;
2 if the patient is truly suffering by his/her own admission and those of his/her near relatives;
3 if he/she seeks help and shows a desire to be relieved of the symptoms.

These procedures, if followed, should rule out social rebels, sex deviants, or criminals from operations performed against their will.

Ethical issues in physical manipulation of behavior

Today direct physical intervention into the brain for purposes of behavior control is probably less important in terms of either its potential uses or potential abuses than the other procedures which are able to manipulate or modify behavior (i.e., drugs). Yet, however narrowly they are practiced, these techniques serve to focus concern on the general area of behavior control. With the new behavioral control technologies it is now possible to intrude directly into the perimeter of a person's conscious defenses. Within the many complex processes which together make up the mind, a single entrance for direct access has been found which circumvents the conventional avenues of the senses. For example, psychosurgery, by directly changing some brain function, bypasses sensory inputs from the environment, the conventional stimulators of behavior.

Also, direct manipulation of the nervous system to effect behavioral changes is completely different from those maneuvers conventionally encountered where aspects of the environment are managed, as in advertising or education. In these latter instances, no great ethical issues are considered to be at stake in terms of the general strategy involved since it is assumed that individuals can continue to operate as free agents; we are free to choose or reject and regardless of our selection, no major psychological scars will be left behind. Because these manipulations have to pass through the sensory system—e.g., vision, hearing, etc.—the individual exercises a level of control. But bypassing the sensory system raises serious ethical as well as social questions. (Subliminal suggestion has been challenged for this reason.)

The brain is still conceived to be the primary repository for humanhood, the source of mentation, emotion, and personality. It is that place wherein are contained the person's most private and intimate treasures. Even legal authority asserts the primacy of the mind by declaring the privacy of the mind to be the ultimate possession.[14] The court extended First Amendment protection to the mind arguing that as the amendment protects the dissemination of ideas and the expression of thoughts, so it must equally protect the individual's right to generate ideas. The argument that freedom of mentation is protected by the First Amendment is argued thusly: The First Amendment protects communication of virtually all kinds—verbal, written, pictorial, etc. Communication, both reception and transmission, necessarily involves mentation on the part of the communicator. Organic therapy intrusively alters or interferes with mentation; therefore, the First Amendment protects persons against therapy that enforces that alteration or interference with their mentation. Breaching the protective barrier of the senses allows entrance inside the final perimeter of defense, possibly changing something very basic. (It is perhaps no coincidence that even among patients suffering behavioral disorders, brain surgery is one of the most feared procedures, although technically this surgery may be relatively simple when compared to some other types.)

Is the brain, then, inviolable? Is it ever justifiable to directly and many times irreversibly alter the very nature of its activity? Dr. Peter Breggin, a practicing psychiatrist, denounced direct intervention into the brain as "blunts" to the highest part of a human and argued for a permanent moratorium. On the other side is the position that there is nothing sacred about the brain any more than there is about the heart, the lungs, or any other organ. The number of ways and the forms of expressing the dilemma are almost limitless.

Gerald Dworkin, a philosopher at Northwestern University, raises the central issue in the matter of behavior control: How ought people to influence one another?[15] The moral side of this question seeks an answer by investigating the autonomy a person is allowed to experience. The reason for this approach is clear when the following definition for the autonomous person is understood:

> The autonomous man, insofar as he is autonomous, is not subject to the will of another. He may do what another tells him, but not because he has been told to do it . . . for the autonomous man, there is no such thing, strictly speaking, as a command.[16]

The autonomous person is one who acts independently. To do this, he must be able to reflect on his/her decisions, motives, desires, habits, and the like. The concept of autonomy allows one the freedom to develop self, to improve one's skills, to lead one's own life, and to choose from among alternative courses of action. The assumption undergirding the concept is that a person so endowed would be more socially competent and valuable.

Obviously, behavioral control methods that destroy the ability of the agent to exercise these capabilities violate autonomy. Dworkin argues that the techniques of behavior control have the potential to deny personal autonomy and, accordingly, they are morally repugnant. He submits the following guidelines for effecting protection of this principle:

1. Methods which support self-respect and dignity are to be encouraged.
2. Methods which are destructive of the ability of individuals to reflect rationally should not be used.
3. Methods which effect the personal identity of individuals should not be used.
4. Methods which rely on deception are to be avoided.
5. Methods of influence which are physically nonintrusive are to be preferred over those which are intrusive.
6. Methods which work through the active participation of cognitive and affective structures in persons are to be preferred over those which shortcut the desires and beliefs of the subject, making them passive agents to change.

It is apparent that Dworkin includes the whole array of behavioral control technologies, not only the physical methods. Whatever technique is employed, the person's right to liberty—the opportunity to be autonomous, authentic, and self-responsible—should be protected and encouraged insofar as it is possible with that person.

A number of related ethical issues are raised by psychiatrist Willard Gaylin which reflect the arguments of freedom and autonomy. (Dr. Gaylin is president of the Institute of Society, Ethics, and the Life Sciences.) He identifies these major categories:[17]

1 *The problem of consent.*

Informed consent is the first concern in every medical procedure, where it many times poses much confusion and dilemma; the principle is compounded more when applied to special cases of behavior modification. As opposed to any other diseased organ of the body (e.g., lungs), the consenting organ in this case *is* the damaged organ. How serious must that damage be before it should be worked on? Who should give that permission? Ideally, it should be the person on whom the treatment is applied. If the damage is so severe that the patient cannot acquiesce, who then is to give the consent—next of kin, relatives, the court? Where social conflict exists, as with prisoners, sexual deviants, and drug addicts, what then?

2 *The distinction between experimental and therapeutic.*

The neurology of behavior is still embryonic. Identical brain operations can produce various effects, even opposite effects. With any of these procedures, there is no real way at present of predicting consequences; in that sense, all of the procedures are experimental. Under such conditions, is free and informed consent at all possible? How reasonable must reasonable consent be? It is difficult enough for laypersons to understand complicated kinds of general surgery when the procedures, risks, and results are well known. How much more difficult it is when explaining equivocal brain surgery. Can a patient ever really know the dangers of the treatment? What are the wider factors involved? May there not be some other less dramatic way to handle the problem in the near future? (The lesson of frontal lobotomy of the 1950s should not be taken lightly.) And then there is another ethical problem: If corrective surgery is designed to benefit overall function, the physical intrusion into the body, even if healthy tissues are destroyed, is justifiable, as in heart surgery. If the overall function is made worse, then the procedure is unjustified. The latter may happen in the case of some forms of psychosurgery.

3 *The organic versus the nonorganic problem.*

In creative or corrective surgery, such as extirpation of diseased tissues or the setting of a broken bone, the intrusion is aimed at an identifiable and abnormal situation. Even in organ transplants, where healthy tissue is removed from a living donor, the object is to improve overall conditions. On the other hand, brain surgery to change behavior has no well-defined, clearly demonstrable focus. In the majority of cases, there is no pathologic focus for the abnormal behavior (an exception is temporal lobe epilepsy), and indeed, after surgery the patient will have a more damaged brain anatomically than before. Behavior itself has more than a single component and some of these components are quite intangible. Should/can organic procedures be used to change a nonorganic problem? Is psychic-disarming a real answer to social problems of sexual inequality, oppression, or environmental stress from whatever source? Do these methods treat the symptoms but not the real causes? Are they too easy a solution to difficult problems?

4 *The distinction between therapy and social control.*

The increasing knowledge and technology of behavior control presents new opportunities for conquering previously incurable diseases, easing human suffering, enhancing the quality of life, and controlling antisocial behavior. But at the same time, there are great opportunities for abuse. The specific dangers are almost self-evident, especially when used as a means of social control. It is for this reason that the earlier mentioned Dr. Breggin, viewing these procedures as a potential method of social control of young people, women, and blacks, called for a complete moratorium. Already, the record is frightening. A host of documents made public by the Senate Judiciary Committee ("Abuse of Psychiatry for Political Repression in the Soviet Union") testified to the use of these methods for purposes of political repression in the Soviet Union.[18] In our country, there have been suggestions of their application in the control of hard-to-manage prisoners under the guise of a new disease designation called *aggressive dyscontrol syndrome* (ECT or neuroleptic drugs are especially effective weapons to force cooperation). Some of these methods have also been used in behavior modification experiments with prisoners (e.g., aversive conditioning). (See Reference 19 for literature on the general area of behavior control in prisons.) Can electrode implantation or surgical ablation of the brain be used as a means of direct political control? Are the dangers of mass abuse sufficient cause to warrant a complete moratorium of these procedures? On the other hand, does their therapeutic value outweigh their potential as a weapon to be used by a malevolent government?

5   *The distinction between therapy and social engineering.*

In matters of physiological function, medicine has little difficulty in determining what is normal: 98.6F. is normal body temperature; 10 fingers and 10 toes are normal; blood pressure is low or high. In mental health, the problem of what is normal behavior is not easily resolved. The problem is more than one of definition; it can pose serious dangers to individual liberty. By defining a piece of behavior as abnormal, we may be subjecting it to certain coercive aspects of law (e.g., enforced confinement, judicial declaration of incompetence, aggressive dyscontrol syndrome). Apparently the Soviets routinely use this judgment to bypass due process and judicial procedure, and institutionalize political dissidents. Furthermore, stigmatization associated with being "abnormal" can also have far-reaching consequences even outside the institutional setting. The labeling of "normal" is a potent force in behavior control which has not been nearly sufficiently analyzed or evaluated (see Gaylin, "What's normal?" Reference 20). Psychiatrist Thomas Szasz is one of the most outspoken critics of a political system which dictates what may or may not be practiced as normal behavior. He asserts that drug abuse, deviant sexuality, gambling, mental illness, abortion, even suicide—activities that harm no one except, sometimes, the person who chooses to commit them—are not questions of ill (i.e., abnormal) mental health at all, but rights guaranteed to every citizen in a free society. Medicine, sociology, psychology, and psychiatry may advise us about such matters, but the individual has the right to decide for himself how he will conduct his life (see Szasz, "Our despotic laws destroy the right to self-control," Reference 21).

6   *Questions of human autonomy.*

The major ethical issue throughout this discussion on behavior control dealt with human dignity and autonomy. Part of human uniqueness is the freedom— however one defines "free"—to be that which we choose to be. Behavior control research is a cut above other kinds since with each advance, the more unfree the recipient of that technique becomes. The commandment "Thou shalt not alter the consciousness of another without his/her consent" still stands as a cardinal principle, at least in those societies where the primacy of the individual is a principal tenet. Should we then not abandon this area before still more subtle ways of behavioral control are invented? Is the fear of living in a controlled society too compelling a reason to continue with this kind of research? Is there any length to which society will not go to suppress behavior it considers deviant?

This study started with the proposition that control means power and behavior control means power over people. The moral issue of behavior control now becomes the problem of how to use the power justly. Human society, at least in the West, in its struggle for control over its own destiny has made the principle of justice its central tenet. It is justice which elucidates the idea that power of one man over men must always be controlled. Without this control, the danger persists that evil manipulators may be given more power. This is an especially sensitive issue in matters of behavior manipulation through direct means.

Even if we accept the fact that research on the human brain so far has not led to a conspicuous diminution in the quality of human life, can we be sure that a greater understanding of brain function would be applied to the benefit of humankind? At the present time it still appears that much good can come from understanding brain mechanisms. We may expect that in the near future understanding will aid in the development of techniques to administer to the needs of the mentally ill and the handicapped; it may even help us to understand ourselves a little better!

REFERENCES

1 John Friedberg, "Let's stop blasting the brain," *Psychology Today* (August, 1975), pp. 18–23; 98–99.

2 José M. R. Delgado, "Psychocivilized direction of behavior," in *New Theology No. 10,* Martin E. Marty and Dean G. Peerman (eds.) (New York: Macmillan, 1973).

3 José M. R. Delgado (in Reference 5), p. 172.

4 Elliot S. Valenstein, *Brain Control* (New York: John Wiley, 1973), p. 266.

5 Elliot S. Valenstein (in Reference 4), pp. 333–334.

6 Jesse B. Newkirk, (Adapted from an unpublished paper presented at the NSF Chautauqua-Type Short Course: Ethical Issues in the Life Sciences, Claremont, Calif., March 1976).

7 Vernon H. Mark and Frank R. Ervin, *Violence and the Brain,* (New York: Harper & Row, 1970).

8 José M. R. Delgado in "Physical manipulation of the brain," *Hastings Center Report* Special Supplement, May 1973. p.11.

9 Peter R. Breggin, "The return of lobotomy and psychosurgery," *Congressional Record,* 93rd Congress (available from Peter R. Breggin, Center for the Study of Psychiatry, 2124 S. Street, N.W. Washington, D.C. 20008).

10 George J. Annas, "Psychosurgery: procedural safeguards," *Hastings Center Report* 7, 2 (1977): 11–14.

11 Barbara J. Culliton, "Psychosurgery: national commission issues surprisingly favorable report," *Science* 194 (1976): 299–301.

12 George J. Annas (in Reference 10), p. 13.

13 William Beecher Scoville, "Only a last report . . . ," *Hastings Center Report* 3, 1 (1973).

14 *Kaimowitz vs. Department of Mental Health,* Civil No. 73-19434-AW (Circuit Court, Wayne County, Michigan, July 10, 1973).

15   Gerald Dworkin, "Autonomy and behavior control," *Hastings Center Report* **6**, 1 (1976): pp. 23–28.
16   Gerald Dworkin (in Reference 15), p. 23.
17   Willard Gaylin, "The problem of psychosurgery," available from *Readings*, Institute of Society, Ethics and the Life Sciences, Hastings-on-Hudson, N.Y., 10706.
18   "Abuses of psychiatry for political oppression," *F.A.S. Public Interest Report* **26**, 8 (1973): 5–6.
19   Helen Blatte, "State prisons and the use of behavior control," *Hastings Center Report* **4**, 4 (1974): 11–13; Peter Steinfels, "A clockwork orange—or just a lemon?" *Hastings Center Report* **4**, 2 (1974): 10–12; *Hastings Center Report* **5**, 1 (1975) "Behavior control in prison." David J. Rothman, "Behavior modification in total institutions," pp. 17–24; Robert A. Burt, "Why we should keep prisoners from the doctors," pp. 25–34; Leslie T. Wilkins "Putting treatment on trial,"pp. 35–37.
20   Willard Gaylin, "What's normal?" *The New York Times Magazine* (April 1, 1973), pp. 54–57.
21   Thomas Szasz, "Our despotic laws destroy the right to self-control," *Psychology Today* (December 1974): pp. 19, 21, 23, 24, 29, 127; and *The Myth of Mental Illness* (New York: Harper & Row, 1974).

CONTROLLING BEHAVIOR THROUGH DRUGS

If the control of behavior by physical means has alarmed, the use of chemical methods may well cause panic for it is with these agents that the most important and significant strides are being made in modifying and changing behavior. Of all the techniques which modern technology has made available for behavior control, drugs are among the most widely disseminated and readily available. Psychosurgery and electrode implantation are, in comparison to drugs, techniques which are extremely limited in the number of people exposed to and willing to use them. In contrast, chemical agents for controlling behavior or mood have always been with us. Alcoholic ferments were probably widely utilized as far back as the dawn of civilization, probably arising about the same time as the domestication of animals and the discovery of agriculture. Hashish, tea, coffee, the opiates, all have played some part in the cultures of South America, the Middle East, Africa, and the Orient. Although the public is accustomed to access to at least some behavior-controlling chemicals, it was not until the psychoactive chemical agents became known and were distributed that a shift in concern over their use and abuse occurred. Now in the public sector as well as in scientific circles, there is widespread interest in the so-called psychotropic drugs—those chemicals which influence the mind and alter behavior, mood, and mental functioning.

Psychopharmacology

Psychopharmacology did not emerge as a distinct science until the decade after World War II, with the synthesis and clinical introduction of chlorpromazine in France in 1952.[1] In the next few years, the pace and development accelerated rapidly. Dozens of new compounds were developed for investigational and therapeutic use. Today, the science of psychopharmacology is rapidly growing, serving as the interface between psychiatry, psychology, pharmacology, and neurophysiology and having important implications in the fields of education, law, religion, and sociology.[2] Psychotropic drugs have the highest rate of entry of any drug in the legitimate drug market. The National Institute of Mental Health lists well over 1000, and the number is being added to. Research and development in the area is being spurred on by newer knowledge of the interaction of molecules with receptor sites on cell membranes and by the ability to synthesize and modify molecular structures in the laboratory so that better-behaved molecular moieties can be produced that have more specificity and direct action while at the same time show fewer side effects.

As knowledge of the relationship between behavior and the brain increases, it is likely that we will develop highly potent and minimally hazardous antipsychotics, tranquilizers, analgesics, antidepressants, euphorics, psychedelics, stimulants, sedatives, intoxicants, aphrodisiacs; in other words, the ability to produce almost any mood state will be ours. It may well be, as some suggest, that the United States and other industrial societies will have to redefine the right to life, liberty, and the pursuit of happiness so it will include the right of absence of guilt, anxiety, tension, depression, and insomnia. If this be the case, profound consequences on values, such as achievements, enjoyment, satisfaction, and the nature of the good life, will bring out immense moral dilemmas.

In the United States, in 1970 alone, 214 million prescriptions were filled for stimulants, major and minor tranquilizers, antidepressant drugs, sedatives, and hypnotics—the main types of psychotropic drugs.[3] These drugs make it possible for many psychotic patients to receive effective treatment in the psychiatric units of general hospitals or in outpatient facilities near their homes instead of at distant mental hospitals. As a result, the number of patients confined to mental hospitals has been decreasing, this despite the fact that the number of admittances is notably increasing. Patients simply spend less time in the hospital than formerly; from six months in 1955 to a little over a month in 1971. The following figures attest further to this change: During the years before 1955 (when the antipsychotic drugs first came into general use), the number of patients confined in mental hospitals rose each year, reaching a peak of 559,000 by the end of 1955. If that trend had continued, the hospitalized population would have risen to about 793,000 by the end of 1972. Instead, the number each year has fallen more and more rapidly—to 276,000 by the end of 1972.[4] Truly, this can be spoken of as a psychiatric revolution.

Psychotropic drugs available today fall into three main groups, depending upon the purpose for which the drug is used:

1 Therapeutic agents (see table).

2 Drugs used for nontherapeutic purposes, for recreation or personal enjoyment: alcohol, hashish, marijuana, psychedelics, various opiates. These drugs have the common capacity to induce a pleasurable state.

3 Drugs to enhance performance and capabilities. At present, only a very few are available (caffeine and amphetamines to counter fatigue). It is suggested that developments in this area will represent the most significant advances of psychopharmacology in the future; there will be drugs to enhance normal performance by improving memory, learning, sexual ability, and intellectual functioning. Experimentation to develop learning-enhancing drugs is proceeding quite rapidly.

Some Common Psychotherapeutic Drugs

Chemical designation	Generic name	Trade name
Antianxiety drugs		
barbiturates	chlordiazepoxide	Librium
benzodiazepine	diazepam	Valium
derivatives	oxazepam	Serax
diphenylmethane derivatives	hydroxyzine	Atarax, Vistaril
glycerol	meprobamate	Equanil,* Miltown*
derivatives	tybamate	Solacen, Tybatran
Antidepression drugs		
psychomotor stimulants	isocarboxazid	Amphetamines
MAO inhibitors	phenelzine	Ritalin
	tranylcypromine	Preludin
	methylphenidate	Marplan
	phenmetrazine	Nardil
		Parnate
tricylic derivatives	amitriptyline	Elavil
	desipramine	Norpramin, Pertofrane
	imipramine	Tofranil, Sinequan
	nortriptyline	Aventyl
Antipsychotic drugs		
The major tranquilizers		
butyrophenones	haloperidol	Haldol
phenothiazine derivatives	chlorpromazine	Thorazine
	fluphenazine	Permitil, Prolixin
	perphenazine	Trilafon
	trifluoperazine	Stelazine
thioxanthene	chlorprothixene	Taractan
derivatives	thiothixene	Navane
Antimanic drugs		
lithium	lithium carbonate	Eskalith, Lithane
		Lithonate
Combination drugs		
tricyclic derivative and phenothiazine derivative	amitriptyline and perphenazine	Etrafon, Triavil

* Subject to the Controlled Substances Act of 1970.

It is with the use of the first of these categories that the major ethical and social concerns arise—at least for the present; hence, the remainder of this discussion will concentrate on psychotropic drugs used for therapeutic purposes.

The therapeutic psychotropic drugs

These major classes of psychotherapeutic drugs—the antipsychotic, antidepression, and antianxiety drugs—are commonly prescribed by physicians.

1 The Antipsychotic Drugs

The antipsychotic drugs, sometimes called the major tranquilizers, are particularly effective against schizophrenia and other psychoses, although they have other uses as well. Chlorpromazine, sold under the trade name Thorazine, was the first of these drugs (1952); more than a dozen other antipsychotic drugs are now marketed.

   a) phenothiazines—largest group and most widely used; chlorpromazine (Thorazine) is the prototype; 12 different phenothiazines are available that are chemically very similar—promazine (Sparine), thioridazine (Mellaril), perphenazine (Trilifon), trifluroperazine (Stelazine), and fluphenazine (Prolixin);

   b) the thioxanthines (Taractan and Navane)—not widely used;

   c) the rauwolfia derivatives—of historical interest, not widely used;

   d) the benzoquinolines—of research interest, closely parallel action of reserpine; not widely used;

   e) the butyrophenones—recently introduced into the United States; useful on some rare forms of behavioral abnormalities (e.g. de Tourette's syndrome);

   f) lithium derivatives—especially effective for the management of manic-psychosis; more often used overseas than in the United States; some debate as to whether these are as effective as chlorpromazine.

   Clinical experience indicates great similarities in effects among the first five classes. They demonstrate sedative, hypnotic, and mood elevating effects and are used in the treatment of major mental illnesses, including schizophrenia, paranoia, mania, and catonia hebephrenia. Neither chlorpromazine nor any of the other antipsychotic drugs cure these disorders but merely suppress symptoms, reducing thereby the period of hospitalization and facilitating the patient's adjustment back into the community. Maintenance therapy is required over prolonged periods of time, often at reduced dose levels. Antipsychotic drugs are relatively safe but a wide range of side effects have been reported. Common side effects include slurred speech, a coarse tremor (often in the hands), uncontrollable restlessness, jerkiness, and tiredness. Often these can be controlled by lowering the dose, changing the medication, or administering a second drug (e.g., Artane to reduce tremors). Although the side effects of the antipsychotic drugs can be serious, the great benefits achieved far outweigh the discomforts and hazards according to most opinions. However, the side effects are sufficiently serious that use of the drugs for calming minor anxieties of everyday living is to be rejected.

2 The Antidepressant Drugs

The antidepression drugs are not tranquilizers. As their name implies, they are prescribed for depressed patients. In general, they tend to stimulate rather than depress the central nervous system.

a) the psychomotor stimulants—amphetamine is the most widely known but has little clinical value in the treatment of depression because changes induced by amphetamine are of very short duration; also it has potential for abuse and a tendency to produce psychic dependence and toxic states. There is a move to ban its manufacture entirely in this country;

b) methylphenidate (Ritalin) and phenmetrazine (Preludin)—widely used but do have dependency and abuse characteristics;

c) monoamine oxidase (MOA) inhibitors—at first widely used but recently their clinical value has been reduced (highly toxic and not as effective as (b)); they are still used in patients who do not respond to other drugs;

d) tricyclic derivatives of imipramine—trade names include Tofranil, Elavil, Aventil, Pertefrane (Norpramine), and Sinequan; most widely used of the anti-depressants; have a broad dose range and are relatively safe;

Depression, although not a dramatic mental illness, is especially widespread in industrialized societies. It has been said that whereas the 1950s was the age of anxiety, the 1970s will be known as the age of depression. It is not clear whether this is actually due to an absolute increase in the incidence of depression or to a greater recognition of the disorder associated with other clinical states.

Although the drugs' usefulness is generally conceded, there are differences of opinion on just how useful they are. Clinicians report generally favorable results in ordinary clinical use; in carefully controlled placebo studies, these drugs usually come out somewhat better than placebos but not dramatically—for example, six or seven out of ten patients might do well on imipramine, while four or five out of ten would do well on inert placebos. The group as a whole is generally effective in relieving endogenous depression (originating from within) but there is little evidence that they are effective in relieving the minor ups and downs of everyday life, or in relieving the sadness from an emotional blow, e.g., the death of a relative.

All antidepressants provoke numerous side effects; most are mild, some are frequent, others are serious but fortunately rare.

3 The Antianxiety Drugs

The antianxiety drugs, or minor tranquilizers, are the most commonly prescribed group of the psychotropic drugs. They have a calming effect for a variety of symptoms including anxiety and nervous tension.

a) Barbiturates—oldest and least effective of the group; low margin of safety; probably the second most widely used instrument of suicide in the United States (auto is first); effective in the treatment of epilepsy; high tendency to produce dependence, habituation, and addiction; withdrawal can be fatal; there is a move to ban their manufacture in the United States;

b) Meprobamate and its derivatives—a middle position between barbiturates and the diazepoxides in terms of effectiveness and side effects;

c) Diazepoxides (Librium, Valium, and Serax)—best in the group for treatment of anxiety, tension, and related states; no known deaths from overdose; less frequent addictions and much less dangerous than barbiturates.

The antianxiety drugs, as opposed to the antipsychotic ones, are not effective in the treatment of psychoses since they do not act upon the autonomic nervous system as do the antipsychotics. Antianxiety drugs are of value in the treatment of anxiety and tension associated with situational states and stress. Hence, they are of special value in the treatment of short-lived episodes of neurotic symptoms. Long-term usage is discouraged since they may produce psychic dependence and have a tendency to be abused which is not true of the antipsychotic drugs.

When antianxiety drugs are tested under controlled conditions, half the patients given diazepam (Valium) were judged to be significantly improved after six weeks on the basis of objective tests and the physician's judgment. A like number given placebos were also found to be significantly improved. In other tests, the reaction of the patient may be strongly influenced by the physician's attitude. Physicians who were enthusiastic about the possible results of drug therapy obtained better results than those who demonstrated a skeptical or pessimistic attitude toward the patient.

A summary of the evidence evaluating effectiveness suggests that the odds are better than 50–50 that a patient *in need* of an anxiolytic drug will be benefited by it. If the physician radiates confidence, the patient is more likely to be helped. The drugs are better than barbiturates and probably somewhat better than placebos. They really do relieve the symptoms of anxiety in a significant proportion of cases.[5]

Valium is the most frequently prescribed drug in the United States as well as in the world. It is given for treatment of a wide range of symptoms vaguely described as "anxiety." Eighty percent of the drug is consumed in *non*institutional settings with most of it being prescribed by local physicians as "something for the nerves." In this regard, it has been called the poor person's psychiatry. Women, mostly those over thirty, outnumber male users two and a half to one (with all psychotropic drugs, they outnumber males two to one), and at all ages women are twice as likely to be heavy users. Doctors generally have assumed it is nonaddictive and impossible to overdose on the stuff. However, a small minority disagrees.

Dr. Marie Nyswander, a New York psychiatrist, contends that it is possible to form an addiction that leads to a patient's building up the dosage to a point where it may be lethal (no deaths have been reported from taking the drug alone).[6]

A study issued by the National Council on Drug Abuse describes Valium as the number one choice of drug abusers.[7] Coroner statistics in Chicago's Cook County indicate that nearly a third of all drug overdose deaths in 1975 involved Valium. The study estimates that four fifths of the soft-drug users and one fourth of those into hard drugs chronically abuse Valium. Drug-control people talk about a "Valium high"—a calm, relaxed feeling leading to sleepiness and stupor. The street price in Chicago in 1975 was three 10 milligram tablets for a dollar.

Roche Pharmaceutical, the manufacturer of Valium, emphasizes caution to prescribing physicians. However, doctors frequently fail to mention anything about caution to their patients. For example, a patient taking Valium may become drowsy, so that it is dangerous to drive a car or operate high-speed or heavy machinery (some authorities correlate the increased number of traffic accidents to the large number of drivers on tranquilizers). The synergistic effects, the "1 + 1 = 3 effect," may also be overlooked. Valium and alcohol do not mix but rather reinforce each other so that two innocent 5 milligram tablets plus two dry martinis may produce a zombie-like condition. (It is reported that Karen Quinlan took Librium prior to going to a party where she drank alcohol; the effect was permanent coma.) Some people at any age, but especially some older people show a paradoxical reaction:

that is, instead of being sedated by Valium, they become highly agitated—just the opposite of what might be expected. It has also been shown to cross the placental barrier where, although its effects are unknown, it may affect the developing fetus. Still another report indicated it interfered with REM sleep.

Valium certainly has been and is still being over-prescribed and abused. Ninety percent of all psychotropic drugs are prescribed by nonpsychiatrists, medical doctors who may not be familiar with the drug's interactions and side effects. This has led to the charge that a large number of these prescriptions have resulted in illness called *iatrogenic disease* (disease caused by the treatment itself).

Ethical and social implications in the use of psychotropic drugs

It is immediately clear that the use of chemical agents to control behavior or mood raises fundamental and controversial issues. Psychiatrist Gerald Klerman identifies two opposing values relative to the use of psychotropic drugs; the one he labels pharmacological calvinism, the other psychotropic hedonism.[8] The first view involves a general distrust and abhorrence of all drugs but especially those used for nontherapeutic purposes. The opinion that "if a drug makes you feel good, it must be morally bad" epitomizes this value. Here any drug is seen as a crutch; abstinence is the higher good. It is this conviction that underlies a good deal of psychotherapy today—mental health is to be achieved by using verbal insights and self-determination rather than through drugs. Drugs may be a lesser avenue but never the primary way to achieve the good life. This has given rise to a split between the psychiatrists who are allowed by law to prescribe drugs and psychologists who because they lack medical certification cannot do so. Psychologists tend to emphasize personal growth as the way to happiness, a variation of the theological view of salvation through good works. Drug therapy is somehow morally wrong and the users are likely to suffer retribution—chromosome damage, dependency, liver problems, etc. The earnest strivings of the whole human being, even in the face of adversity, are to be preferred over any shortcuts to happiness offered by drugs.

Personal achievement is seen as a valued component of humanness and a reliance on drugs to attain it is regarded as wrong in any moral or value sense. It is worth noting that the position of abstinence over indulgence undergirds the popular media's attempts to curb the use of illicit drugs, too. Hence, if a drug makes you feel good (e.g., marijuana), there has to be something wrong with it. The potential (and often unsubstantiated) hazards of addiction and physical and mental deterioration are paraded before young people in attempts to discourage their use of drugs, especially the illicit ones. On the basis of results so far, this kind of educational program has not been a stellar success.

Psychotropic hedonists, the other extreme, view this whole argument as nonsense. Just as it is foolish not to utilize the benefits of technology designed to make life easier—for example, very few people still resist vaccination against disease or refuse to wear eyeglasses to correct defective vision—so it is utterly senseless not to profit from drugs which can assist in relieving some of life's unpleasantries. Therapies which prescribe drugs are much more humane and effective than the old-fashioned approaches to mental illness that meant much mental anguish for the persons involved, long periods of institutionalization, unending therapy sessions, and frequent relapses. Not to use drugs is like refusing to set a broken bone when the wherewithal exists for doing so—and this is immoral!

Willingness to tolerate discomfort is less a sign of moral strength and virtue than of stupidity and lack of sensitivity. The administration of drugs in cases of mental illness is consistent with the Hippocratic Oath which says, "I (the physician) will follow that system of regimen, which according to my ability and judgment, I consider for the benefit of my patients." The beneficial effects of psychotropic drugs is clearly obvious. Also, one of the major long-run effects of psychotherapeutic drugs has been a change in public attitude toward mental illness.[9] When a drug abolishes psychic symptoms (e.g., hallucinations), the wall separating mental from physical disease is no longer tenable. Psychoses can now be viewed as real diseases amenable to medication instead of them being viewed as mental, mysterious, and menacing as they were in former times. A change in attitudes of this kind by both the medical profession and the general public can go far in effecting cures or long-term adjustments for persons afflicted with mental illness by making them once more acceptable to society. Besides, there is an ironic ring to our espoused values of abstinence and actual behavior. Society's stance on tobacco and alcohol is in sharp contrast to its proscriptive position on drugs, an inconsistency that has not escaped the purview of young people when they are admonished not to use certain (those labeled illicit) drugs. The advertising media also glamorize the use of drugs as a way to vanquish unhappiness and/or pain. Although the drug industries' motivation is economic, the result often softens people's attitude concerning "pill-popping." The press has had another effect in relation to disseminating information about drugs. Headlines such as "Doctors Announce New Asthma Cure" or "New Wonder Drug for Pneumonia" undoubtedly have an impact on people's thinking.

One aspect of this impact is that society's conceptions on the use of drugs are undergoing profound change. Resistance to drug use has been likened to the attitude of those who have opposed flying, or vaccinations, or abortions, or anything else that was new. Young people of today seem to be at the forefront of this change. The use of drugs to enhance oneself and one's relationships is not being regarded as wrong on any moral or value scale. Efforts to decriminalize and even legalize marijuana use dramatizes this change in attitude. Given the likelihood that further advances in psychopharmacology are inevitable, and the availability and use of these drugs will become even more widespread, the discord in values between the old and the new is likely to become more intensified.

Robert Veatch focuses on this conflict by posing two issues; the right to control one's own body chemistry and the right to control the body chemistry of others.[10]

The Right to Control One's Own Body Chemistry

Within specified limits, does the individual have the right to determine his or her own life style? Does this include the choice to change internal body chemistry or refrain from changing it through the use of drugs? What effect will private control have on that already fuzzy boundary between genuine psychosis and psychopathological forms of upset associated with the stresses of everyday life? Is free accessibility to drugs the easy solution to problems of living? Is some stress and normal discomfort good? Is a "happy pill" a worthy substitute for "activity in accordance with virtue," Aristotle's definition of happiness? Will achievement be affected? Will the drive to succeed and motivation be blunted by drugs? What about social progress? (It has been said that slaves would still be slaves if behavior control drugs including "happiness pills" were available in the 1800s or women would still be captive in the Victorian sense if tranquilizers had been discovered earlier.) Is it better to be a happy slave than an unhappy Socrates? Is Aldous Huxley's "soma society" to be preferred over one marked by conflict and strife? But are drugs simply palliatives, "band-aid" therapies that merely mask underlying problems whether they be social or individual? Dr. Jonas B. Robitscher gives this reason for minimizing dependence on drugs to reduce pain, both physical and psychic:

> It is a mistake to think that those hesitant about drugs want suffering perpetuated. Suffering can be useful not because it is character-building, but because it indicates something wrong in the system.[11]

Again, the previously mentioned Thomas Szasz asserts, "I believe that just as we regard freedom of speech and religion as fundamental rights so should we also regard freedom of self-medication."[12] On the other hand, is the judgment "any drug is a crutch" a more acceptable one? Is it morally wrong to rely on drugs for happiness, security, pleasure, or escape? Does this detract from the nobleness that has made us human? Does a humanizing life-style have moral limitations placed upon it to wit that simply because something can be done does not carry with it the justifying sanction that it should be done? Psychiatrist Louis Jolyon West makes the following comment on this proposition:

> Let us assume the development of a "happiness drug" which is relatively safe. It would make it possible for a human being to go from birth to death without having encountered suffering, tragedy, and anxiety. Trauma could be swiftly counteracted by drugs. What kind of people are those going to be, those who grow up without undergoing the trauma of "normal life"—as *we* know it? To what extent are our ideas of maturity, nobility, sympathy, and so on, dependent on the experience of suffering? That after all, is the point of Huxley's *Brave New World*: that the nonsufferer is somehow inhuman.[13]

Furthermore, it can be asked, is it wrong for society to dictate a single ethic for all citizens, i.e., abstinence? But then again, can we afford the chaos of each individual choosing for him/herself? What are the limits to individual freedom and autonomy in matters of drug taking?

The Right to Control the Body Chemistry of Others

"Thou shalt not alter the consciousness of another without his consent" is a commandment that holds just as true with drugs as it did in matters of physical intervention. The control of the behavior of others raises first-level questions of freedom. Psychiatry does have the legal power to coerce treatment if commitment of a patient to an institution has been legally transacted. The institutional staff and psychiatrist may assume responsibility for the treatment of the patient, the principle here being that self-determination and free will stops when antisocial and disturbed behavior begins (e.g., suicidal behavior, depression, etc.). The whole concept of informed consent becomes confused when the patient becomes irrational. Drug control of behavior judged to be socially deviant is rapidly becoming one of the most feared uses of this new technology. According to reports filtering out of mental hospitals and prisons, those drugs are being administered for custodial rather than therapeutic reasons. In hearings held before a Senate judiciary subcommittee, cases of "chemical strait-jacketing" were recounted by a number of witnesses who themselves were former inmates at mental institutions.[14] Statements like these pervaded the testimony: "one injection every week or two and you have a nation of zombies, easily controlled"; "the nightmare of being a psychiatric druggie"; it "felt like (my body) was being twisted up in contortions inside by some unseen wringer."

Drug use for custodial reasons is especially widespread in facilities for the elderly where understaffing and other institutional inadequacies require conformity if any semblance of efficiency and order are to be maintained. At the change of daytime to nighttime staff, those confined are frequently sedated with a variety of concoctions to render them manageable until the next morning when the daytime (full-strength) staff returns to duty. In many penal institutions persons have been selected for drug treatment on the basis of frequent fights, deviant sexual behavior, unresponsiveness, and noncooperation, while in other cases drug treatment is designed simply to break the will of the individual, especially if he is judged "incorrigible."[15] Again, by medically labeling the behavior a disease, aggressive dyscontrol syndrome, one can define social nonconformity (in or out of prisons) as a mental illness and then treat it with medication. By going directly into the brain, all resistance is destroyed (e.g., Haldol, a drug developed for the treatment of schizophrenia, has been used effectively in persons for control of behavior). Aversive conditioning using the drug anectine (succinylcholine IV), which produces muscular paralysis, including paralysis of the respiratory system, has been experimentally tried for purposes of conditioning. According to some reports, chemical destruction of the brain is employed on those judged to be politically dangerous in the Soviet Union. State diagnosis like "creeping schizophrenia since childhood" is enough to merit long-term institutionalization (and isolation) where sulphur injections and other mind-bending psychotropic drugs can be administered at the discretion of the state. (Whether or not the same practice has occurred in the United States is an open question, but there have been accusations that it has.) The debate about the use of amphetamines and methylphemidate to treat children judged to be hyperkinetic is often seen in this light, using drugs for behavior control to induce social (school) compliance. Some fear this is a dangerous precedent. If Ritalin is good for a hyperkinetic child, would it be good for a hyperkinetic town or even a hyperkinetic culture?

Another issue under this general heading is the control of drug traffic, both licit and illicit, by the federal government. Delegated government officials attempt to eliminate free accessibility to those drugs presumed to be of harm to society. To be sure, society must place some limits on standards of production of drugs, on labeling, and on access to certain of these. Perhaps such restrictions cannot be avoided. But the unresolved issue is how high a value do we place on individual freedom, including the right to control one's own body chemistry?

An interesting case study considers the complete prohibition, both its manufacture and sale, of amphetamines (and Preludin) in this country (they, along with Ritalin, are banned in Sweden and Japan). The reason behind this prohibition is the abuse potential of these drugs, in both legal and illegal ways. In hearings held before the Senate Small Business Committee in 1976, reports of amphetamines and related drugs (methamphetamine and phenmetrazine, otherwise known as Preludin) being used for treating obesity were described; and in fact, the major application of these drugs is for the control of obesity.[16] Over 25 million prescriptions were written in 1975 for amphetamines and similar drugs, virtually all for weight loss. There are 2.25 million Americans who regularly take prescribed amphetamines; this does not count the untold number of users who buy these drugs on the street. Their widespread use continues despite the fact that they are ineffective for weight-control and they are unsafe. Dr. Lester Grinspoon, of Harvard Medical School, explained that amphetamines can cause a three to four week euphoric "high" that may have as one of its side effects a diminished appetite and consequent weight loss. After this period, these drugs are no longer effective as weight reducers unless the user increases the dose, thus initiating a pattern of abuse. Prolonged use of amphetamines can result in psychosis, panic, and confusion; also, some studies associate these drugs with birth defects.

Physicians, testifying before the subcommittee, recommended that because the abuse of amphetamine is so widespread, it and related drugs should be banned altogether. On the other side are the millions of overweight people in the country who every day are reminded that their problem is real and diet pills offer the hope for relief. (In 1971, 12 billion diet pills were manufactured, an all-time high.) What are the limits to freedom in this case? Should physicians have the option of prescribing a medication that in their best judgment may benefit their patients? (See the above reference to the Hippocratic Oath.) Should these drugs be available to patients if patients are made fully aware of the benefits and consequences? Is this part of informed consent? Do we really and truly have a right to use any drug we choose? Does the federal government have a right to legislate in the area of drug use?

Certainly the host of ethical and social issues raised by recent advances in chemical control of behavior remain unsolved. It is by no means clear where and if any controls on these substances lie. We know that these agents exist, with unquestioned good in some cases and with unsuspected as well as known dangers in others. Given the fact that the mechanism whereby many of the psychotropic drugs effect their dramatic changes on behavior is largely unknown, as well as their potential for exerting power and control over others even against their will, the question remains, How shall these agents be regulated?

Values pertaining to the physical and chemical control of behavior

1 One should not affect the brain of another so that he/she lacks the capacity to react.

2 It is morally unacceptable to invade the patient's ultimate perimeter of personhood with therapies that leave the brain permanently damaged unless there are compelling reasons for doing so.

3 Bypassing the sensory system raises ethical questions because it removes control over one's own behavior by preventing freedom of choice.

4 Individual freedom to consent to treatment of mental illness is questionable for the reason that the organ which gives the consent is the diseased organ.

5 Informed consent in cases of mental illness is difficult to obtain since the therapeutic procedures have a measure of uncertainty connected with them.

6 The treatment of a behavioral disorder (that may have an environmental cause) with a brain-altering therapy is unethical since the brain itself cannot be shown to be pathological.

7 The danger of abuse of physical mind-altering techniques overrides any therapeutic value obtained from them and should therefore be generally banned.

8 The identification of what is called normal behavior can lead to political, social, or economic abuse.

9 "Thou shalt not alter the consciousness of another without his/her consent."

10 Within limits, individuals have the right to control their own body chemistry.

11 Drug taking is too easy a solution to a variety of life-related problems.

12 Some physiological and psychical stress is good.

13 Individual achievement and motivation will be blunted by drug-taking.

14 Social progress will be blunted by drug-taking.

15 Persons will be less human if they freely use drugs.

16 The physician-psychiatrist is in the best position to determine proper treatment for mental disorders.

17 The exercise of free will stops when antisocial and disturbed behavior begins.

18 Coerced treatment is allowable if the person is dangerous to himself (herself) or to others.

19 Coerced treatment is allowable even if the treatment is not likely to result in positive gain (e.g., therapeutic versus custodial care).

20 The brain is the ultimate privacy.

21 The brain as being something special is only a social construct, like nudity.

22 The government has the right to intervene in those areas where the practice of a behavior is likely to result in personal harm.

23 Social forces rather than biological factors are the most direct cause of socially deviant behavior.

24 Under the guise of medical treatment, potent methods of altering behavior are being used for social control rather than for the best interests of the individual who has been given the label deviant (or sick).

25 The power for manipulating behavior delegated to the medical profession can be too easily abused and must, therefore, be subject to some kind of external review process.

REFERENCES

1 Gerald L. Klerman, "Psychotropic drugs as therapeutic agents," *Hastings Center Studies* 2, 1 (1974): 81.

2 Gerald L. Klerman (in Reference 1), p. 82.

3 *The Medicine Show* by the Editors of *Consumer Reports* (Mount Vernon, N.Y.: Consumers Union of the United States, 1974).

4 *The Medicine Show* (in Reference 3), pp. 271–272.

5   *The Medicine Show* (in Reference 3), p. 262.

6   Marie Nyswander, in "Is Valium's value voided by risk?" by Gilbert Cant, *Chicago Sun-Times*, (February 21, 1976).

7   "Experts cite Valium as top substance for drug abuse," *Champaign-Urbana News-Gazette* (October 20, 1975).

8   Gerald L. Klerman, "Psychotropic hedonism vs. pharmacological Calvinism," *Hastings Center Report* **2**, 4 (1972): 1–3.

9   *The Medicine Show* (in Reference 3), p. 275.

10 Robert M. Veatch, "Drugs and competing drug ethics," *Hastings Center Studies* **2**, 1 (1974): 68–80.

11 Jonas B. Robitscher, "Comments on suffering," *Hastings Center Reports* **2**, 5 (1972): 6.

12 Thomas Szasz, "Our despotic laws destroy the right to self-control," *Psychology Today* (December, 1974): 19, 21, 23, 24, 29, 127.

13 Louis Jolyon West, "Comments on suffering," *Hastings Center Report* **2**, 5 (1972): 6.

14 "Woman fears 'zombie nation'," *Champaign-Urbana News-Gazette*, (November 19, 1976).

15 Daniel E. Travitzky, "Volunteering at Vacaville," *Hastings Center Report* **7**, 1 (1977): 13.

16 Constance Holden, "Amphetamines: tighter controls on the horizon," *Science* **194** (1976): 1027–1028.

BIBLIOGRAPHY

Dalton, Elizabeth, and Kim Hopper, "Ethical issues in behavior control: a preliminary investigation," *Man and Medicine* **2** (1976): 1–40.

Klerman, Gerald, "Behavior control and the limits of reform—the use of new technologies in total institutions," *Hastings Center Report* **5**, 4 (1975): 40–45.

London, Perry, *Behavior Control* (New York: Harper & Row, 1969).

Shore, Milton F., and Stuart E. Golann (eds.), *Current Ethical Issues in Mental Health* (Rockville, Md.: National Institute of Mental Health, 1973).

Toulmin, Stephen (ed.), Mental Health—entire issue of *Journal of Medicine and Philosophy* **2**:3 (1977).

"Introductory note: the multiple aspects of mental health and mental disorder," Stephen Toulmin, pp. 191–196.

"The concept of mental health and disease: an analysis of the controversy between behavioral and psychodynamic approaches," Theodore Mischel, pp. 197–219.

"Mental illness, the medical model, and psychiatry," Gerald L. Klerman, pp. 220–243.

"The mad and the bad: an inquiry into the disposition of the criminally insane," Leonard V. Kaplan, pp. 244–304.

SOME RELATED ISSUES

Overmedication

Americans have become a culture of people who want instant cures for everything so they pop pills at an alarming rate and try almost anything that promises hoped-for relief. Most of us believe in better living through chemistry. More than 75 million Americans consume some kind of drug every day, or at least once a week and each year $11 billion is spent on prescription drugs (Valium, Librum, and

Darvon are the best sellers) and an additional $2.6 billion is spent on over-the-counter pharmaceuticals, the so-called OTC's.[1]

Three million people every year experience severe reactions, sometimes fatal, to the drugs they take. Four percent of all hospital admissions in the country are the result of drug-induced illnesses. In Chicago's Cook County alone, 42 drug-abuse deaths were reported by the coroner for the month of March (1975). Heroin accounted for only seven of these, while the others involved prescription drugs. These consisted of a variety of common sedatives, barbiturates, and tranquilizers; Darvon, Valium, Librium, and Doriden were most represented.[2]

Only a few years ago the number of truly effective drugs available was very limited. Today, there is a prodigious array of potent drugs that can cause marked physiological changes—drugs capable of doing great good or great harm. The popular media swamp us with messages from the makers of analgesics, minor tranquilizers, sleep inducers, cough suppressants, energizers, stomach acid neutralizers, and the like. Estimates on the total number of OTC's vary from 100,000 to 500,000; no one knows for sure. These huge numbers, however, may be misleading for only about 200 significant active ingredients are used over and over again in these drugs, either alone or in varying combinations.

Since the introduction of tranquilizers in the mid-1950s, the use of psychotherapeutic drugs has increased at an accelerating rate. In 1970, some 210 million prescriptions were filled in American drugstores for stimulants, major and minor tranquilizers, antidepressants, sedatives, and hypnotics. These drugs, in the same year, accounted for seventeen percent of all prescriptions (including refills) filled in drugstores in the United States. There is a definite trend toward even greater use of psychoactive drugs.[3] The impact of these drugs on the medical expectations of many in the general public has been described in a government study as follows:

> While physicians might define good health as simply the absence of bad health, many laymen see good health as a state beyond the mere absence of any disorders, encompassing feelings of unlimited energy, freedom from anxiety and depression, and the presence of contentment and happiness.[4]

What we seem to have here is the application of the judgment of the French revolutionary St. Just, "We have invented happiness."

Many demand that they be given access to this form of happiness. Patients come to the doctor expecting to receive medication that will make them feel better and if it is not prescribed they seek it elsewhere, usually from a more cooperative physician (and such physicians are easily found). The story is told of a New York doctor who routinely included antianxiety drugs in over fifty percent of his prescriptions without the patient's knowledge. If the prescription didn't work, at least the patients felt better! Heaviest drug use is found in the forty–fifty year age bracket, although other age groups are also heavy users. An interesting age division by use can be observed in males: Men in their thirties emphasize stimulant drugs; those in their forties and fifties prefer tranquilizers; and those in their sixties and older gravitate toward sedatives. (What does this reveal about our society?)

Physicians are pushed into overprescribing not only by patients but at the urgings of the pharmaceutical industry as well. According to the HEW report in 1968, between sixty and seventy percent of physicians receive their first information on a new drug from the manufacturer, by means of medical journal advertising, through direct mail, or through the manufacturer's representative.[5] A great number of physicians rely on manufacturers' information almost exclusively. Consider the following advertisements:

Serentil—"for the anxiety that comes from not fitting in";

Milpath—"to keep the constant complainer from becoming an office fixture";

Navane—the goal is "a working schizophrenic";

Ritalin—for the hyperkinetic child who is in "constant, purposeless activity . . . he's bright, yet does poorly in school." (CIBA, the producer of Ritalin, grosses $13 million per year or fifteen percent of its total profit from this one drug.)

Many pharmacists are aware that by just looking at the new prescriptions that come in each day, they can tell which pharmaceutical house representative has been through town.

Of course, no physician can be adequately informed on the intended use, safety, and efficacy of the thousands of drugs presently on the market. Ninety percent of all psychotherapeutic drugs are prescribed by general practitioners and internists who may or may not be familiar with the action of these drugs or the dangers attending their use. Even specialists are unable to keep up with new products in their own area of speciality.[6] Furthermore, the average physician lacks adequate knowledge of practical pharmacology.[7] According to HEW, few medical schools educate medical students in the practical use of pharmacologic agents beyond a basic formal course. Adding still more confusion is the fact that prescripton drugs are available to the physician in 14,250 different dosage forms and strengths. For example, phenobarbital ". . . is available in at least 9 different colors (one supplier sells the drug in five shades), 18 different strengths, 5 dosage forms, 7 bottle sizes for standard tablets, and at least 6 sizes for the drug in solution."[8]

In 1974, there were approximately 800 drug companies in the United States (no one is sure of the actual number); 135 were members of the Pharmaceutical Manufacturers Association which together controls about 95 percent of all prescription drugs in the country. The top 30 of these companies corner 70 percent of the market.[9]

As mentioned earlier, huge quantities of nonprescription drugs are used every year. Although not as powerful as the prescription drugs, they are more readily available. But they are not at all harmless. A form of drug misapplication is called polypharmacy or "therapeutic shotgun." These drugs are combination medicines containing several different drugs. Cough syrup is a good example of polypharmacy. Most "shotguns" are of the OTC variety. The problem with these is that by including a number of drugs, only one of which *may* be effective in the treatment of the target condition, the others may cause unnecessary harm to the body.

The consumption of OTC's is spurred on by the great barrage of advertising encouraging their use; the factor of suggestibility may be as important as a genuinely felt need, and probably in more cases than not, the placebo effect is more important than the drug itself. The person swallowing the drug thinks himself/herself better as a result of the very act itself. Millions are daily led to believe that the relief of headache, tension of everyday life, insomnia—all are but a pill or two away. One in ten persons surveyed uses OTC *psychotropic* drugs, usually tension-relievers, in any one year.[10]

Currently the FDA is reviewing the efficacy of all marketed drugs, especially the OTC's. Independent panels of experts rate drugs as effective, probably effective, possibly effective, or ineffective. Drugs in the last two categories cannot be marketed unless conclusive evidence of effectiveness is submitted by the drug company to warrant reclassification.[11] As one drug company lawyer remarked in regard to this new FDA policy, the review marks "the beginning of the end for the proprietary (money-making) drug industry as we now know it."[12]

Certainly figures such as those cited are impressive. There is an increasing trend toward using drugs—both prescription and nonprescription—when none may be needed. The question of whether or not overmedication constitutes a moral crisis in our society is under debate. On the one hand are those who argue that drugs are to be used only for therapeutic purposes (the so-called medical model), and then only under strict professional supervision. Drug use is a crutch; it weakens the will and is a poor method for dealing with life's complexities. Further, the complete avoidance of suffering is beyond the bounds of human living. Human life is such that no persons are free from a measure of anxiety on at least some occasions during the course of their lives. Also, pain under certain circumstances is beneficial (see Robitscher, p. 291). It indicates a disorder in the body. Intellectually and spiritually it can spur on great achievement in many areas of human endeavor. The richness of human relations is sometimes enhanced through shared suffering. Suffering cannot be judged an evil without first qualifying the statement.[13]

The opposing view reasons that happiness is an end in itself. Indeed, it is safe to presume that to avoid needless suffering is a legitimate objective for living. There is surely nothing morally or humanly wrong with avoiding suffering when it is possible to do so. To many in this school of thought, psychotropic drugs—at least the more common varieties—are simply adjuncts of comfort and utility. Cocaine, by some reports, is being accepted as a recreational drug even among the most elite of society. This behavior is defended by Szasz who contends that it is nobody's business but the individual's as to what he or she may take as long as it harms no one else. If one has the right to control one's own body, then this includes the privilege of accepting or rejecting the use of drugs. Probably somewhere between these two extremes—suffering ought always to be avoided and, suffering ought never to be avoided—is a more moderate view. The capacity to bear physical pain and anxiety is relative to the persons involved. The ethicist James Gustafson is of the opinion that persons are not under a moral obligation to undertake voluntarily most forms of suffering that they can avoid.[14] The crucial question is, Where is that fine line between avoidance because of real suffering (either physical or mental) or avoidance because of inconvenience? And does it make any difference?

REFERENCES

1   Barbara Varro, "Pills-a-popping," *Chicago Sun-Times* (October 13, 1976), p. 65.
2   "Drug-death data points to medicine," *Champaign-Urbana News-Gazette* (April 23, 1975).

3   M. O. Kepler, "The physician and drugs: professional misuse and personal abuse," *Man and Medicine* 1, 2 (1976): 162.
4   Hugh J. Parry, Mitchell B. Bolter, Glen D. Mellinger, Ira H. Cisin, and Dean I. Manheimer, "National patterns of psychotherapeutic drug use," *Archives of General Psychiatry* 28 (1973): 769–783.
5   M. O. Kepler (in Reference 3), p. 164.
6   Harry L. Williams, "Statement on U.S. Senate, select committee on small business, sub-committee on monopoly," *Present Status of Competition in the Pharmaceutical Industry* 2 (U.S. Government Printing Office, 1967), pp. 460–461.
7   M. O. Kepler (in Reference 3), p. 164.
8   Milton Silverman and Philip R. Lee, *Pills, Profits and Politics* (Los Angeles: University of California Press, 1974).
9   Milton Silverman and Philip R. Lee (in Reference 8), p. 137.
10 Hugh J. Parry et al. (in Reference 4), p. 221.
11 M. O. Kepler (in Reference 3), p. 162.
12 "FDA to review over-the-counter drugs," *Chemical and Engineering News* (Jan. 17, 1972): pp. 10–11.
13 James M. Gustafson, "Genetic screening and human values," in *Ethical, Social and Legal Dimensions of Screening for Human Genetic Disease*, Daniel Bergma et al. (eds.), (New York: Stratton Inter-Continental Medical Books, 1974), p. 217.
14 James M. Gustafson (in Reference 13), p. 219.

Societal policy toward mental illness

The introduction of effective psychotropic drugs for the clinical treatment of mental illness has had immediate and direct effects upon social policy toward mental illness. The need for prolonged hospital care has been minimized and in some instances eliminated. Many mental patients who in the past were removed from the family now remain at home undergoing therapy in local psychiatric units. Such large numbers of patients are being discharged from mental hospitals into the community that the number of patients hospitalized at present has fallen to the pre-1950 level. Figures show a continuing decline in hospitalized mental patients from a high of near 600,000 in 1955 to 215,000 in 1974. If the trend continues, the inpatient population may drop to 100,000 by 1980.[1] Taking patients out of mental hospitals and placing them in the community has virtually become a national policy. The policy is encouraged for several reasons: Better care can be provided in small community facilities rather than large isolated institutions; the federal constitutional right to adequate treatment in state institutions is forcing a change in policy away from mere custodial care to therapeutic care;[2] the cost of institutional care has increased seven-fold from 1959 to 1974;[3] and the widespread use of psychotropic drugs has greatly reduced the time spent in institutions.

While a few hospitals have been closed outright, patient populations within others have been reduced. But releasing patients who do not need custodial care to community-based, privately operated facilities that offer regular access to the every-day world has become a point of controversy for several reasons.

In the first place, it has been contended that this large number of discharged patients does not represent a true gain in the treatment of mental illness; rather, it is but a statistical artifact, for these patients in the community are frequently left emotionally blunted, occupationally impaired, and socially isolated.[4] Because, as mentioned earlier, the chemical agents simply suppress symptoms, the social impairment is still there, especially in those with severe disturbances. Furthermore, the practice of early release has created a major misunderstanding in the general public which is quick to jump to the conclusion that persons discharged from confinement are "cured". Community-based programs in the form of halfway houses, sheltered workshops, emergency protective resources, and community treatment centers are urgently needed if those discharged are to be assisted in their rehabilitation. These aids must provide follow-up therapy to facilitate the reincorporation of former mental patients back into society as useful members. We are very far behind actual need in the provision of these facilities—witness the wholesale reduction and elimination of state-supported budgets for community-care facilities. So derelict has society been in this regard that psychologist Franklyn Arnoff contends that we may be producing more psychological and social disturbance than we correct. Arnoff claims that the reorientation from hospital to community-based treatment has had profound iatrogenic effects (disease produced by the treatment), arising from unnecessary stress placed on the individual by the family as well as a society unprepared to respond to his/her needs. This problem can only be exacerbated by the phasing out of the public mental hospital as part of official policy at the federal, state, and local levels. The Supreme Court added still more reason for concern when it ruled in July 1975 that a state may not confine involuntarily for mere custodial care any mentally ill patient who is not dangerous and who can function on the outside.[5] This and other court decisions has established the principle that state mental hospitals cannot operate as purely custodial-care facilities but must provide active treatment. Since the right to treatment is now established by law, a number of questions arise about the adequacy of resources available for treatment as well as workable alternatives for handling patients when they are released. Other problems related to this policy include local residents who resist the establishment of board-and-care facilities in their neighborhoods out of fear for their safety which is, of course, unfounded, or the effect that these facilities will have on property values; who, after all, wants to live next to a house full of former mental patients? On the other side are those who worry about the economic impact with loss of jobs and closing down of facilities in communities when a reduction in public funding results in their being phased-out.[6] The dollar costs of mental-health reform will be enormous. Governor Wallace estimates $110 million for the state of Alabama alone. The social cost of the present system is devastating to the patients and the community. Can a balance be struck?

REFERENCES

1   Roger M. Williams, "Are they closing the mental hospitals too soon?" *Psychology Today* (May, 1977): pp. 124–127; 129.
2   "Freeing mental patients," *Newsweek* (July 7, 1975): p. 45.
3   Roger M. Williams (in Reference 1), p. 124.
4   Franklyn N. Arnoff, "Social consequences of policy toward mental illness," *Science* **188** (1975): 1277–1281.
5   *Newsweek* (in Reference 2), p. 45.
6   Roger M. Williams (in Reference 1), p. 127.

MBD

An issue sharply dividing public and professional opinion is the use of psychotropic drugs (notably Ritalin and Dexedrine) to treat children reported to have serious learning difficulties because their behavior is unmanageable. Two major points of controversy are these: (1) Does this behavior result from some kind of brain malfunction? and (2) Should powerful mind-affecting drugs be used in an effort to control the behavior?

To the first of these questions, we can answer that there is a lack of solid proof as to a causal relationship between hyperactivity and brain malfunction; and in fact, doubt has been expressed that the condition even exists. There is no objective test (neurological, intelligence, or behavioral) that positively identifies the condition. This uncertainty is reflected by the multiple names that have been assigned this behavior in children, including hyperactivity syndrome, hyperkinetic disorder, minimal brain damage, and minimal brain dysfunction (MBD). A typical list of hyperactivity indicators are excessive rocking, wriggling, and climbing; the rapid wearing out of furniture, toys, and clothes; experiencing close calls repeatedly; being overactive, easily distracted, excitable; talking in a silly and immature way; having trouble sitting still; not getting along with classmates; being impatient; showing marked ingratitude; being difficult with auditory discrimination; being clumsy. Most individuals thought to have the disorder are unhappy, have low self-esteem, and feel bad about their behavior.[1] These indicators—all of which are termed neurological "soft signs"—may be present in whole or in part, to a greater or lesser degree. They may be present throughout the day, only in the morning or at nighttime, or after meals.

According to some, hyperactivity is rapidly reaching epidemic proportions in this country with some estimates putting the number of afflicted children at about five percent of all American school children or almost a million and a half youngsters. Some estimates go even higher, suggesting that ten to fifteen percent may be the more accurate figure.[2] It can occur in both sexes but is more prevalent in boys, showing a boy-girl ratio of 10:1. It is thought to be more than age-limited, extending into adolescent years and even into the twenties and thirties, where affected individuals may demonstrate under-achievement, have a greater tendency to become psychotic, and frequently operate on the fringes of legitimate society, often turning to illicit drug use.[3]

There are two sides to the question of the reality of MBD's existence for the reason there are no neurological "hard signs" that identify it. Any or all of the indicators described above can be observed in varying degrees in about every "normal and healthy" child. In the past, it was thought that the cause of MBD was subclinical brain damage, undetectable by available diagnostic techniques and thus called minimal brain damage. A more recent theory suggests that it is not caused by true brain damage but by fetal maldevelopment or possibly by genetic factors. Other researchers do not accept an organic etiology at all, preferring instead environmental and/or social causes. Still another causative factor, according to some, might be (at least for some cases of hyperactivity) an allergic reaction to certain kinds of foods.[4] In the latter instance, allergic irritation from certain foods might possibly cause localized swelling in the brain. If the swelling occurs in areas that are involved with aggression, the behavior typically associated with the hyperactive syndrome is triggered. Identifying and removing the offending food or foods from the diet would theoretically reduce or eliminate the symptoms.

Why has a disorder, the nature and even existence of which is still very puzzling, achieved such notoriety in the past few years? There are at least two factors to consider here: (1) the concern of interest groups (i.e., drug companies and schools), and (2) diagnosis of the disorder.

Almost all children medically diagnosed as hyperactive are treated with psychoactive drugs—Ritalin, Dexedrine or Cylert. Nationally, between 500,000 and 2 million school children take one of these drugs for hyperactivity; the exact figure is unknown.[5] Ritalin, an amphetamine-like drug, accounts for about eighty percent of the prescription and Dexedrine, also an amphetamine, a large portion of the remainder. In terms of dollar costs, the typical pharmacy price for Ritalin (1975) varies from $9.90 to $16.00 for one hundred 20-milligram tablets. CIBA, the manufacturer of Ritalin, grosses $30 million annually or fifteen percent of its total profit from this one drug. There is a large profit to be made in the sale of psychoactive drugs.

At the heart of any successful product lies a vigorous promotion campaign and this is true in the case of Ritalin, too. Up until 1971 CIBA was promoting Ritalin at PTA meetings by means of a traveling display and speakers who asked, "Is your child overactive?"[6] When Ritalin was placed on the government's schedule for hard narcotics (Class II) in 1972, the advertising strategy changed. However, the basic theme persisted: The child who is overactive in school and experiencing learning difficulties can benefit from Ritalin. Specially prepared pamphlets by the drug company on hyperactivity are distributed to parents and physicians, and conferences for physicians are sponsored by the pharmaceutical houses. Through the efforts of these companies, much of the information concerning MBD has been brought to the attention of the public.

A second interest group that has played a leading role in the diagnosis of hyperactivity is the school. Schools frequently suggest to the parents that their children are hyperactive and should receive medication. The literature is filled with stories relating efforts by school personnel to compel parents to put their children on psychoactive drugs.[7] In some cases when parents refuse they are intimidated with threats that their children will be kept back a grade or transferred to special classes for the "learning disabled." In some school districts ten to fifteen percent of the children are taking these drugs by prescription from a family doctor, frequently at the urging of school authorities. A Rhode Island physician told a mother of a second-grader that her child did not require medication but that she should give the youngster the drug anyway "to please the school." The fear of some is that drugs may be replacing other forms of discipline at the grade-school level. Many teachers believe that they can pick out hyperactive children (one California teacher personally "diagnosed" nine of her 28 students as hyperactive).[8] Schrag and Divoky state that between 88 and 96 percent of grade-school teachers think they can spot hyperkinesis. So common has this become that "stimulants and other drugs are now a fact of life in the management of hyperactive children in schools."[9]

Turning attention to its diagnosis, hyperactivity is not easily determined since it has no hard neurological signs. It can be expected that misdiagnosis will occur. Schools frequently refer their pupils to those physicians who are known to prescribe psychoactive drugs and avoid those physicians not sympathetic with the school's diagnosis. Because hyperactivity has become such an easy label, the busy physician may overlook more serious illnesses that may be the cause of it, or cannot expend the time to evaluate the total environment of the child.[10] The general practitioner or pediatrician often lacks the training or inclination to get at the root of the child's problem. The expedient approach is to conduct a cursory examination and then prescribe Ritalin. In cases of thorough examination, both physical and environmental, the actual incidence of MBD was determined to be much smaller :han the numbers previously given. The tentative conclusion at this time is that MBD probably does in fact exist, but it is not nearly as prevalent as earlier estimates indicated.

The second major question asks whether or not powerful psychoactive drugs should be administered to children. Most of the medications are administered in tablet form, usually by the mother in the morning before the child goes to school, then by a responsible person at school, such as the nurse, the teacher, or the principal, or in some cases, by the child himself or herself. The usual dosage is twice a day although 3 or 4 pills may be taken daily in serious cases.

Amphetamines, or "pep pills," known popularly as "speed," are typically used as stimulants. In children they demonstrate a paradoxical reaction, that is, they suppress symptoms of hyperactivity in some unknown way. But like most psychoactive drugs, these stimulants merely mask the symptoms; they do not cure the disorder. Amphetamine maintenance makes a large number of children agreeable to educational and counseling programs, possibly by enabling them to better focus their attention and channel their energies. Those favoring this therapy insist that children are not drugged into submission as the scare literature would have the public believe. About one fourth of those treated are not aided at all; the others show varying degrees of alleviation, with a large percentage experiencing dramatic change. These latter show immediate psychological growth, increase in attention, lower impulsivity, decreased bullishness, and experience success rather than failure.[11] According to some, these latter changes are among the most dramatic in the entire field of psychiatry—an almost immediate and abrupt reversal of behavior.

To the critics of drug therapy for children, using drugs is the simple and easy solution. For those diagnosticians who are willing to take the time and effort, the child's real problem can almost always be identified as a functional organic disorder, an allergy, a reaction to an adverse social environment in the home, the school, playmates, or whatever. A major cause of critics' alarm is the scanty nature of long-term effects of drug taking. This is particularly alarming when one considers the young age of the "patients" and the many productive years that presumably remain. Ritalin can cause complex changes in the central nervous system; among some of the side effects may be nervousness, insomnia, hypersensitivity, loss of appetite, nausea, dizziness, weight loss, stunted growth, etc. (Ritalin cannot be prescribed in Sweden or Japan.) Does chronic administration result in a higher likelihood of drug use later? Again, no evidence exists, although one preliminary study suggested that treated MBD children have a lower risk for subsequent drug abuse largely because the new-found success they experience makes them less apt to join deviant subgroups later in life. However, it is well to keep in mind that toxic manifestations of drugs have an unpleasant way of surfacing only years and millions of patients later.[12] Another cause for concern arises from the observation that dependence is widely recognized as a problem in adults who take amphetamines for weight contol. It is for this reason, among others, that the Food and Drug Administration recommended that amphetamines not be prescribed for obesity control. Those opposed to widespread prescription of amphetamines for hyperactivity have difficulty with the public attitude that allows these drugs to be administered to children in cavalier fashion while at the same time takes a violently antagonistic position to even the casual use of illicit drugs (e.g., marijuana). Perhaps the answer lies in the observation that society does believe in drugs—but only on the condition that they are taken as medicine!

The moderate view between the two extremes of always and never submits that careful stimulant medication should be used in those cases diagnosed to be truly MBD and then only as one *part* of a total treatment plan. Drugs should never be the first or only therapeutic tool. All productive avenues should be pursued to diagnose and treat the disorder, and continuous evaluation of those on drugs must be made so that errors can be avoided. Above all, this position insists that there are no easy answers to MBD. Stimulant medication can be truly beneficial in helping some children (but not all) find a way to cope with their problem.

The question, Does extended treatment produce psychological or physiological damage? has no straightforward answer either. There is no hard data. One attempt to conduct a scientifically controlled experiment was tried in mid-1972 in Boston. Because of violent community criticism, the study was terminated in 1974 while it was still in the preliminary stages.[13]

Opponents of the experiment identified the following ethical and public policy objections:

1 The study was one of behavior control and it was to be conducted by the state (it was funded by the federal government; supervised by agents of the state—teachers and professors—and carried out in public institutions—the schools). This has the potential of establishing a dangerous precedent in behavior control.

2 There was not adequate distinction made between individual and environmental causes of behavior. Subjects were to be identified, at least initially, by the school and the intervention was to be entirely medical. No consideration was to be given to the school environment itself as possibly being causative.

3 The question of whether medication was required at all was overlooked. It was assumed that everyone in the study was a likely candidate without a primary diagnosis.

4 No provision was made to try alternative approaches, only medical. For example, changing classrooms, teachers, or other kinds of school reform were not part of the protocol.

Although the list is not all-inclusive, it does set the tone for the ethical and social concerns arising from this issue. Another set of considerations inquires into the problem that children may be harmed in the process of labeling. Stigmatization, designating persons who exhibit a kind of behavior thought to be different or judged to be undesirable, was discussed on another occasion in this text (i.e., under mass genetic screening programs, see p. 143). Are the same risks incumbent here? Is the self-fulfilling-prophecy idea applicable in cases where children, even the very young, are identified as being behaviorally aberrant?

Does the easy solution of stimulant medication divert attention from the inadequacies of a social environment, for example, schools, and obstruct the apparent necessity of social change? Is this but another instance where medical solutions are applied to social problems? Is there a danger that the easy acceptance of medication therapy in one area of social control will lead to applications in others as well? Employing nothing but benevolent motives, the state can already force its help on individuals judged to be too disordered to act for themselves—wayward youths, the mentally handicapped, drug addicts, and those convicted of crimes. Using psychotropic drugs in the name of mental health lends itself quite nicely to social control.

It was reported by a psychiatrist on the floor of a recent conference discussing the issue of mass behavior control that as many as twenty percent of the black children in the Los Angeles section of Watts are regularly prescribed Ritalin. If this figure is nearly accurate, the danger that drugs will be used as the simple solution to everything is a real threat to freedom and social justice. We may be lulled into the acceptance of chemical solutions to social and political problems through education, propaganda, or advertisement. If the use of drugs, legitimized under the label of health-producing, is approved for the control of children judged to be abnormal, what is to prevent the drugs from being used to modify and control the behavior of political dissidents, prisoners, mental patients, and demanding minority groups? All such abuses would preclude addressing the real problem and would thereby bring to a halt further, or at least seriously retard, social progress. If, as has been claimed, social dissatisfaction is the prelude to innovation, what would the widespread administration of drugs do to change malfunctioning social systems?

There is the argument that the treatment of MBD by medication serves as a model for future applications of newer and better drugs yet to be compounded whose design is to force social compliance. For example, if a hypothetical new drug is developed in the future that is very effective in promoting learning, should it be administered to children? Or only to those who experience difficulties? Or to all? And adults?

Finally, on a more practical level, several more questions could be asked: Would the hyperactive child have improved without the administration of drugs? What are the drug's effects on personality development? Is the probability of later mental disorder decreased? Is the likelihood of creativity or of innovative thinking enhanced or diminished by drugs? Is there the potential for excessive compliance? The verdict again to all of these is that we do not know!

From these few observations it can be seen that studies on hyperactivity are another example of science intermeshing with social systems. The issues raised are not to be taken lightly. Again, only an informed and concerned public can guard against abusive use of the powerful tools arising from scientific innovation.

REFERENCES

1 Paul H. Wender, "The case of MBD," *Hastings Center Studies* 2, 1(1974): 94–102.
2 Sydney Walker, "We're too cavalier about hyperactivity," *Psychology Today* (December, 1974): 43–46; 48.
3 Paul H. Wender (in Reference 1), p. 97.
4 K. E. Mayer, "The physiology of violence, allergy and aggression," *Psychology Today* (July, 1975): pp. 77; 79.

5 Carole Wade Offir, "Are we pushers for our own children?" *Psychology Today,* (December, 1974): p. 49.
6 P. Schrag and Diane Divoky, *The Myth of the Hyperactive Child* (New York: Random House, 1975).
7 Carole Wade Offir (in Reference 5), p. 49.
8 Carole Wade Offir (in Reference 5), p. 49.
9 P. Schrag and Diane Divoky (in Reference 6), p. 92.
10 Sydney Walker (in Reference 2), p. 43.
11 Paul H. Wender (in Reference 1), p. 99.
12 Paul H. Wender (in Reference 1), p. 100.
13 "MBD, drug research and the schools," (Special Supplement) *Hastings Center Report, 6,* 3 (1976): p. 32.

BIBLIOGRAPHY

Kolata, Gina Bari, "Childhood hyperactivity: a new look at treatments and causes," *Science* **199** (1978): 515–517.

Psychotherapy

Psychotherapy, the third method of behavior modification, is less intrusive than the other two: physical manipulation and psychopharmacology. In this approach, the objective is to influence another's behavior through psychological means. Throughout the process, the patient, or client, is more-or-less free to accept or reject the therapy to which he/she is exposed.[1] Although there may be exceptions to this belief, as in hypnosis or when one is under deep distress, psychotherapeutic approaches are more easily defended against since the channels to the brain on which they rely are still the sensory system and we do exercise more or less control over them.

The term *psychotherapy* encompasses a diverse number of approaches to promoting changes in personality and behavior such as psychoanalysis, behavior therapy, client-centered or Gestalt therapy, sensitivity training, transactional analysis, EST, the primal urge, and many more. Many types of therapy come and go, depending on the vogue of the day. The use of psychotherapy is more widespread in modern society than it has ever been before. With this increasing popularity must come an increasing concern with the ethical issues associated with its practice.

A first concern relates to the profession itself. Psychotherapy has experienced astounding growth in recent years; an increasing number of persons now call themselves therapists and many new philosophies and techniques have emerged. Despite this growth there has been relatively little research to determine the effectiveness of various types of therapies. There is practically no assistance available to people searching for help through psychotherapy as to which of the many available kinds offers the most hope in affecting the sought-for relief from some psychological distress. To the afflicted person it is essentially a trial-and-error matter. And although it may be a matter of selection or personal choice, not all are equally good and some leave the person worse off.

Allen E. Bergin warns that psychotherapy can be dangerous to your (mental) health.[2] In studies carried out by him and his colleagues, it has been determined that while therapy helps many, substantial numbers of people are hurt by it. The attitude of the therapist was the primary determinant of success or failure, not the kind of therapy involved. Therapists who showed high levels of empathy, warmth, and genuine concern had much better results than those who were impatient, authoritarian, and aggressive, who frequently challenged clients to immediate self-disclosure and emotional expression.

The profession has virtually no rules regulating its practice and nothing prevents unlicensed persons from practicing their own versions of psychological therapy under such titles as psychotherapist, sex therapist, group leader, interpersonal relations consultant, and the like. Although most states license practicing psychologists, social workers, and psychiatrists, enforcement is often lax. Anyone who can find a patient can be a psychotherapist providing she/he is sufficiently adept at circumventing certain legal strictures. In a system as open as this one, the danger of unqualified practitioners wreaking deep psychological harm on some is inherent.

Psychologist Thomas J. Cottle cautions against one of these perils.[3] The free expression, or "let it all hang out" school, which is rather universal to a diverse number of psychotherapies stands as a threat to individuality and privacy. In the first place, it might be best to shelter a few secrets about ourselves. Although it is desirable and frequently necessary for a disturbed person to reveal ideas and emotions that trouble the inner-self, complete self-revelation can have an untoward effect on one's psyche. A world which strips away our privacy and individuality, a world of complete openness, can also deprive us of those most cherished values of all: individual freedom, the right to be one's own person and in the final analysis, the privacy of one's own mind. There may be some things about me that I prefer not to be known even if they are only fantasies.

And then there is the problem of confidentiality. Exposing information about oneself can too readily be used for purposes other than that for which it was originally intended. Professional therapists are especially vulnerable to this threat. Confidentiality has always been a problem where the psychiatrist or psychologist has been employed by an institution.[4] Those on the payrolls of private or public mental hospitals, public schools, and private corporations can be too readily persuaded or coerced into releasing information to potential employers, insurance companies, police, federal investigators, or whoever else might find it helpful to obtain private vitae about a person. The 1971 burglary of Daniel Ellsberg's psychiatrist's office is a most vivid demonstration of this search for information, but there are countless numbers of less dramatic cases where invasion of personal privacy has been practiced in recent years. With the coming of National Health Insurance (Chapter 9), the problem will be magnified still further since government then will have some if not full access to one's health records including one's mental health.

Accountability to society is still another concern, for the therapist in effect is called upon to serve two masters: his patients and the greater society which he may be in a position to protect if he has access to certain kinds of information. Secret Service agents routinely check on threats against constitutionally elected officials in California.[5] Also in California, the State Supreme Court ruled in favor of a murder victim's parents who sued the psychologist and the University of California for not informing them of the threats made against the victim by the murderer while under hospital care. What are the limits of confidentiality? Should patients be warned that anything they reveal in therapy sessions may be used against them? (A medical version of the Miranda clause.)

Next, there is the issue that psychotherapy is essentially geared to accommodate the middle and upper classes.[6] Psychotherapists themselves are usually of middle and upper class standing and this may be one of the reasons why the profession has taken an implied negative stand toward the poor.[7] Therapists tend to adopt an authoritarian or superior position in dealing with the poor whereas they treat middle-class patinets more as their equals. Another factor contributing to the elitism of psychotherapy is a monetary one. Treatment, especially when it extends over a long period of time, can be expensive. It is a luxury which poorer people simply cannot afford. Halleck summarizes the condition this way:

> It is deplorable enough that psychiatrists do not offer the poor the same quality treatment that they offer the affluent; it is even worse when, in situations where ability to pay is not a crucial factor, psychiatrists tend to offer more prestigious . . . treatments, such as psychotherapy, to middle-or upper-class people and to use potentially repressive treatments, such as drugs and other somatic therapies, for lower-class people.[8]

If psychotherapy is effective, than certainly the poor are in as much need of its services as are the wealthy. It would seem that those offering psychotherapy ought to be in a position to respond to this need even if it involves a reorientation of the traditional methods for delivering that service.

Leaving behind the issues that are related to the general practice of psychotherapy, an entirely different set of concerns demands attention, namely, patient/therapist interactions. The matter of confidentiality has already been briefly discussed but it is worth emphasizing once more that the client seeking professional help is in a vulnerable position. The revelation of intimate thoughts and feelings does represent a deep disclosure of the subject's privacy. If the information gathered is going to be used for other than counseling purposes, the client at least deserves to know this and he/she ought to be so informed before the interaction begins. It is the ethical therapist who will honestly make clear the "rules of the game."

The conditions under which a person approaches the therapist may vary; it may be involuntary or voluntary. Included in the involuntary category are cases in which a family member or friend pressures the person into counseling. Society acting through the courts may also coerce an individual to undergo psychotherapy. The basic ethical consideration here is a familiar one: informed consent. The same arguments that apply in the whole matter of human experimentation and behavior control can be advanced here, e.g., "thou shalt not alter the consciousness of another without his consent." It is not at all clear whether or not it is ethical to treat a person who has not come of his/her own accord and may not be capable of informed consent. Alternatively, should treatment be withheld from or coreced on a person who may be a threat to society?

The problem of informed consent does not arise in the case of voluntary patients. Persons who willingly come into the counseling session seek relief from some troublesome problem. But, the subjectivity of the therapist will necessarily intrude. The desirable goal is that as a result of the therapy, the client can make an independent choice to effect a behavioral change. The ethical concern here is with the extent to which the therapist forces his/her values on the patient. It is probably unethical to manipulate the patient in any way and this includes forcing personal values on the client. The therapist may convey his/her values to the client and the situation remains ethically acceptable as long as the client is allowed free choice. That therapy which clarifies the choices and the potential effects the choices may have on the person and society, allowing the individual to make more rational decisions, may be considered ethical. To be sure, there is a fine line between manipulation and free choice in these matters particularly in cases of the severely distressed. It is the responsibility of the therapist to remain on the ethically acceptable side.

This brief description of psychotherapy has done little more than glimpse at the ethical and social implications of its practice. A detailing of them would require much more space than is available here. But, the overriding concept relates once more to values—those of the client, of the therapist, and of society. Accommodating all three without creating conflict is perhaps an ethereal goal, but if ethical behavior is thought to be of any worth, then responsible action must prevail.

Psychotherapy is potentially a strong force, capable of influencing the beliefs and actions of other people. The ethical concerns, although not as intense as with other procedures for behavioral control, are nonetheless salient. If psychotherapy expands to become a major service component in society as it well might, then the ethical and social implications of its practice will demand more study than it is presently receiving.

REFERENCES

1 Robert Michels, "Ethical issues of psychological and psychotherapeutic means of behavior control", *Hastings Center Report* **3**, 2 (1973): 11–13.
2 Allen E. Bergin, "Psychotherapy can be dangerous," *Psychology Today* (November 1975) 96; 98; 100; 104.
3 Thomas J. Cottle, "Our soul-baring orgy destroys the private self," *Psychology Today*, (October, 1975): pp. 22–23; 87.
4 Fred Powledge, "The therapist as double agent", *Psychology Today* (July, 1977): pp. 44; 46–47.
5 Fred Powledge (in Reference 4), p. 46.
6 Enrico Jones, "Psychotherapists shortchange the poor," *Psychology Today* (April 1975): pp. 24; 26; 28.
7 Seymour L. Halleck, *The Politics of Therapy* (New York: Science House, 1971).
8 Seymour L. Halleck (in Reference 7) p. 94.

BIBLIOGRAPHY

"In the Service of the State: The Psychiatrist as Double Agent." Special Supplement, *Hastings Center Report* **8**, 2 (1978): 24 pp.

Deprogramming—A misuse of psychotherapy?

Psychotherapy leading to behavior modification can be a subtle form of brain control if it is misused. Ideas like man's social or political control via behavior modification appear to most people a scenario more properly relegated to the realm of science fiction, or if not there, then at least projected into some society far-off in time and place. But today throughout the United States and Europe, a form of behavior modification is being practiced on hundreds of free citizens against their will in the form of *deprogramming*. Deprogramming as it is presently practiced is coerced change of behavior and beliefs of devotees of many so-called cults, religious organizations judged to be undesirable.

Two sides of the issue can be discerned: (1) that of the parents and close relatives of the subject, along with lawyers, ministers, and some within the judicial system that interpret deprogramming as an ethical means to combat the alleged brainwashing and mind manipulation used by cults to attract and secure members; and (2) that of the cults themselves, along with other judges who view deprogramming as an affront to First Amendment freedoms.

Because deprogramming has been carried out within a religious context and instigated by parents of the follower, this questionable practice has been largely ignored by society. However, there are social and ethical ramifications here that demand attention. The important questions may not be religious at all but, rather, strike at the very core of our conceptions of human dignity and individual freedom!

What is deprogramming? Michael Mewshaw described it this way:

> the process amounts to little more than a methodical and sometimes violent attempt to exorcise, not Satan, but unpopular, misunderstood, and inarticulate notions about God.

Deprogramming as it is practiced is generally a three-step process: (1) bodily capture of the individual to be deprogrammed; (2) transportation of that person to some prearranged site, often across state-lines; and (3) the deprogramming session where the seized individual is held prisoner, isolated in a single room while deprogrammers work him/her over psychologically and emotionally. This part of the "therapy" is an effort at intense counter brainwashing and continues until the individual is "broken," i.e., deprogrammed. This may require several days or weeks to effect. The deprogrammed person then recants his/her former beliefs and is welcomed home again. Sometimes, they are enlisted to assist in the deprogramming of others.

Deprogramming of mainly young adults began in 1971 by Ted Patrick, former representative of community affairs for the governor of California. The effort has been formalized as the Freedom of Thought Corporation located in Tucson, Arizona(the organization was awarded tax-exempt status in 1976). The corporation charges between $10,000 and $25,000 to deprogram a single individual, defending its rather costly therapy on the grounds that a number of people are involved and a variety of physical facilities are required, including transportation over sometimes long distances.

Deprogramming has been given the name legal kidnapping because existing laws are used to carry out this nefarious procedure. However, these laws are being used for purposes other than their original intent. For example, conservatorship papers are used to obtain legal custody of persons to be deprogrammed. Conservatorship was initially designed to protect the aged and senile who were no longer able to conduct their own affairs or responsibly oversee their possessions (e.g., real estate). The law allowed next of kin or other responsible persons to act in their behalf. Persons under conservatorship are legally under the will of those given conservatorship. This can mean that such persons can be subjected to therapeutic treatment; in this case, deprogramming.

A second and higher law has also been implicated by deprogrammers—the law of proclaimed necessity. It is written by private parties and has precedence over statutory law. The defense offered by deprogrammers is that they are motivated to act in behalf of parents who have errant children and, therefore, whatever action is necessary to correct the errant behavior should be excused from legal constraints. Under this claim, kidnapping is permissible. It is well to understand, though, that these coerced individuals are not children, at least not legally; the majority are between the ages of twenty and thirty. The legal age in most states is eighteen years of age.

The legal issue involved with deprogramming is much unsettled. The First-Amendment right—to practice a religion of choice—is at stake. In a California case, the judge ruled that deprogramming was legally acceptable since he doubted that parents would willingly permit their children to be harmed. (The decision was later reversed by the State Appellate Court). A New York judge ruled quite the opposite, asserting that any attempt to circumvent the right to freedom of religion presents a clear and direct danger to Constitutional guarantees.

The means used to effect the deprogramming is another debatable concern. The deprogramming process involves long sessions of confinement and constant verbal bombardment, including abusive language and loud shouting. The psychological condition of the victim has been described as "learned helplessness" reinforced by the belief that counteraction or resistance is futile; he/she is trapped. Finally, the cult member begins to accept what is being told him/her in order to alleviate the helplessness. The philosophy of deprogramming is best described by Ted Patrick when he asserts that the purpose is to "bring the victim to the point of hysteria, anger, and hatred." Working to enter the mind through the emotions, the latter being placed in a state of turmoil, the victim can be told the "truth." Later, this is reinforced by rehabilitation.

Deprogramming is not only questionable legally but also ethically. Deprogrammers misuse the law to meet the desires of particular interest groups. They rely on coercion, hence, there is no voluntary or informed consent. The therapy that is administered is not the required medical treatment, at least not as it is practiced in the traditional form; conservatorship law allows medical care when dispensed for the welfare of the person. Deceit is often employed to entice the victim away from protective surroundings to facilitate the kidnapping. The marathon counter-brain-washing sessions affect the brain of the deprogrammees so as to block their capacity for reflection and exercise of freedom of choice. Personal autonomy is violated repeatedly. Deprogrammers are not trained physicians or psychiatrists and they lack an understanding of the potential for inflicting profound psychological damage either in the short- or the long-term. The whole deprogramming effort is to inculcate "right thinking." To allow one group to decide for another what constitutes correct thoughts is a dangerous precedent to be tolerated in a democratic society. Deciding for the group what is normal can have far-reaching consequences such as social engineering directed by a few for the many. The complete breakdown of human dignity during the period of interrogation is also an affront to some of our most highly prized human virtues.

Deprogramming also violates a person's right *not* to be a patient. Coerced treatment cannot be justified under the circumstances of deprogramming since the subject is not dangerous either to himself or others. The alleged charge that subjects are mentally incompetent has been rejected by the courts on several occasions.

As a free country, commitment to the absolute right of freedom to worship is a fundamental principle, the first guarantee included in the U.S. Constitution. Kidnapping for any reason is a serious crime, but kidnapping for the purpose of coercing a person to change his/her religious beliefs and behavior violates not only the person's right to worship as he/she chooses but the right to think and believe without coercion. If it is accepted that persons may be forced to change their religious beliefs, then no liberties of any person will be safe. When do persuasive methods become mind control with the correlated loss of freedom to choose? In the words of one analyst: "Deprogramming would revoke the Reformation, the Enlightenment, and the Bill of Rights."[1] A group with a different opinion on a subject, whether it be religious, social, political, or economic, is protected in the expression of that view by the Constitution. To insist that some things are normal and others are not, is to invite those bent on doing mischief into society's tent. It is best that we bury the idea before it buries our freedoms!

REFERENCE

1   Edd Doerr, "Deprogramming and religious liberty," *The Humanist* **37**, 1 (1977): 44–46. Much of the information for this section was obtained through personal interviews and listening to recorded tapes of persons who have either undergone and/or expressed themselves on the issue of deprogramming.

I especially wish to thank Scott Higdon, a member of "The Way Biblical Research and Teaching Ministry," founded by Dr. V. P. Wierwille.

BIBLIOGRAPHY

Other references that are related to this topic are the following:

Mewshaw, Michael, *Earthly Bread,* (New York: Random House, 1976).

Mewshaw, Michael, "Irrational behavior or evangelical zeal?" *Chronicle of Higher Education,* (October 18, 1976).

Patrick, Ted, *Let Our Children Go!,* (New York: Dutton, 1976).

Wierwille, V. P., "Our Times", *The Way Magazine,* (March/April, 1976).

9

MEDICINE
AND THE
PUBLIC INTEREST

HEALTH CARE IN AMERICA

The crisis in American medicine

We have heard a great deal during the last few years about the crisis in health care in the United States. This is a difficult concept to evaluate. Today, there are more persons working in health occupations than ever before, the increase even outstripping population gains. The delivery of health care today involves nearly 5 million people, making it the nation's third largest industry in terms of the nation's workforce.[1] There is an excess of hospital beds in the United States which according to some estimates may be as high as 200,000 on any given day.[2] It would seem that hospital facilities are more than adequate, ensuring every American almost any of the professional services required. Added to this is the observation that each year more persons have insurance coverage for some part or all of their medical bills. Nearly nine out of ten Americans are now covered by private health insurance as compared to seven out of ten in 1966.[3] Over 50 million people are now covered by Medicare and Medicaid. In 1950, funds spent for health were $12 billion. In 1972, over 80 billion dollars was expended, accounting for some 7.6 percent of the GNP. In 1975, health-care spending reached $118.5 billion. For the year 1976, $139.3 billion or over 8 percent of the Gross National Product was poured into the delivery and procurement of health care so that this single activity has become the number one consumer of financial resources in our country, surpassing even defense spending (which was 6 percent of GNP in 1976). The annual per capita cost for medical care now averages $547, or $1 out of every $9 of the average worker's salary.[4] A recent Department of Health, Education, and Welfare study projects our nation's health costs up nearly 40 percent to an astronomical $224 billion a year in 1980.[5] Such enormous expenditures for health might easily exceed 10 percent of the Gross National Product in the future. Indeed, the United States spends more money on health care than any other nation in the world; our national investment has increased at a spectacular rate over the past several decades. Today, medicine stands at its highest peak of achievement. Infant mortality in the United States has declined 12.7 percent since 1950; the death rate from heart disease has decreased 15 percent in the last six years. Yet, despite these impressive statistics and others that could be cited, it is commonly accepted that our medical system is in a state of crisis.

The emergency is not that the system faces imminent collapse but rather, is in the following: (1) The number of physicians and other personnel is still too few in many areas of the country. For example, the nationwide patient to physician ratio is about 550:1; in certain areas of Chicago the number is 1600:1. (2) The delivery of health care—again in certain areas—is grossly inadequate. A health study comparing poor and nonpoor areas in a metropolitan area found the poor had a 60 percent higher infant mortality rate, a 200 percent higher incidence of premature births, 200 percent more cases of TB, and a 100 percent higher incidence of cervical cancer.[6] (3) The inequality of health care—ours has been described as a system designed for the middle and upper classes (usually white middle and upper classes). Several studies have shown that blacks get worse treatment than whites even when they pay their own bills or have health insurance identical to that held by whites. The poor on Medicaid get even worse than the blacks who can pay.[7] (4) The costs of health services are rapidly rising. Health-care costs have been going up at nearly twice the rate of the government's Consumer Price Index, according to a recent report of the government's Council on Wage and Price Stability, an "extraordinary inflationary behavior that cries out for controls."[8] (5) The most important contemporary problems in modern medicine are philosophical and ethical rather than scientific or technological. Examples of the latter have been discussed throughout this text; other questions raised are: Whose life should be prolonged? How are the costs of medical care to be funded? Is health care a right or a privilege? Do physicians have the right to practice where they choose?

According to Rosemary Stevens, these problems are of recent origin.[9] In earlier times it made relatively little difference to the outcome of many conditions whether or not the patient obtained medical help. It is only fairly recently that medicine could deliver a product which was unambiguously beneficial. Ivan Illich selects the year 1913 as a turning point in the history of modern medicine. Around that time a patient began to have more than a 50–50 chance that treatment from a professional medical practitioner would provide any specific benefit.[10] What, after all, could the physician accomplish for anyone, rich or poor, a hundred or so years ago? Now, the scientific understanding of diseases, their origins and control, and the accompanying technological revolution has brought medicine into the public domain. The extension of medical care to the general public, even those in out-of-the-way places closely parallels the recent advances in medicine. Today, the problems that health care confronts lie not in the lack of achievement but in the widening gap between what *can* be done and what *is* being done. The crisis is in the delivery, not the potential for health care.

The reasons cited for this crisis are many. To name a few: shortage of primary care facilities for timely treatment of less severe medical problems; uneven distribution of services; ineffective use of allied health professionals to reduce the burdens on the doctor; the fee-for-service principle practiced in this country; the increasing number of third-party payment plans; the rise in malpractice suits; and the like. However, it is the cost of health-care delivery that has become the single most prominent battleground, and the financing of health care is one of the significant political issues today. A national health policy, including national health insurance, is a high priority government item. President Jimmy Carter is clearly committed to some form of national program with little or no out-of-pocket cost to the patient. Vice President Walter Mondale has long been identified as a supporter of national health insurance. The Democratic platform pledges expanded health care with federal assistance.

The rising cost of medical care

The growth in prices for health care are by now well known. Patients are getting less for their money than before. Medical care now consumes 8.6 percent of the nation's total output of goods and services, compared with only 5.9 percent in 1966 and 4.5 percent in 1950. Although the cost of living went up about 4.5 percent for the year 1976, hospitals raised their charges 11.8 percent and doctors boosted their fees 10.7 percent.[11] The average stay in a hospital today is from $154 to $175 a day compared to $48 in 1966 and $16 in 1950. This is a total increase of as much as 1000 percent in a little over twenty years—seven times the inflation rate when compared to the rest of the nation's economy!

But the most remarkable increases have come only within the past ten years. Figures reveal an extraordinary rise that picks up enormous momentum in 1966, just after the passage of Medicare programs for the old and Medicaid payments for the poor. Ever-rising costs for medical services have made necessary some alternative system to the one presently in operation. Some politicians are warning the medical profession that a public backlash is building that could give an added push to a government take-over of the medical industry. Much recent debate has centered on some form of national health insurance that would reduce financial burdens borne by many. But insurance by itself promises little relief to the many problems facing our health-care system, and in fact, may have little impact upon improving the quality of care. The immediate beneficiaries will be the profession itself for insurance is not a guarantee of service but a guarantee of payment. By further encouraging expenditures and by reducing still more the constraints of market mechanisms for holding down costs, the fires of inflation will be fueled all the more intensely. The system will also feed a federal and local bureaucracy who must maintain it.

In the past, the patient's pocketbook served as a brake on the demand for health care, especially the expensive kind; the quality of medical care one received was pretty much determined by the extent one was willing to pay for it. What the patient can afford for medical care acts in much the same way that a housewife's limited budget forces her to start buying chicken when the price of beef becomes too high, thus driving down the price of beef.

The practice of modern medicine in the United States got its start in the early part of this century and is still wedded to the dominant pattern of professional behavior begun in those early days—fee for service; independent private and solo practice; and very few public restraints (the doctor-knows-best policy). That kind of medical system encouraged the seller (the doctor) to tell the buyer (the patient) how much the buyer would have to pay and it also set many of the prices. Gross abuse from severe exploitation of this essentially monopolistic system was limited by the integrity of doctors, compassion for patients, and the fact that high prices would drive the patient to another doctor or to no doctor at all. Current medical practice, in many respects, preserves this earlier character, especially the *fee-for-service* principle under which the profit motive continues to control costs. Also, there exist within the medical profession many doctors who insist that they control their own destiny. The argument is that government or any other outside regulation stands contrary to good health care delivery. But to many these traditional views no longer fit the new conditions.

This is especially true in the case of ever-rising medical costs, where as a result of recent changes, largely brought about by private and federal health insurance plans, the traditional market restraints are being eliminated by so-called third-party payment of medical bills. Increasingly, one party gets the service, one party provides the service, and a third party gets the bills. When the major fraction of medical costs is borne by someone other than the patient, the demand for care is practically infinite. Doctors, hospitals, health equipment suppliers, pharmaceutical companies all are human, and it is far too easy to submit more charges and services than was the rule in former times. The current and widely publicized Medicaid scandals suggest that foxes are not very trustworthy at guarding chicken coops. Furthermore, fearing malpractice suits, many physicians are forced to practice medicine defensively, ordering more tests and procedures than they otherwise would. Insurance coverage also induces more and more people, on the basis of sometimes trivial symptoms, to opt for highly expensive and elaborate treatments such as extra tests, unnecessary surgery, and elaborate terminal care. Virtually no market constraints are left and prices continue to skyrocket. Without some control system to replace market mechanisms, continued inflation will make it more and more difficult for the vast majority of Americans to obtain adequate health care. Money still usually buys medical care in the United States today.

A second factor contributing to accelerating costs is medical technology itself. The explosion in medical technology has changed the very character of modern medicine. Growth in knowledge of the causes of disease has been a key element in the development of new technologies to intervene in the disease process. American engineering ingenuity has risen well to the task in developing a huge array of sophisticated medical gadgetry, such as computerized axial tomography, scanners, cobalt therapy units, blood gas analyzers, multiphasic screening systems, portable blood dialyzers, etc. There are probably few limits on technological development. Of course, all these processes require highly trained medical specialists and specialized technicians whose services are expensive.

The producers of medical equipment have done a superlative job in persuading health-care providers of the merits of their engineered and expensive merchandise. So that now, these represent a significant capital investment to the institution purchasing them—one axial scanner costs $500,000—and operational costs can only be reclaimed by using the machines and the services they provide. For example, it is hard to escape the conclusion that a significant proportion of surgery is attributable to the presence of surgeons rather than to the presence of disease. Less expensive services may be by-passed to increase utilization of the other more costly therapies. The operation of third party payments makes this whole affair palatable and, in fact, many times encourages the consumers to seek out this esoteric technology, as long as they do not have to pay for it![12] And besides, there is a psychological edge associated with complex technology. One would rather have his/her ills attended to by the newer technologies; they have a reassuring ring to them in this Space Age of sophisticated gadgetry.

Academic medicine also shares in promoting technological innovation. Substantial prestige follows the announcement of a new technique. The result has been a proliferation of new approaches and the development and/or acquisition of all kinds of sophisticated devices even when applications may not be practical or desirable. The principle seems to be that what is technologically feasible in medicine will be done, regardless of consideration of costs, utility, or ethics.[13]

Bureaucratization is a third factor providing impetus to the rise in costs without commensurate gains in quality. "The most mismanaged businesses in the country are hospitals" says Dr. Joseph H. Skom, president of the Illinois State Medical Society.[14] The ratio of administrative personnel to patients continues to rise; according to Dr. Skom, as many as two thirds of the people in administration are not needed. The proliferation of other hospital employees who provide no service to patients also is accelerating, for example, pharmacists at every nursing station and nurses who do nothing but paperwork. Hospital red tape and the cost of compliance to federal and state regulations absorb still more health care dollars; by one estimate the hospitals in the state of Florida spent $50 million to comply with one particular safety statute.

In general, what is perceived here can be expected to continue in the future. The collision between capitalist medicine, the growth of medical technology, and the enlargement of a medical bureaucracy, on the one hand, with the demands of the public for quality medical services at reasonable prices, on the other, is a forecast which is hard to escape and will probably occur during the next decade.

Health-care delivery and federal responsibility

It is quickly becoming evident that the government has a responsibility to ensure that all citizens have the wherewithal to meet rising costs, that health care be more equitably distributed, and that steps be taken to halt inflation. The means for doing so are, however, highly controversial. Debate over health-care financing and control of its delivery seriously challenge the historical prerogatives of the medical profession. The traditional position of medicine functioning as a part of the private market system is interpreted by many to mean the privilege to regulate itself and dictate its own destiny. Most of the medical profession stubbornly resists any change in the system that would involve departure from an item-by-item purchase of services on a fee-for-service basis or any alteration that would question the decisions of physicians. However, the system is being caught on all sides by forces calling for change, for example, the stratification of the profession into professional specialities, group and clinical practices, pay-in-advance health programs, more skeptical attitudes of patients toward physicians, changing social attitudes emphasizing among other things equal accessibility and distribution of health-care facilities, etc. These concerns are challenging the limits of medical professionalism; most especially the question of who should control the medical care system. The increasing rift between organized medicine and the public interest has led many, both in this country and abroad, to conclude that the delivery of health can no longer be a private matter to be purchased as any other market commodity. Rather, health care must be considered a necessary *social* resource like education or police protection. According to this view, the overall well-being of a nation depends on its measure of health; therefore, medical care must be open equally to all who need it and controlled by those who use it, i.e., the public.

A number of nations of the world have incorporated some of these ideals into their health-care systems. In this country, the most recent solution focuses on the issue of financing health care in the form of a national health insurance program. Needless to say, the issue of national health insurance raises heated debate between proponents and opponents, especially those opponents who contend that it would lead to sure and certain ruination of medical care in this country if we had "socialized medicine."

A Short History of Health Care Delivery in the U.S.

National health insurance is not a new issue; it has been under consideration in one form or another for more than fifty years. As early as 1910, even the American Medical Association was concerned with the financing of a national health insurance program. In 1916, its committee on social insurance recommended a system of national health insurance and drafted legislation for that purpose. However, soon after that, the AMA was taken over by a different group of physicians who adopted the long familiar stance of complete opposition to federal involvement in medical care delivery. From that time on the organization began to function as a special interest group for the profession, assuming almost complete control over the delivery of its services in the United States.[15]

With the world-wide Great Depression following World War I, many European countries enacted provisions for free medical care for its citizens or reimbursement for its costs. But because of the AMA's opposition, health insurance was never included in the package of social security legislation pushed through by Franklin Roosevelt in 1935. It is of historical interest to note that this legislation originally included provisions for national health insurance. Social security legislation that did pass made limited exceptions for welfare or charity benefits to those with special medical needs (i.e., the poor and the medically indigent).

In the long debates over health-care financing, dating from the early part of this century, the medical profession continued its strong defense of private practice in opposition to proposals for government-sponsored health insurance. The word *private* as used here had two meanings: (1) private practice as the opposite of government control or socialized medicine, and (2) professional privacy, or the privilege of a responsible profession to regulate itself and dictate its destiny. The official stand of the AMA, based on continuing support for these two propositions, was endorsement of voluntary and private health insurance. In the early 1940s, the Blue Cross and Blue Shield plans were developed, largely by physicians who recognized the importance of these plans both to themselves and to their patients. The American Hospital Association set up the Blue Cross plan while local physicians' societies sponsored Blue Shield plans. These plans covered only specified medical expenses and were available to those who paid for them, either personally or through employee benefit plans. Neither plan opposed the rising charges of hospitalization and doctors fees and, in fact, the plans were a major force encouraging cost increases. The poor were forced to depend on public welfare institutions, as they had done in the past. The public voice continued to raise the issue of health service costs and financing as year after year technological advances in medicine pushed costs inexorably higher.

There were a few efforts at facing the problem during and immediately after World War II. These were based largely on group practice prepayment plans and were among the first of the present Health Maintenance Organizations (HMO). Under HMO, for a fixed fee payable in advance, a local group or union contracts a medical facility for needed medical care. Included in this is around-the-clock services of a physician, emergency care when needed, in-patient and out-patient hospital services, etc. The name Health Maintenance Organization was given to prepaid medical plans during the Nixon administration. The Kaiser-Permanente Health Plan, centered in California and established during World War II, was the first major private prepaid group plan of medical care in the United States. It currently enrolls over 3 million people and serves as a model HMO. With this plan, doctors earn a yearly fee for the number of patients in their care under a system called capitation, whether the patient is sick or well. The efficiency and economy of the system is shown by the following statistic:[16] Kaiser plan patients spend an average of half a day in the hospital a year; the national average is double that, 1.2 days. Although the plans have had widespread promotion and a few have been around for sometime—the Kaiser-Permanente Plan has been in existence now for more than 35 years—there has been little nationwide acceptance of HMO's.

The movement toward a more comprehensive health-care strategy at the national level lost momentum in the 1950s. A major factor was the reluctance of physicians to develop or even participate in prepaid group practices (i.e., HMO). Many doctors justified their opposition to these programs on several grounds: (1) they were a threat to the face-to-face relationships between physician and patient that were felt necessary for good treatment; (2) the closed-panel characteristics of contractual group practice denied the patient a free choice of physicians; (3) there might be less incentive to try new therapies in group prepaid practice since efforts to economize might be the guiding principle; (4) the overall quality of health care would suffer in the production-line medicine of the HMO. Furthermore, the AMA warned physicians practicing in a group that they would be subject to closer ethical and professional scrutinizing by colleagues and the contracting organizations than would be the case in private practice.

Several court cases challenged the AMA advocacy of the free-choice principle. It was argued successfully before the courts that free-choice implies free-market competition. Free-market competition presupposes well-informed consumers who can make enlightened choices. In both cases these requisites did not hold, for the health-care industry as it was constituted was in fact a closed system; competition between practitioners was judged professionally unethical. Advertising is not permissible nor is consumer information generally available. Comparison shopping is not possible in a closed system. Further, it was held that the industry is monopolistic. Doctors themselves control almost all of the decisions, including most of those related to patient care costs. It was concluded, therefore, that if there is no free-market, then the principle of free choice of physicians cannot be upheld. These judgments led to a change in the official position of the AMA in 1959, to one that was more generally supportive of group practice. AMA's endorsement of group plans encouraged a new interest in their development in the mid-1960s.[17] However, most remained rather small in the number of people served.

In 1974, former president Gerald Ford signed the Health Maintenance Organization Act which aimed at encouraging the development of HMO plans through a system of federal grants. To date, fewer than a dozen have received federal approval and none have proved as effective as the Kaiser-Permanente Plan. The current lack of interest among most physicians and the public suggests that although these plans are likely to slowly undergo future growth, the reform of American medicine does not lie with HMO's.[18]

Another factor limiting the development of a national health policy during the 1950s was the political atmosphere of that time. The 1950s was the cold-war decade where the superiority of American individualism was set up emphatically against the absence of any freedom under Communism. In keeping with this, efforts were made during the Eisenhower years to upgrade the effectiveness of private health insurance plans rather than initiating new federal programs. However, for the poor, a public-private mix of funds was tried. The middle class was encouraged to rely on private health insurance, this in spite of the growing awareness that private health insurance could not adequately protect the population against rising medical costs. Several hundred million dollars were given to states in so-called "vender payments" under the Social Security Administration to provide medical services for the poor and the medically indigent. It was thought that further government intervention was unnecessary (the-best-government-is-the-least-government principle). Under this policy, so the government thinking went, most of the population would have some form of medical coverage.

As one might guess, this strategy did not work, largely because of the insurance gap, that gap between the actual cost of medical services and the portion covered by insurance policies. Even at its most efficient level, private health insurance managed to cover no more than a third of the total medical bills of private patients. Exclusions and restrictions, the economic havoc on a family of catastrophic illness, and the inflating effect of third party payments hindered millions of citizens from obtaining adequate health care. As annual medical costs rose from $84 per capita in 1950 to $250 in 1967, out-of-pocket expenditures assumed a greater and greater proportion of the load. This especially handicapped low income and fixed income (i.e., retirement) households—an inequality that is characteristic of any inflationary spiral.

By the beginning of the 1960s, it became more and more apparent that something had to be done. The issue of federally sponsored health insurance was still in the government mill. A different tactic was initiated in the late 1950s by both Republicans and Democrats. The strategy chosen was not intended as a general solution to the economic quagmire of pay-power outstripping cure-power but was another patchwork job aimed to assist only those who suffered most, namely, the elderly living on fixed incomes.

It turns out, of course, that the elderly are twice as likely to suffer from chronic health problems as younger people; they experience two and a half times more restricted activity; and they endure substantially more acute illnesses. Yet, fully half of the elderly were not covered by any type of health insurance and others were only partially or inadequately insured. Between 1957 and 1959 a national survey of old people, excluding those in institutions, found that half of those suffering from bronchitis and visual impairments were not under medical attention; 43 percent of the cases of paralysis were unattended; and over 40 percent of the hearing impairments were not under medical supervision.[19] It is of interest to note that as late as 1958 the AMA officially condemned health payments through Social Security as "unwise, unnecessary, and not in the public interest."[20]

So rather than restructuring a badly inadequate health system, the country selected the option termed income maintenance. This protected the economic circumstance of those who lived on retirement incomes by assuming for them a part or all of the cost of medical care. In practice this was nothing more than the old welfare routine polished up a bit and extended to cover more of the eligible elderly.

By 1960, compulsory national hospital insurance for the aged became a major political issue. A spate of bills was introduced into Congress (e.g., the Forand bill, HEW proposals, etc.), from which emerged a compromise measure, the Kerr-Mills Act of 1960, the forerunner of Medicaid. This legislation provided both federal matching grants to states for medical payments under Old Age Assistance programs and services to the elderly medical indigent who met specified qualifications. In practice, this act also was simply an extension of long-practiced, existing welfare medical programs. (The Kerr-Mills Act was supported by the AMA.) The procedural details set up by the legislation destined it at best to only partial success and at worst as an unhappy failure. But then, no one seriously pretended that this law was the final answer to meeting health needs of the elderly. The best that it could accomplish was a temporary holding action until more effective legislation could be enacted. The broader question of adequate health care for all Americans was not even touched.

President Kennedy strongly endorsed hospital insurance for the aged in his message to Congress in 1961, but again congressional efforts to enact it were unsuccessful. Major health insurance legislation was not passed until the burst of social reform which followed the assassination of President Kennedy and Lyndon Johnson's election to the presidency. With the Democratic landslide in 1964, the composition of Congress changed dramatically in favor of federally supported domestic policies. Included here was a turning in favor of some form of compulsory hospital insurance under Social Security. Such a proposal became an important inclusion in President Johnson's Great Society program. Once more, strong efforts were made to minimize direct government intervention. The AMA, in a last-ditch stand against hospital insurance through Social Security, developed its own Eldercare proposal. This called for a state-federal program to subsidize private insurance policies and hospital, doctor, and drug bills for the elderly. Bettercare (under Republican sponsorship) submitted a federal program whereby the elderly would be encouraged to contribute part of the premium of a voluntary health insurance program with public funds subsidizing the remainder. Various other bills suggested tax-credits, deductions for health insurance premiums, expansion of the floundering Kerr-Mills program, and the like. The struggles between those who wanted health insurance as part of a general social insurance for all as a matter of right and those who wanted it to be a form of welfare for those who could qualify, between those who wanted it federally administered and those who preferred local control, and between those who wanted universal coverage and those who thought only specific groups with genuine need should be protected was partially resolved with the enactment of amendments to the Social Security Act in 1965. This brought into being Medicare and Medicaid programs. Medicare offers compulsory hospital insurance through Social Security, subsidizes voluntary health insurance for medical bills for those 65 years and older, and provides expanded programs of benefits for the medically indigent. This program was in large part federally administered. Medicaid is a form of welfare for low-income younger persons and is administered by the state, supported with federal matching funds. As a result of these two programs all elderly became beneficiaries and the poor had some portion of their medical costs paid for by the government. The two programs are basically financing methods which reimburse the patient or pay his medical costs directly to the provider. For example, under Medicare, for a single illness a patient has 60 days in the hospital free, except for a $124 deductible, and 30 additional days at $26 a day. For physicians' services, Medicare pays 80 percent of all reasonable charges except a $60 deductible each calendar year (1977 schedule).

The enactment of these amendments has been hailed as landmark legislation for in the long debates leading up to their passage, the general public, not the professional voice, determined how health services were to be financed. The political position of the AMA from the 1940s to the mid-1960s did effectively delay legislation and, in fact, stood in opposition to the political and social climate of the times. But the passage of Medicare and Medicaid, at least in theory, marked the beginning of a new era—direct federal intervention in health care programs in the United States, including involvement in the development of health-care facilities, educational institutions, and payment plans for certain segments of our population. All of these have set precedents for continuing federal involvement. Accompanying the increasing governmental role in health care was a resurgence of various human-rights movements (e.g., women, blacks, special problem groups, etc.). There were efforts to establish as rights certain concepts of medical care and public health that formerly had been seen only as privileges. Among other things, the federal government funded neighborhood health centers in poor and rural areas as part of this movement. In 1971, the continued shortage of medical care, especially in rural areas, led to the development of a National Health Service Corps under the U.S. Public Health Service.

Entering the decade of the 1970s, the major movement has been toward attempting to control costs while maintaining quality. In January of 1975, former president Ford signed a broad form of health planning legislation: the Health Planning and Resources Development Act. The objectives of this legislation were the following: (1) to promote equal access to comprehensive quality care for all Americans; (2) to use public financing insofar as is necessary to achieve this goal; (3) to reorganize the health care system as consistent with the first objective and at reasonable costs; and (4) to accomplish planning under consumer, not professionally dominated agencies. The law also established a network of local health planning agencies across the country, each serving up to three million people to oversee the use of federal health funds in each area. One of the aims of the local agencies is to implement some sort of cost control over medical costs. The bill also creates a set of guidelines for health care which the localities, with the prodding of the new local agencies, would try to achieve. Although not explicitly stated, the new program is intended to provide a framework to review federal spending for national health insurance that is expected to be enacted soon. It is hoped that by having a monitoring program set up and ready to go, the gross abuses of the kind accompanying start-up of the Medicaid and Medicare programs can be prevented.*[21] The intent of the National Health Planning Act was not to close the gap between what is and what ought to be done, but rather, the intended function was to bring about planning which would begin to close the gap; it was at best a beginning.

The federal government is in the midst of yet another experiment, this one to determine how the country can cope with the costs of catastrophic illnesses. The experiment started in July of 1972 with an amendment to the Social Security law giving Medicare coverage to virtually anyone in the throes of end-stage renal disease. The program expenditure for the first year was about $250 million and included dialysis services for about 13,000 patients at a cost of from $10,000 to $40,000 per patient. It is estimated that 8000 to 10,000 persons may be added annually. Some have guessed that the National Renal Dialysis Program, when it is fully operational in 1983 aiding some 60,000 people, will involve an outlay in the neighborhood of a billion dollars per year. The thinking in many circles expects that the issue that started with the kidney will expand to take in other catastrophic illnesses, too. Hemophilia groups have pressured Congress for complete coverage of treatment at a possible annual cost of $150 million. The perfecting of artificial hearts at a price of $35,000 apiece could add another $1.75 billion or so. The question foremost in many minds will be how to do this without going bankrupt.

It is of course true that we operate in a system of finite resources. The trade-offs here are such that money funneled into expensive, high medical technologies which save few lives would not be available for other purposes; for instance, for less-costly medical treatment or preventive care that might save many lives, or for important areas of research that would get at the causes of these diseases and that would result in medical intervention that would be less expensive.

Opportunities for complete reappraisal of the health delivery system are being offered to the country. However, in the overall, our national leaders have been slow in doing anything about it. The problems still persist, problems such as the continuing rise in the cost of health-care services and deficiencies in its delivery in various sectors of our population. The conclusion is still glaring: there remains no national health policy of the kind enjoyed by many European countries for several decades already.

---

* Medicaid, the state-run program of medical insurance for the poor, was originally to cost the government $258 million in a single year; but the estimate proved to be woefully wrong. For example, in 1974 alone the federal government paid half of the total cost of the $10.5 billion program. Medicare, which offers benefits to the nation's elderly, cost much more than expected and stimulated a sharp rise in the expense of treatment. It has become the target of much misuse as instance after instance of cheating is uncovered. As one critic pointed out, "fraud is a way of life with Medicaid." Hopefully the country can learn from that experience, and the National Health Planning Act may preclude a repetition of these events.

The delivery of health care—the options

Deficiencies in American health services are evident everywhere: the low- and middle-income family going into hock to pay hospital bills in cases of catastrophic illness or accident; self-serving expansionism of hospitals in pushing for further capital developments without consultation with other institutions or assessing local needs; the lack of home-care facilities; the social discrimination of large city outpatient clinics; the inadequate care of the poor and some ethnic groups; the use by the middle and upper classes of independent specialists and facilities, thereby commanding a disproportionate share of medical resources; great amounts of resources lavished on costly equipment and facilities which save few lives but deprive many others of simple medical treatment or preventive care; absence of any medical care in some rural areas; the wretched conditions and lack of staff in many municipal hospitals and public institutions where hospital services, particularly in some major cities, are reaching the breakdown point; the lack of definition of who is eligible for public hospital care that varies from community to community; accusations against pharmaceutical companies which promote and profit from drugs which are overpriced, useless, or even harmful; surgeons performing unnecessary surgery as reported by the House Oversight and Investigations subcommittee to the effect that approximately 2.4 million needless operations were performed in the country in 1974 at a cost of about $3.9 billion; some unscrupulous physicians and related health care personnel who have depleted the coffers of Medicaid, Medicare, and other insurance plans in unethical and sometimes illegal ways; and so forth.

These details could be increased many times over but a single theme would still sound through: The reform of the health system runs headlong into the entrenched interests of a great number of powerful constituencies, including physicians, hospitals, health insurance agencies, and the pharmaceutical industry. Most state and local governments have demonstrated little capacity for effective planning in the provision of health services; the real power still resides in the nongovernmental spheres mentioned above. Doctors themselves control almost all decisions, from the decision about hospitalization to the decision whether to prescribe drugs by brand or generic name. Most patient-care costs are generated by doctors' decisions.

Much current thinking insists that these conditions can only be alleviated if the federal government takes decisive action. Congress is in a position to legislate with respect to health. Precedent has been set, for example, by Medicare and Medicaid legislation which enlisted the federal government as an active participant in the delivery of health care as well as a number of other government health-care programs described earlier.

Those who believe far-reaching changes in the organization of health services are necessary not only to control costs but also to ensure equity insist that these four broad components must be included:

1 Every citizen, whatever his/her economic status, place of residence, color, age, or other considerations, will have guaranteed access to adequate medical care.

2 Guaranteed access is a public responsibility with the ultimate responsibility residing at the federal level.

3 Substantial funding by the federal government will be required.

4 Individuals within the program have a responsibility to maintain, insofar as possible, their own health, necessitating the establishment of a strong health education program (It is worth noting here that a recent study conducted by the Institute of Medicine reveals that the educational level of parents is the single most important ingredient in the health status of children).

However, the current political attitude at the federal level still favors a considerably more conservative strategy taking the form of some sort of national health insurance (NHI). Although several attempts have been made to write this legislation, especially in the 1974 Congressional session, differences between the executive and the legislative branches, between Republicans and Democrats, and among interest groups have so far stalled enactment. Critics of National Health Insurance submit that it is simply a method of collecting funds and disbursing them on a country-wide basis. Its purpose is obstensibly to reduce *financial* barriers to access; the old inadequacies and problems would remain. Any NHI law passed would address primarily two issues: financial coverage for catastrophic illness and some broadening of entitlements for ambulatory care (i.e., outpatient facilities). It could continue to sit on the top of a chaotically organized health-delivery system without changing or modifying a thing; the old inequities can continue unperturbed!

A common component in the several plans already submitted in Congress makes health insurance compulsory for everyone. Funds would be collected from the employee and/or employer and matched with funds from the public treasury. The government would act as the insurer. In effect, the government simply replaces or supplements the services now provided by private companies. Several of these bills contain proposals for making health services more widely available, assigning physicians to underserved areas, reducing inequities, emphasizing health-maintenance organizations (HMO), establishing professional standards review organizations (PSRO), and giving the federal government a voice in regulating some aspects of the health-care system, such as quality and cost. It is not very likely that many of these latter propositions will meet with legislative or executive approval, although PSROs were brought to reality by the passage of Public Law 92-603 in 1972. However, the effectiveness of professional review has not as yet been overly successful in controlling costs or ensuring quality either, probably because the control of the practice of medicine still resides essentially in the hands of physicians. It still remains to be seen whether or not PSROs can be an effective agency for regulation.

The opposition to NHI, however, is concerned not with the matter of regulation *per se* but whether regulation is best exerted by the private or the public sector. This is a resurfacing of the old question, Who should control the medical care system? Consumer protection and public accountability have become the by-words in medical matters as they have in many other areas of public concern; this is exemplified by Ralph Nader's Public Citizen's Health Research Group. Repeatedly, they, the popular press and congressional subcommittees led by Senator Edward Kennedy's Senate Health Subcommittee, call the public's attention to overbuilt hospitals, unnecessary surgery, overpricing of pharmaceuticals and unethical or illegal practices of physicians and health institutions. The medical profession counters with last-ditch efforts to preserve its historical status of independence as exemplified by a recent House of Delegate's action (December 1976). In that action, the AMA, after deep and controversial debate, endorsed a national health insurance program. The program, among the most conservative of the several health insurance proposals suggested, included using the existing private insurance industry and making participation voluntary for employees. It reflects AMA thinking by calling for minimum federal involvement, no added Social Security tax for funding, and voluntary participation. AMA president Dr. Richard Palmer warned the delegate that the election of Jimmy Carter could mean trouble for American medicine based on the president's known support for a national health insurance program. He emphasized that the AMA must have its own version to fight for its point of view, which is minimum federal control.[22]

Some have concluded that even if NHI is enacted, such legislation will have only a minimal effect on how the health-care system operates and will result in only a marginal improvement in the quantity and quality of the national health picture. In the final analysis, NHI still only addresses itself to the purchase of health care from the providers who can continue to deploy themselves and act pretty much as they did in the past. The national experience with Medicare and Medicaid does not inspire confidence. If NHI were enacted, the prospect is that more pressure would be put on the health-care system for more cost increases. The price tags of several bills introduced into Congress range from under $10 billion to over $80 billion, with some estimates going as high as $100 billion annually. Further, it isn't likely that any new legislation can correct the severe maldistribution of health manpower.

We have a medical system that is highly technical, disease-oriented, largely fragmented and uncoordinated, and that uses methods of organization that often seem to be based on private gain rather than on the most effective or efficient attainment of the public good. To provide insurance coverage for continuation of the present system will perpetuate existing inadequacies and will not provide a mechanism for improvement in the health-care system. In both instances—attempts at regulating cost and the deployment of manpower—runs counter to the free enterprise system.

Still another objection to NHI states that it will continue to foster a dual system of health care by setting baseline standards of payments. Any citizen still may privately purchase additional care over and above what is established as baselines. Under such a system, the old inequities will continue to exist.

It has been argued that anything less than complete federalization will not result in the basic reforms required. The suggested alternative to NHI is National Health Service (NHS), and here we are certainly not without precedent. The world trend is toward putting the health-care system under more and more government control. Table 9.1 shows the systems which exist in sixteen countries for payment of general practioners and specialists in the context of health insurance or a national health service. NHS is characterized by large contributions from the general treasury, nationalization of some or all of the health facilities (e.g., hospitals), and some systemization of the health delivery system. Proponents insist that NHS will provide both financing of care as well as regulation of the structure of the system. Public monies will be put to the task of providing adequate health care for all, something that private money and health-care professionals have not been able or willing to accomplish. Anthony Lewis' words describing the English nationalized system admirably sums up the view of those favoring a NHS:

Table 9.1

	Type of System*	Payments of specialists		Payment of general practitioners	
		Unit	Method	Unit	Method
Cyprus	Service	Salary	Direct	Salary	Direct
Egypt	Service	Salary	Direct	Salary	Direct
France	Insurance	Fee	Reimbursement	Fee	Reimbursement
Germany (Federal Republic)	Insurance	Fee	Direct	Fee	Direct
Great Britain	Service	Salary	Direct	Capitation	Direct
Greece	Insurance	Salary	Direct	Salary	Direct
Israel	Insurance	Salary	Direct	Salary	Direct
Italy	Insurance	Salary	Direct	Capitation, fee	Direct
Lebanon (until late 1960s)	None	Fee	Private	Fee	Private
The Netherlands	Insurance	Fee, case	Direct	Capitation	Direct
Poland	Service	Salary	Direct	Salary	Direct
Spain	Insurance	Capitation	Direct	Capitation	Direct
Sweden	Insurance	Salary, fee	Reimbursement	Fee	Reimbursement
Switzerland	Insurance	Fee	Direct, reimbursement	Fee	Direct, reimbursement
Turkey	Insurance	Salary	Direct	Salary	Direct
U.S.S.R.	Service	Salary	Direct	Salary	Direct

* Payment Plans for the Delivery of Health Care, in Special Issue on National Health Insurance 27 (4) April, 1974. Reprinted by permission. (F.A.S. 1974)

At its best, American medicine is superb, as British doctors often admiringly remark. But too few Americans get the best. That is why the United States is down further than might be expected in world health tables, not only in comparison with Britain. In infant mortality, for example, a 1969 United Nations report showed twenty-two countries with a lower rate than ours.

The characteristic, generous answer to such evident national failings is to spend more money. But we know by now that in the medical field, that alone is no solution.

What needs to be changed is the system of delivering medical care to the individual American. It is, as a British medical writer put it, "a desperately inefficient as well as a heartless way of bringing the benefits of modern medicine to the population; despite its wealth the health of America is poor."[23]

In spite of its technological superiority, the United States does lag behind other Western industrialized countries in major health indices. The rate of infant mortality has not fallen as rapidly in the United States as in other industrialized countries: The U.S. rate of approximately 17 deaths per 100 live births in the first year of life ranks far below Sweden (10/1000) and the Netherlands (11/1000) and the U.S. rate for nonwhite infants is still at the high figure of 30/1000. Life expectancy at birth in the United States is 67 for males and 75 for females while in Sweden, life expectancy is at 72 and 77 respectively. This ranks the United States seventeenth for male longevity and tenth for female life expectancy. In heart disease, Americans rank twentieth worldwide.[24]

There are forces within our society which lead to the hope that some of the problems observed can be addressed more effectively. To return to a point made earlier: Health care is a valuable and necessary *social* resource. Medicine, contrary to professional opinion and as recent legislation submits, is "not above politics." It seems worth emphasizing the oft-used axiom: Society never moves backward in time. In the matter of health benefits, once full services are offered, resistance from the majority prevents reduction or moderation. The significance of this observation for the present debate is substantial. Numerous precedents have been set by federal decree. Any health service which offers less than a decent standard of care for every American is simply no longer acceptable, nor is it feasible. Even if more federal control is instituted, the fact remains that we would be among the last major industrial nations to socialize a vital function like health care. For all our fears about socialized medicine, no major nation who has enacted one has yet to disassemble its socialist health-care system or face a health crisis with which it could not deal.

The ethical and social issues

To this point, the chapter has described the historical context for pending and future legislation dealing with the delivery of health care in the United States. The objective is to provide the student a background to more effectively follow events related to this very sensitive issue and to better judge their ethical worth. The history behind present efforts can provide valuable insights. There are, naturally, a host of ethical and social issues related to these historical changes. A few of these are:

1　Is health care a right or privilege?

2　Do physicians have the right to practice where they choose?

3　How much public accountability should be required?

4　Will a regulated system interfere with the traditional patient-physician relationship?

5　Will quality suffer?

6　What new challenges might federal health-care delivery present to the concept of humanness? of individual freedom? of justice?

Another important issue is the question: Will national health policy with rigid government control bias medical care and research? According to the Institute of Medicine the immediate effect of making services freely available to the public is that more and more people opt for highly expensive and elaborate forms of treatment (e.g., extra lab tests, unnecessary surgery, expensive terminal care, etc.). This would place a demand on these services requiring their expansion. In the long run, medical care could be biased in favor of technology-intensive procedures. These activities, in turn, would drain away funds and manpower from lower-cost primary care. A further skewing of medical practice may occur if money funneled into the development of these technologies would preclude research into the causes of diseases, where a not infrequent payoff is the discovery of less-expensive therapies. (For example, one can only wonder how many billions of dollars the nation would now be spending on iron lungs if research for the prevention of polio had not been done.)

Turning our attention to but one of these issues, the matter of health care as a right versus health care as a privilege, we find that much controversy continues to abound. It can be considered a first-order consideration for the reason that the national response to the proposition will determine in large measure the health policy that will be adopted.

Gene Outka writes in "Social Justice and Equal Access to Health Care" that at least five positions can be distinguished in terms of the delivery of health care.[25] These are:

1. to each according to his/her merits or desserts;
2. to each according to his/her societal contribution;
3. to each according to his/her ability to acquire whatever is freely available to others in the open market place of supply and demand;
4. to each according to his/her essential needs;
5. similar treatment in similar cases.

He concludes that the most desirable societal good is the assurance of comprehensive health services for every person irrespective of income and geographic location (number 4). Each of the other positions listed present difficult problems of judgment and/or the danger of ethical abuse.

In order to discuss the question of right to health care, the concept of rights must be evaluated, for a position on the nature of rights will specify an attitude. Robert M. Sade defines right as "freedom of action" and submits the right to life as the beginning point to all other rights; each has a right to his/her own life.[26] Three corollaries are implied here: (1) the right to select those values one deems necessary to sustain personal life; (2) the right to exercise judgment over courses of action required to achieve these values; and (3) the right to dispose of these values once acquired in any way one chooses. In a free society, one can exercise these rights by selecting a means of producing economic values (goods and services). He/she is free to exchange these with others who are similarly free to trade. For example, the bread baked by the baker belongs to him and he is free to dispose of it in any way he sees as appropriate without others infringing on this right. Translating this interpretation of rights to health services, the concept of medical care as a right is immoral because it coerces the dispenser (the physician) to a course of action which may not be consistent with his/her own values. The medical practitioner is denied his/her own life and the freedom of action to support it. Accordingly, Dr. Sade suggests, medical care is neither a right nor is it even a privilege; it is a service that is provided by doctors to people who wish to purchase it. He contends that if health care is a right, then people own the service without their being given it by the only ones who could bestow it, that is, the doctors. If health care is a service, then doctors are free to dispense it in a manner they judge appropriate much like the baker who dispenses the fruits of his labor—bread.

Rebuttals to Dr. Sade's argument were fast and furious following its publication. Essentially, opposition insisted that medical care is not like any other professional service for several reasons. Rising public expectation will not accept a "pay or else" position any longer. It may have been palatable in long-ago times but it certainly is no longer true today. Also, the doctors themselves are not self-educated but obtain a great deal of financial aid from the state in the form of medical schools and professional opportunities. Neither are physicians today autonomous individuals free to do as they please; a variety of corporate bodies play major parts in medical care for example, hospital boards, medical societies, accrediting bodies, insurance companies, labor unions, businesses, health and welfare funds, and citizen's groups. Even bakers of bread are not completely free to follow any action they choose, and it must necessarily be so if we desire a stable society. Further, Dr. Sade's view of rights are bourgeois freedoms and rights reserved for the ruling class. Free enterprise as a freedom of the ruling class to do what they want to do is no longer acceptable; profit motives and marketplace mechanisms are totally out of touch with the contemporary philosophies of equity and humanitarian concern.

Examining another position on the right to medical care, lawyer Charles Fried points out that rights invoke entitlements, by which he means that persons not having the stated entitlements can demand them regardless of others' opinions or desires.[27] Included here is the concept of equality, that is, whatever entitlement one individual or group can claim, others can too. Thus, the right to health care means that all can obtain that which only the most wealthy can afford. And, of course, he submits that this is nonsense for no country can finance a medical care system where this is practicable. For example, he cites the instance of artificial hearts. If they are perfected, they will certainly be very expensive to install and maintain. Then, will the thousands who could benefit from them be entitled to this therapy under the principle of equal access? The answer is clear for no government has the wherewithal to provide them. Rather than complete accessibility to health care, Fried offers as an alternative the right to a *decent standard* of care for all, which does not insist on the best available principle. As with education, housing, or legal assistance, rights do not imply the best; persons are free to purchase more solely determined on their ability to pay; and we do not find this morally repugnant in a free society as long as adequate provisions are made for those who are in a lesser economic position. Rather than obscuring the issue by debating only the two extremes—rights without qualification and medical care as a privilege—it would be in our best interests to determine what is a decent minimum of health care available to all and a way to provide this. David Mechanic, medical sociologist, is of the opinion that a decent standard of care for every American is possible without a complete revision of the present system or by excessive federal spending but it cannot be done within the context of our present system.[28]

It is clear that the issue of health care in America is far from resolved. The road before us is a difficult one between antagonists and proponents of a more satisfactory system. As in most legislation directed toward social policy, change will come slowly. It will be important for the public and for a variety of specialists to become knowledgeable and involved about this issue so that whatever policy is adopted will help reduce the societal gap between medical knowledge that is known and medical knowledge that is applied.

COST-EFFECTIVE HEALTH CARE

Money and health

Since the beginning of the Industrial Revolution there has been a tremendous increase in the mass of knowledge (science) and in the development of new products and methods (technology). In medical practice, too, as noted earlier, no aspect has escaped scientific attention, and for virtually all human diseases there are improved modes of diagnosis and therapy that have transformed medicine from an art to a sophisticated complex science. These methods have resulted in the most expensive medical tradition and the most advanced medical technology (with the possible exception of Sweden) in the world.[29] Despite the many remarkable achievements— or perhaps because of them—there are problems. What has been produced is a medical care system which has been characterized as hospital-centered, highly technological, disease-oriented, and therapy-focused rather than one that is health-oriented. Dr. Mary Culhane McLaughlin, upon becoming health commissioner in the city of New York in 1969, described the situation this way:

> We haven't been able to do effective preventive care and early treatment, so over and over we spend thousands when for a couple of hundred dollars we could have kept the patient out of the hospital and helped him more besides.[30]

If the present patterns of medical care are followed, there will be increasing emphasis on technological medicine with rapidly escalating costs but with little or no increase given to primary care or preventive medicine. The problem throughout this strategy is that there is a limit to the portion of the GNP that can be allocated to health care. Financial crisis is a very real threat if our national program involves only the infusion of additional federal dollars to support larger coverage. Economizing in health care is probably possible only by radically reorienting the pursuit of health. Herman M. Somers, a Princeton economist who has testified extensively in Congress on the economics of health insurance, says "every other country in the world with NHI (National Health Insurance) has found that unless they control costs, their medical bills can take up the entire GNP."[31]

There is an extremely important lesson coming from the discussions of cost and National Health Insurance. The proposals for NHI frequently create the impression that individual health is a commodity to be purchased just like one buys groceries or a TV set. NHI, by making medical services more generally available by paying the cost will somehow bring about a healthier America. This is only partly right. Certainly, if minor ailments go unattended, all too often a major illness follows and the chance for a cure may be reduced or lost. But the thrust of opinions of a number of experts is that plowing still more money into our present health-care system will effect at best only a marginal improvement in the quality of life and the improvement of health. The task force on consumer health education of the National Conference on Preventive Medicine in June of 1975 corroborated this judgment:

> It appears that therapeutic medicine, important as it is, may have reached a point of diminishing returns. The 12 to 15 percent increases that we are adding to our hundred billion dollar health care bill each year—even the portion that is not caused by inflation—apparently have only a marginal utility.[32]

The public opinion that still larger expenditures for health care as a way to achieve greater health is a questionable assumption. Consider: During the early part of this century life expectancy in the United States increased, but it reached a plateau in 1954. In 1967, W. H. Fortes explored the relationship between national expenditures for health and actual results. He concluded that the country could halve or double total expenditures without changing longevity appreciably.[33]

Not only will simply pumping more money into the present health-care system be ineffective in creating a healthier America, but the present disease, crisis-oriented approach is likely to have far less significant impact on health status than is generally assumed. Rene Dubos, among others, emphasized that while the physician does heal through such processes as reduction of fractures, the surgical removal of diseased or malfunctioning tissues and organs, and the use of drugs ranging from antibiotics for the treatment of infection to major tranquilizers for mental illness to synthetic hormones, much disease is, in fact, self-limiting. Perhaps as much as eighty percent will correct itself given a conducive environment. Virulence, it seems, depends not solely on the ministrations of the health-care practitioner but in great part upon social, economic, and cultural conditions. The delivery of health care is most effective when applied to certain identifiable conditions of disease for which there is information as to efficacy. But contrasted with socio-environmental factors which affect health, medicine plays a minor role though it continues to be cast for the lead.

To a large extent, we are today approaching the logical limits of curative and restorative medicine as noted in Fig. 9.1. Since 1967, most of the deaths in the age range 10 to 70 either are due to degenerative diseases or are fatalities arising from accidents, suicide, or homicide. Having dealt with the infectious scourges of a previous generation effectively, the big killers today are coronary heart disease, cancer, and stroke. The current frontier of medicine lies in dealing with the chronic diseases, but it is among these diseases that the practice of medicine has had the least impact and treatment of them is often very costly. Medicine has contributed much to the preservation of life and human longevity by successfully combatting infectious diseases and by stressing the importance of proper nutrition, but in contrast it has not been able to do much more than maintain persons afflicted with what some have called the diseases of civilization (heart disease, cancer, stroke). The easier infectious diseases whose treatment has been proven cost-effective have been brought under control; on the other hand, the treatment of degenerative diseases is not only costly it is not uniformly successful. If our direction continues to favor sophisticated therapies, with concentration of resources on expensive equipment and facilities where relatively few lives may be prolonged, then medical breakthroughs in the years ahead can have no other effect than forcing the costs of medical care even higher and encouraging physicians to still more specialized practices requiring new modes of treatment and highly technological hospital care. According to a recent Rand Cor-

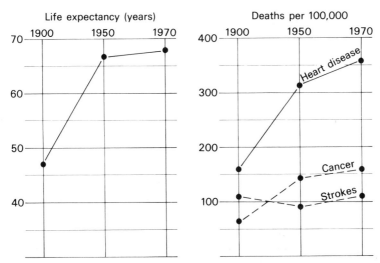

Fig. 9.1 *A comparison of the causes of death in the United States at various times during the twentieth century. (From Ralph C. Greene, "Ethical culture and physical culture." Reprinted by permission from* The Humanist, *March/April 1977, p. 37.)*

poration report, "It is clear that decisions on investment in biomedical research (and new modes of therapy) will have important implications concerning investment in a national health insurance program. Such cross-linkages deserve more attention than has been given to them in the past."[34]

The proposals presently being considered, for example NHI, take for granted the wisdom of our current approaches to the pursuits of health and thereby advocate that in the future we will get more of the same. The programs almost entirely ignore the question of whether what we now do in health is what we should be doing. By embracing without qualification the "no fault" principle—I can't help it if I get ill— the important proposition of personal responsibility for the status of one's own health is ignored. Further, to spend thousands of dollars on medical care that attempts to rescue an individual from the results of a faulty living pattern may actually contribute to a worsening rather than an improvement in our nation's health for it tends to foster the belief among the public that doctors can cure anything from hangnails to cancer. As has been stated doctors and public health officials have only limited power to improve our health. Health is not a commodity which can be delivered in discrete units nor is it something one purchases, especially after it becomes malfunctional. Medicine can help only those who help themselves. Pursuing the best health policy for the American people may mean striking a proper balance between government guarantees of an efficient health-care system to everyone and encouraging, if not insisting upon, individual responsibility for health maintenance. Such a system must involve total treatment, with an emphasis on both prevention and treatment.

Personal responsibility for health—An ethical imperative

In a new, long-range health-care blueprint issued by HEW, the *Forward Plan for Health, Fiscal Years 1977–1981*, it is urged that far greater attention be given to the preventive aspects of medical care.

> . . . . . only by preventing disease from occuring, rather than treating it later, can we hope to achieve any major improvement in the nation's health.

The authors of the plan go further to state:

> Many of today's health problems are caused by a variety of factors not susceptible to medical solutions or to direct intervention by the health practitioner. This poses a dilemma for health professionals in defining a proper role for themselves in prevention of disease and a practical problem for those concerned with setting the boundaries of health planning.

Dr. Frederick C. Swartz stated before a U.S. Senate Subcommittee on Aging that "our greatest health problem is in the physical fitness of the nation. Here the answer is the simplest and cheapest, has the greatest application and its reflection on the reduction of morbidity and mortality rates would be immediate and tremendous. It is entirely possible that a well-practiced physical fitness program begun early in life would increase life expectancy by 10 years. . . . "[35]

A powerful bloc of opinion and expertise now supports the proposition that, since socio-environmental factors are the single most important determinants of health status, relatively small sums could be spent which would sharply reduce disease, morbidity, and death. In the matter of environmental clean-up, for example, Lester Lave and Eugene Seskin make the following claim: It is likely that a 50 percent reduction in air pollution can reduce mortality from lung cancer by 25 percent; cardiovascular mortality by 25 percent and reduction in the overall incidence of cancer by 15 percent.[36] It is frightening even to consider what diseases, unknown to us now, are gestating in our contacts with environmental hazards.

The cancer story is a classical example reflecting this change in strategy toward curbing disease. In the mid-1960s, there was a great deal of optimism about curative cancer research and the frequently expressed objective "to cure cancer in your lifetime" was widely broadcast. Huge sums of both federal and private money were committed to the crusade against cancer (see for example " 'Moonshot Medicine' and the Conquest of Cancer", Reference 37). However, in spite of much diligent effort, the researches did not fulfill expectations so that in the mid-1970s, the cancer control movement shifted away from imminent cure toward working to protect the environment. Increasingly, observers now consider cancer to be seventy to ninety percent environmentally induced and in this regard it has been said that western technological societies live in a sea of potentially carcinogenic chemicals. The vast majority of cancers are now thought to be associated with chemical, physical, social, dietary, and cultural factors. Some of the causative agents are obvious, producing clearcut effects. For example, it is estimated that about thirty percent of cancer deaths in U.S. males are attributable to cigarette smoking alone. In other instances, the causative agents are not definitely known but there are indicators. For instance, about 27 percent of all cancer deaths are connected with disease of the digestive organs, suggesting that the effects are dietary in origin, hence, subject to some level of conscious control.³⁸ All in all, the notion that cancer is a preventable disease has more promise than the one that science may provide a cure. Far more likely than not, the cure is not around the corner. And as likely as not, it will not be cheap. In any case, the present conception of cancer informs us that the largest number of lives will be saved by taking preventive measures rather than by trying to cure the already ill.

Much the same picture holds for the medical care of diabetes. One of America's foremost diabetes researchers, Dr. John Galloway, told a diabetes symposium that the big problem in treating the disease "is the life-styles we have. The health-care system can't do much about it until we change. We have spent billions of dollars on health-care delivery but the problems needing most attention are obesity, smoking, drugs, and the stress of our lives." He further stated that trying to straighten out the diets of diabetics involves two opposing forces: (1) obesity as a function of advanced civilization, and (2) a philosophy of life. "Many of us don't have a philosophy which would give us discipline to do what we know is best for us," And this is the central issue in initiating an ethic of responsibility that includes one's health.³⁹

Studies have shown that health and longevity depend on a combination of factors, most especially those related to life-styles. Most chronic lung diseases, much cardiovascular disease, most cirrhosis of the liver, many gastrointestinal disorders, numerous muscular and skeletal complaints, venereal disease, nutritional deficiencies, obesity and its consequences, and certain kinds of renal and skin infections are in large measure self-induced or self-caused. To these conditions must be added the results of automobile accidents, suicidal attempts, as well as accidental poisonings, drug abuse, and burns. These observations impress upon us something we are altogether willing to forget—that we are in important ways responsible for our own state of health.

Dr. Ralph C. Greene presents the following list as preventable risks to health:⁴⁰

A. Drugs

    1. a) Alcohol addiction: causing cirrhosis of the liver, brain damage, cancer of the esophagus, malnutrition, and heart damage (frequently fatal).

        b) Social excess of alcohol: increasing motor-vehicle accidents, and obesity.

    2. Smoking: causing lung cancer, emphysema, chronic bronchitis, coronary disease, stomach ulcers, and cancer of the lips, mouth, tongue, nasal passages, sinuses, and larynx; increasing stillbirths and premature deliveries; hastening aging and wrinkling of facial skin; greatly increasing hazards of home and forest fires and motor-vehicle accidents; the annoyance to nonsmokers and unsightly littering.

    3. Abuse of prescribed pharmaceuticals: leading to drug dependence and tolerance to the necessity for increasing dosage and drug reactions; of exceeding prescribed dosage—if one pill is good, two (or more) are better—leading to poisoning and other adverse reactions (drug reactions are the tenth leading cause of hospital admissions—300,000/year).

    4. a) Psychotropic drug addiction: leading to suicide, homicide, malnutrition, and accidents.

        b) Social use of psychotropic drugs: leading to social withdrawal and acute anxiety attacks.

B. Diet and exercise
1. Overeating: leading to obesity and its consequences.
2. High animal-fat intake: leads to atherosclerosis and coronary heart disease; when combined with low fiber increases the risk of bowel cancer, diverticulosis, and appendicitis.
3. High sugar intake: as above, plus contributing to tooth decay.
4. Fad diets: leads to malnutrition.
5. High salt diets: leads to hypertension.
6. Sedentary life: aggravates coronary heart disease, hypertension, and obesity, and causes poor physical fitness, lack of endurance, and slovenly appearance.
7. Undernourishment: numerous health problems, weakness, vitamin and mineral deficiencies, slow growth, and mentally deficient offspring.
8. Lack of recreation and excessive work pressure (workaholism): associated with peptic ulcers, hypertension, and coronary heart disease.
C. Careless driving and vehicle maintenance and failure to fasten seatbelts: leads to accidents resulting in injuries and death.
D. Promiscuity and sexual carelessness: leads to syphilis, gonorrhea, and other diseases caused by close contact, such as hepatitis and mononucleosis.
E. Neglected pets: transmit numerous bacterial, parasitic and viral diseases too numerous to list here (e.g., dogs alone can carry as many as 50 different infectious organisms).

The message of this list is clear: The most insidious agent for disease today is ourselves; the only truly effective treatment is prevention; the only prevention is a change in life-style.

For five and a half years, Dean Lester Breslow and his colleagues at the UCLA School of Public Health have conducted an important series of studies on health using some 7000 adults.[41] [Note: He studied health, not disease as is traditionally studied at medical schools.] Developing a method of crudely quantifying the state of one's health and well-being, he investigated the effect of living habits and routines on physical health status. He identified seven independent rules which correlate well with good health and longevity. These were:

1. Eat three meals a day with special emphasis on breakfast.
2. Don't eat between meals.
3. Don't smoke cigarettes.
4. Get seven or eight hours of sleep a night.
5. Moderate use of alcohol.
6. Keep weight down.
7. Moderate daily exercise.

Breslow's group reported that a 45-year old person who practices three or fewer of these habits can expect to live to be 67. The person who practices six or seven of them has a life expectancy of 78. In the words of Dr. Anne Somers, testifying before a Senate health subcommittee, "where else, in the entire field of health care can you expect to get a payoff of 11 years life expectancy?"

Other dramatic results of the study conclude that people who follow all seven rules are healthier and live longer than those who follow six, six more than five, and so on, in perfect order. Also, the physical status of those over 75 who followed all the rules was about the same as those aged 35 to 44 who followed fewer than three. Moreover, these differences in physical status connected with life-styles persisted at all economic levels, and except at the very lowest economic levels appeared largely independent of income. (It is interesting to note that not once does the study give the conundrum to see one's doctor regularly.)

Breslow's findings certainly are nothing new. Everyone knows that sedentary living, poor diet, obesity, smoking, and heavy drinking is not good for your health whereas eating right, exercise, and being moderate in all that we do will make for health and long life. The implications for a public health policy are however, frequently overlooked in our rush to throw more money at the problem. The facts of astronomical health-care costs and the perceived limits of what therapeutic medicine is capable of doing can combine to set the stage for a new approach to health policy. One example might be to build either positive or negative inducements, or both, into a national health insurance plan by measures such as reducing or refusing benefits for chronic respiratory disease care to persons who continue to smoke. As far back as February 1971, in his health message to Congress, President Nixon declared, "In the final analysis, each individual bears the major responsibility for his own health," and one form of this responsibility might indeed be a penalty on those who voluntarily abuse their health (as some health and accident policies presently do).

The chief problems of preventive medicine are two:

1. To prove beyond doubt that such practices as exercise, proper diet, and a 55 mile-an-hour speed limit do have positive payoffs in terms of physical health.

2. To persuade a pleasure-loving, affluent, and undisciplined society to accept the necessary good-health practices.[42]

In regard to the first, there is a lot about preventive medicine that we simply do not know. In some cases, information about how to prevent a disease is elusive. In others, cause-effect relationships are difficult to establish with convincing certainty, since in many instances the wages of poor health habits may be paid for much later in life. As Leon Kass states it: "If it isn't likely to rain for 20 years, few of us are likely to repair our leaky roofs." In all cases, there is a lot of room for research, but only a small group of people is presently lobbying for the necessary spending. Much more is still spent on biological research of causes and treatment of disease than on preventive medicine. This challenge to medicine comes at a time when it is increasingly committed to an esoteric technology of disease-treatment. The paradox is obvious.

Regarding the second, it takes no special powers of observation to see that most people do not follow preventive advice. In spite of all that has been said, no one really knows how to persuade people on a mass scale to change their behavior in ways that will be good for their health. It is interesting to speculate what the effect on the nation's health status might be if Breslow's seven rules became part of every school curriculum. Just to communicate the concept of responsibility is no doubt a most difficult task to accomplish. It is but one more instance of the age-old challenge: how to get people to do what is good for them without tyrannizing them. Ethics can make a contribution here. For example, to make one's health someone else's duty is unfair to the society of which we are all a part. To inculcate the concept that each individual has a duty to preserve his/her own health can be elevating to human dignity and wholesomeness.

Although some prefer to take their chances rather than facing the prospect of giving up presumed pleasures, many could be encouraged to follow a more prudent course if specific efforts resulted in an increase in their life span. Supporters of this approach to a national health policy argue that effective health education programs should be required at hospitals, schools, local public health information centers, and through the popular media.

Nationwide, there has been in recent years a growing interest in health and health education, including a greater concern for proper nutrition, adequate exercise, dental hygiene, and the hazards of smoking. Simple safety precautions can reduce the number of victims of the leading killer of young people, the automobile; good nutrition appears to prevent a variety of diseases; and controlled exercise may promote health. People can begin to emphasize these subjects in their homes and communities. There is evidence that, at least among some groups, this attention is paying off.

Health—A form of morality

Jeffrey Salloway, medical sociologist, describes a growing interest in health as a form of morality.[43] One criterion of personal worth is the effort practiced to achieve good health. Daily joggers, bicyclists, natural food fadists, vitamin C and E munchers, the avoiders of butter, eggs, and marbled steaks, the emphasis on the appearance of youth; these and others are the characteristics of this new morality. The message rings clear: "People who don't take care of their health are not nice people." If there is a negative side to this remarkable change in attitude and behavior it is twofold: (1) it may be an attribute still pretty much practiced by middle and upper class whites, suggesting it may be an elitist preoccupation reserved for the affluent rather than one of genuine concern ("its something the rich can afford to do"), and (2) it is the consumer, not the health practitioner, who has caused the rediscovery in his/her own abilities to maintain personal health. The medical professions pay lip service to the general idea but so far at least, they have done little to promote its coming to fruition. More often than not crisis-response continues to mark health-care delivery.

If the above observations are true, then health is seen not to be the exclusive product of medical care. Our medical system has less impact on health than social and environment factors do. We must start over in our efforts to achieve health. Substantially better health cannot be bought for the American people as a whole with several billion more dollars. People must relearn how to take care of themselves and one another. There must be a *community* conscience that places value on individual life and health. Preventive measures are inconsistent with the spirit of "every person for him/her/self." Unlike present-day crisis-focused medicine, we will then not have to rely on profound and costly interventions when health has been lost. Isn't it time the nation began to pay more attention to approaches that promise great improvement at smaller cost? The moral responsibility for maintaining one's personal health is not a far-fetched idea. Only then will a national health-care program be truly effective and cost-wise efficient.

VALUES PERTAINING TO THE DELIVERY OF HEALTH CARE

1 The proper role of medicine is to administer to the needs of the suffering without discrimination.

2 Society has a moral obligation to care for the suffering.

3 All citizens should be guaranteed access to adequate and necessary health care.

4 Health care is a social service.

5 The government must regulate the structure and cost of health care.

6 Individual citizens have a responsibility to maintain their own health.

7 The health-care industry is more properly administered as a private enterprise.

8 Quality will suffer if the government intrudes into the health-care delivery system.

9 Health care is a right.

10 Some form of public accountability should be required of all medical personnel.

11 Medical practitioners should be protected against public abuse.

12 More attention and resource commitment should be given to preventive medicine as opposed to expensive, high-technology therapies.

13 Health care is an earned commodity.

14 Health care is neither a right nor a privilege but a service that the professional may dispense according to his/her own set of values.

15 Health care is primarily a community or social rather than an individual concern.

16 State medicine has worked better in other countries than free enterprise has worked here.

17 Opposition to national health legislation is tantamount to being opposed to progress in health care.

18 "People who do not take care of themselves are not nice people."

19 Government involvement in medical-care delivery is coercive and violates the free society of physicians and patients.

20 Physicians, as fellow humans, have needs that must be accommodated.

REFERENCES

1 J. B. Oakes, "Clinical engineering—the problems and promises," *Science* 190 (1975): 239–242.

2 James Mann, "Uproar over medical bills", *U.S. News & Business Reports* (March 28, 1977), p. 36.

3 James Mann, (in Reference 2), p. 45.

4 Robert B. Griefinger and Victor W. Sidel, "American medicine", *Environment* 18, 4 (1976): 6–18.

5   Sylvia Porter, "National health insurance likely congress priority," *The Champaign-Urbana News-Gazette,* (January 11, 1977) p. 10-A.

6   R. Feldberg, "Health care in America—a social approach," *Science and Society Series: Issues of Health Care,* (November 1973).

7   Lawrence D. Egbert, in "Hospital favors affluent whites," *University of Illinois Daily Illini,* (July 15, 1977) p. 8.

8   "Astronomical costs seen in U.S. health take-over," *Chicago Sun-Times,* (December 23, 1976).

9   Rosemary Stevens, *American Medicine and the Public Interest,* (New Haven: Yale University Press, 1971) p. 433.

10 Ivan Illich, "Two watersheds: the American public health system," reprinted in *Moral Problems of Medicine,* Samuel Gorovitz et al (eds.), (Englewood Cliffs: Prentice-Hall, 1976).

11 James Mann (in Reference 2), p. 37.

12 Jeffrey Colman Salloway, "Health problems and policies for the 1980s: putting the people back in," (unpublished paper, 1976), University of Illinois, Urbana-Champaign.

13 Jeffrey Colman Salloway (in Reference 12), p. 4.

14 Ed Borman, "Hospitals are 'most mismanaged'," *The Champaign-Urbana News-Gazette* (February 14, 1977).

15 Robert B. Griefinger and Victor W. Sidel, (in Reference 4) p. 14.

16 "AMA endorses insurance plan", *Chicago Sun-Times,* (Dec. 8, 1976).

17 Rosemary Stevens (in Reference 9), p. 423.

18 Eli Ginsberg, "What next in health policy?" *Science* 188 (1975): 1184–1186.

19 Rosemary Stevens (in Reference 9), p. 433.

20 Rosemary Stevens (in Reference 9), p. 435.

21 Deborah Shapley, "Health planning: new programs give consumers, Uncle Sam a voice", *Science* 18 (1975): 152–153.

22 "Memo to medicine", *Chicago Sun-Times,* (Nov. 29, 1976), p. 35.

23 Rick J. Carlson, "About Kennedy's health insurance plan," *Center Report* 6, 1 (1975): 26–30.

24 Robert B. Griefinger and Victor W. Sidel (in Reference 4), p. 14.

25 Gene Outka, "Social justice and equal access to health care", *The Journal of Religious Ethics* 2 (1974): 11–32.

26 Robert M. Sade, "Medical care as a right: a refutation," *New England Journal of Medicine* 285 (1971): 1288–1292.

27 Charles Fried, "Equality and rights in medical care", *Hastings Center Report* 6, 1 (1976): 29–34.

28 David Mechanic, "Rationing health care: public policy and the medical marketplace," *Hastings Center Report* 6, 1 (1976): 34–37.

29 Robert B. Griefinger and Victor W. Sidel (in Reference 4), p. 16.

30 Allan Chase, *The Biological Imperatives: Health, Politics and Human Survival,* (New York: Holt, Rinehart and Winston, 1971), p. 40.

31 Deborah Shapley (in Reference 21), p. 152.

32 Barbara J. Culliton, cited in "Preventative medicine: legislation calls for health education," *Science* 189 (1975): 1071–1072.

33 Philip H. Abelson, "Cost-effective health care", *Science* 192 (1976): 619.

34 Deborah Shapley (in Reference 21), p. 152.

35 Philip H. Abelson (in Reference 33), p. 619.

36   L. B. Lave & E. P. Seskin, "Air pollution and human health," *Science* **169** (1970): 723–728.

37   Glenn W. Geehold, " ' Moonshot medicine' and the conquest of cancer," *Man and Medicine* **1**, 1 (1975): 51–56.

38   "Cancer and the environment," *F.A.S. Public Interest Report* **29** (1976): whole issue (1–8).

39   "Diabetes expert sees life style an answer," *Chicago Sun-Times*, (November 25, 1976).

40   Ralph C. Greene, "Ethical culture and physical culture," *The Humanist* **37**, 2 (1977): 35–37. Reprinted by permission.

41   Nedra B. Belloc and Lester Breslow, "Relationship of physical health status and health practices," *Preventive Medicine* **1** (1972).

42   I. H. Page, "Preventive Medicine," *Science* **193** (1976): 837.

43   Jeffrey Colman Salloway (In Reference 12), p. 15.

[Note: Portions of this chapter appeared in *The American Biology Teacher* **39**, 4 (1977): 227–236. "Medicine and the public interest," by George H. Kieffer.] Reprinted by permission.

BIBLIOGRAPHY

Carlson, Rick J., *The End of Medicine*, (New York: John Wiley & Sons, 1975).

Ehrenreich, Barbara, and John Ehrenreich, *The American Health Empire: Power, Profits and Politics* (New York: Random House, 1971).

Illich, Ivan, *Medical Nemesis* (London: The Trinity Press, 1975).

Kass, Leon R., "Regarding the end of medicine and the pursuit of health," *The Public Interest* 40 (1975).

Kennedy, Edward M., *In Critical Condition: The Crisis in America's Health Care*, (New York: Simon & Schuster, 1972).

Ribicoff, Abraham, *The American Medical Machine* (New York: Harper & Row, 1973).

Wechsler, Henry (ed.), *The Horizons of Health* (Cambridge: Harvard University Press, 1977).

III

NONMEDICAL ISSUES

III

NONMEDICAL USES

10

OBLIGATIONS TO FUTURE GENERATIONS

FUTURE ETHICS

Responsibility for the future forms the central element and constitutes the first consideration to the solution of the many issues raised in this text. The distinguishing feature of the many innovations in biology and medicine is that they can contribute mightily to the betterment of the human condition now and in the future, or they can generate massive evil even for generations yet unborn. Countless examples have been cited which illustrate that we have now the power to make the world much better; on the other hand, it can be made a much less pleasant place not only for ourselves living in the present but for our descendents as well. More than ever before, we must be alerted to the fact that our moral obligations extend beyond ourselves to generations that will follow us. It is necessary that society strive hard for a positive future orientation, defining goals for future life and responsibly choosing those actions necessary to achieve those goals. The main responsibility of an ethic regarding the future is to pass on to coming generations a world where there is a reasonable chance of being able to confront successfully the problems that we will have bequeathed to them.[1] Not only does this stipulation apply to the obvious cases of population and environment but also to the suggestions of genetic intervention, medical engineering, behavioral control technologies, and the like. Many of these are more than one-generation phenomena. Modern technological activity has injected a new factor of moral significance calling for what might be termed an ethic of long-range responsibility. It is evident that what we exhaust of the earth's limited resources will not be available for use by future generations; any process we innovate which might be irreversibly harmful for human life will have its greatest effect upon them. Thus it must become one of our highest ethical imperatives to order our lives and actions in such a way that entitlements of generations to come are not seriously jeopardized.

There is a very close link between images of the future and ethics. Ethics deals with the realm of what *ought to be* and this automatically presupposes a picture of the future in a way that contrasts with the present. Ethical decisions are normally conclusions for guiding future actions in terms of future consequences. Ethics lives in future communities through symbolic conjecturing of that future.[2] However, traditional ethics, according to philosopher Hans Jonas, is not suited to the task of dealing effectively with the far-off future (e.g., fifty to a hundred years from now). It has almost entirely ignored the claims of long-range posterity. Human actions are viewed as having a small effective reach, hence, limited accountability and the presumption of short-range appraisals over consequences judge the ethical rightness of courses of action. The historical notion of causal responsibility is limited by the narrow vision of causal chains of events.[3] Negligence and moral liability are judged on the basis of immediate or near-term outcomes and measured by past experiences. Even now, customary standards for ethical behavior are oriented to the past as many of our previous discussions demonstrate. The good and evil consequences of an action lay close to the act, frequently derived from previously established normative traditions. Proper conduct had its past and immediate criteria. The long-run consequences are left to chance, fate, or providence depending on one's preference. The traditional view of ethics is summarized in this observation of Jonas: "an ethical universe of contemporaries"[4] or by biologist Garrett Hardin as "I–Thou, Here and Now!"[5]

No previous ethics had to consider the global condition of human life and the far-off future, much less the fate of the entire species. However, we clearly now have the power to affect the lives of those yet to come by contributing to the conservation of the total environment in which we live and which our posterity will occupy someday. Since traditional ethics leans backwards for its sanctions, it is ineffective in coping with actions which bear heavily on the destiny of coming generations. The new circumstances demand a new concept of duties and rights, new values and new social systems, embodying a new vision of the future as well as motivating the will to actualize them. If we indeed have an obligation to posterity, what is the basis of this moral imperative? The question, at least, is not senseless anymore. The world in its broadest sense has become a human trust and something of a moral claim is made on us not only for our own ulterior sake but for those generations yet to be.[6]

But traditional ethics is not alone in its inability to respond effectively to futuristic concerns. Time-bound deficiencies pervade most of everything we do. The recent and controversial Club of Rome report—*The Limits to Growth* (Donella Meadows et al, 1972)—submitted that as many as ninety percent of all decisions made in the commercial and political worlds are predicated on a time span of six to twelve months. The average duration of governments worldwide is only three years. Under these circumstances, the horizon of the forseeable future is quite myopic as even a casual observation of governmental actions testifies.

It could be argued that evolution did not prepare us to conceptualize in the distant future. For much of human history, the real urgencies were taken up with events of the moment. Life, for the vast majority, was violent, severe, and mostly short. A futuristic preoccupation is a luxury of those who have plenty; those less well-off have few reasons to identify with generations beyond their own. Even to this day the poor and the disadvantaged cannot afford the future.

Unbridled self-indulgence on the part of one generation without regard to future ones was and still is the modus operandi of biological evolution and may even be regarded as rational behavior. Human beings are interested in what is coming up next and what is going on immediately around them. The majority of people care about the next few days, the next few weeks, perhaps about the next few years; and they care about themselves, their families, their jobs, their neighborhoods, occasionally their own race, and sometimes their own nation. They do not look far ahead in time nor do they really care much about what is happening far away. In any culture, the number of people who can think in terms of the far-off future are few indeed. Even in societies exhibiting a preoccupation with features as far forward as heaven, hell, "happy hunting grounds," or reincarnation, the symbolism is not designed to make the present or the future physical world any better. The hoped (and prayed) for outcome was to leave a life of travail behind and escape to one beyond which was free of sorrow, suffering, and inequity (e.g., "The poor you will always have with you." John 12:8). Nor did these inventions even consider the physical world as being very important anyhow since one's destiny was to be realized only in the afterlife. A good existence after death was seen as the reward for even a miserable life endured before death.

But our ineptness to deal with the future is not hopeless. Biologically we do possess *some* capacity to transcend the here and now and, in fact, humans may be the only animals that can pass the limits of present reality. The development of this sense of futurity no doubt contributed much to the growth of human civilization for from it the nurture of nature became possible. The invention, refinement, and spread of the processes of logic, mathematics, alphabet, literacy, and methods of science contributed to the emergence of human biocultural adaptations. Worlds Two and Three of Karl Popper require that persons be able to look forward in time (see p. 14). Both in the realms of objective and subjective knowledge, perceptions are based not only on the past and present, but on future considerations as well. According to Joseph Fletcher, in the earlier referenced "Profile of Humanhood,"[7] we cannot be truly human nor can we attain the summit of humanhood if we are unable to elaborate a mental picture of another world in a coming time. A "sense of futurity" was suggested as an important criterion for determining humanhood.

Unfortunately, the images of the future usually conjured up—at least until very recently—were eschatological or Utopian, and seldom dealt with changing the reality in which persons lived. The effective extension of foresight when applied to the real world was limited to time dimensions of one generation or less. The result has been a sharp cleavage, with the "idealists" on the one side and the "realists" on the other.[8] The idealists say no to the present and yes to some chosen future construed to be much better than the present time. The deficiency here is that no workable prescription is given to get from here to there. It might be reassuring to some to project a utopian future when one is knee-deep in mud but it is quite another matter to submit a prescription for attaining it. The realist, on the other hand, says yes to the present and has little traffic with the future. As problems or crises arise, solutions are generated. Why be concerned with the future when we have problems enough in the present? The proponents of the here and now seem to hold the fort, characterizing the spirit of our times.

What has been said so far may be all rather abstract even a little detached from the problem at hand, but it has some important and practical implications. The majority of humankind in its present state is not predisposed to the long-range future. If what has been stated is even close to the real situation, then it would seem that we are ill-equipped biologically, culturally, politically, or even ethically to deal effectively with the future. However, that does not dismiss us from a future's responsibility for countless numbers of examples point to the conclusion that in spite of the marvelous achievements of human knowledge and power, we are susceptible to error, to mistakes in judgment and action, which can lead to unintended and far-reaching harmful consequences. This means that the rationale of human actions with respect to what we do cannot be based on short-term expectations only, but must be based on some other, more general principle—not as individual or as a generation, but as a species in time. And this requires a totally new moral orientation!

RIGHTS OF THE PRESENT VERSUS FUTURE GENERATIONS

Before postulating an ethical system that suggests guidelines for a resolution to this conflict, a first order of business concerns itself with the more basic question: "Do we, in the first place, have a moral obligation to deny ourselves certain advantages in the present in order that those who are not yet born may live better?" This question poses the old issue of why should we feel moral obligations to those who will follow us? The easy answer was given by Joseph Addison way back in 1714 when he wrote "we are always doing something for posterity, but I would fain see posterity do something for us," or John Trumbull in 1782, "what has posterity done for us?" There are several other ways one can dispose of this problem:[9]

1. The belief in a divine plan that includes care for all who populate this globe, now and in the future.

2. The belief that we will be rewarded in the afterlife so we must not become overly concerned with worldly cares; we will always have evil with us anyway.

3. Beneficent natural law will automatically bring the inhabitants of any age to their maxium well-being; the future will take care of itself through the operation of natural law.

4. Western civilization, if not the world, is in its death throes; it is a circumstance which cannot be fundamentally changed—our only hope is that the kingdom will outlive us. Since this position leaves no hopeful prospect for the future of humankind on earth, there is no point in being concerned with it—in fact, some would even say, the sooner it ends the better.

5. Circumstances and systems evolve over time as part of cultural mechanisms; consequently, the future is not approachable in terms of present-day needs and desires (who afterall can see the future?); a moral concern for the future is a nonissue (this is probably the prevailing view of the majority).

What all of these have in common, of course, is a flat rejection of future responsibility. Martin Golding has made the remark that if we have any obligations at all to future generations, they amount to no more than an obligation not to plan for them.[10] Robert Heilbronner in *An Inquiry into the Human Prospect* asks, "On what private 'rational' considerations, after all, should we make sacrifices now to ease the lot of generations we will never live to see?" And, in fact, for want of a strongly felt and defensible moral stance, sacrifices for the future may be rejected much as we seem to neglect a moral obligation toward suffering in distant parts of the globe today. That which cannot be seen cannot be experienced. And so the fundamental issue is this: Can an obligation for the future be rationally defended? The only possible answer to the question, according to Heilbronner, "lies in our capacity to form a collective bond of identity with future generations." Christian ethicist James Gustafson in an unpublished paper makes the following argument:[11] All thoughtful people would agree that what one generation inherits from the generation that preceded it is not merely an accumulation of past products. Rather, each generation receives the aggregation of past changes increased or reduced and they bequeath to the next generation a world still further changed by themselves. Observations of the geological record as well as the many evidences of biological evolution demonstrate that change is driving toward irreversible ends. This is the nature of our world. Humans can influence some of these changes or modify their pace and direction but they cannot halt them; they may accelerate some and decelerate others, but they cannot stop them. Since it is we who must use the resources of the natural world, whatever they may be, our activities contribute to and participate in change and, in varying degrees, are the determinants (often the major determinants) of the kind and range of changes that occur. In view of this inescapable circumstance in which we find ourselves, we have imposed on us a *moral obligation to the future*. And this because human beings can cause change!

It has become increasingly clear that the human enterprise cannot be given a carte blanche to do what it pleases. Human actions must not only serve the essential needs of present-day existence but must anticipate in wise and responsible ways the needs of future generations so that they are not deprived of the necessary conditions for sustaining human life and those experiences which enhance it. It is of the utmost importance for the continued survival of our kind, therefore, to recognize and accept this obligation, to base policy on the certainty that change will occur, that our interventions can effect these changes, and that we, to some degree, can predict the consequences of our own actions. To be sure, humankind of today cannot make the decisions for those living tomorrow, but what our generation does with the earth is rather decisive for what future generations will be able to do. Actions of one generation can have profound effects on the options available to future generations. We can be reasonably certain that the proper interests of posterity cannot be met or fulfilled if our actions today deprive them of the conditions with which to fulfill them.

ENTITLEMENTS OF FUTURE GENERATIONS

What specifically are future generations entitled to? This is a particularly difficult question, largely because the rights of the future unborn have never been philosophically, legally, or ethically analyzed in any great depth. But whatever our obligations might be, the present knows very little about the life conditions of the future; therefore, the present cannot articulate specific priorities for the future. However, it is possible to develop plausible guidelines which can define the limits of intergenerational responsibility.

Ethicist Ronald Green proposes three basic guides to our thinking about obligations to the future; he labels these "axioms of intergenerational responsibility."[12]

1. "We are bound by the ties of justice to real future persons." Since we live in a world of finite resources and space, there is a physical limit to what we can do with it. Present environmental and population concerns emphasize that the potential to harm those now living through unwise environmental perturbations do exist. It is morally unjust to willingly cause harm and suffering in the present world. Furthermore, adherence to a moral system provides ways for adjudicating possible conflicts between persons and for facilitating noncoercive solutions of social disputes. Reasoned commonsense replaces the play of force and power in guiding human affairs.

   Postulating a future world with actual persons living in it is an assumed reality. Since the future will embody real persons, then a link between them and us is established. Even as our wishes and behavior can conflict with extant persons, so they can conflict with future persons, and moral reasoning can be employed to settle the dispute. For this reason, the requirements of justice insist that we must consider the needs of future generations. As we must equitably distribute goods and opportunities in the present, so we must do so over time. If we fail to do so, we neglect our moral duty. The test of the Golden Rule can be applied here: Could I be satisfied if the policy or action were applied to me? In this instance it is required that one place him/herself into a future world.

2. "The lives of future persons ought ideally to be better than our own and certainly no worse."
   Each of us receives something from our predecessors and profits generally from what was done before us. It is reasonable, therefore, to suggest that we are duty-bound to better the conditions for those who will follow us. The Abbot of the Benedictine Congregation of Vallombrosa observed this simple truth back in 1804 when he wrote:

   > . . . . no one who plants a fir tree can hope to fell it when it is fully grown, no matter how youthful the person is. In spite of this the most sacred obligation is to replant and husband these pine forests. If we sweat for the benefit of posterity, we should not complain as we reap the results of the efforts of our forefathers . . . Not one of our forebears survive now nor shall we when those who follow on cut down the trees that we planted for them.[13]

   Although providing a better life for our followers, the delineation of the conditions required to attain it is a worthy value; it is not easily done for it hinges on the question of what constitutes a "quality life" for future generations. Though it cannot be specified in detail, at least these three considerations should be included: (1) human emotional health, (2) cultural richness, and (3) environmental quality. Determining how these can be directed or influenced positively is difficult but it is relatively easy to identify those actions which will worsen any of them. If we in the present generation squander, decimate, dissipate or otherwise misuse our natural and cultural environment that we have inherited, future generations will be worse off than we, regarding these assets.

3. "Sacrifice on behalf of the future must be distributed equally in the present with special regard for those presently disadvantaged." This relates directly

to the Rawlsian theory of justice (see p. 58), in which inequalities are to be arranged so that they are to the greatest benefit of the least advantaged. This means that in practice, as we institute policies for the future, we do not disproportionately harm our least advantaged citizens. The less affluent can least afford the necessary sacrifices, hence, equal justice requires that burdens be shared by all, even to giving the burdens to those who can better afford them. Although this axiom does not speak in terms of moral obligations for the future, it does specify guidelines for dealing with it in the present. By emphasizing what is frequently overlooked by those who propose futuristic considerations, namely, the involvement of all classes of society including the poor, the principles of equity and justice are seen to be applicable both for a present and a future ethic. Failure to recognize potential injustices against the less privileged members of our community by causing them to bear a larger share of our intergenerational responsibility may endanger efforts to protect future generations through resentment and resistance by that segment of society.

What is required to implement these as well as any other axioms that deal with the future is some sort of predictive capability. Predictive knowledge assumes ethical importance when it assesses moral liability and blameworthiness. Sumner Twiss identifies two particularly important components of an ethic for long-range responsibility which deal with conjecturing futuristic implications of scientific innovation.[14] These are as follows:

1. There is a moral imperative of acquiring relevant predictive knowledge *before* implementing a technology which carries some wide-ranging scale of action.

2. Ignorance about delayed and/or indirect consequences of an action, particularly when these may be irreversible or harmful, constitutes moral reason for restraint in developing and implementing a technology.

The question of moral liability relating to some future consequences will be discussed more thoroughly in a later chapter (Chapter 13, the section on An Ethos of Science). The point to be made here is that there may be significant ethical constraints that determine which courses of action may or may not be permissible. We must evaluate our actions in terms of the best available estimate of their consequences. The *ethical* question must go beyond merely asking, Have we done the right thing? Rather, do we have the *right* to do such and such? And the answer to the question is not measured in terms of its conformity with the moral standards of the past. Instead, rightness is dependent upon whether or not the course of action brings promise of a future well-being insofar as we can determine it.* Ethical deliberations must take into account all obtainable information and then propose a decision. As a very minimum, the living have an obligation to refrain from actions that would endanger future generations' enjoyment of the same rights that the living now enjoy.

---

* Expressions such as "future well-being," "interests of future generations," "quality of life," etc., may seem to leave the door wide open to ambiguities, equivocations, and unforeseen circumstances, yet it can be contended that the conditions basic for physical survival as well as those that contribute to the aesthetic human experience can be known in accordance with our present conception of them.

Thus, a futures ethic must be an ethic of promise.[15] To cite an example: Much has been made of the social benefits to be derived from a plutonium economy, namely, the reduction through utilization of troublesome and dangerous radioactive wastes, the exploitation of abundant supplies of uranium-238, lower energy costs, an expanding economy with a high standard of living, etc. The difficulties with this proposition are clear, namely, plutonium is extremely toxic to humans, it is extremely long-lived (half-life of 24,000 years), the dangers of theft, sabotage, and nuclear proliferation, the special safety factors of liquid metal breeder reactors, etc. In view of this balance sheet which pegs the present against the future, one is compelled to ask, Do we have the right to seriously jeopardize the health and lives of countless future generations? Future generations may well curse us for having made a Faustian bargain which did not adequately consider the risks to their lives and health for a small gain in ours and perhaps the next one or two generations. Using Twiss's criteria, it is unacceptable to embark on programs that pose great foreseeable and unforeseeable dangers merely on the faith that these will be solved in the future. We have obligations to govern our interventions into nature in such a way that the human species in future time is not deprived of the necessary conditions for its physical and spiritual well-being. This obligation might well require restraints upon our actions, indeed, restraints upon our freedom to act in those ways that are predictably harmful to those who follow us.

Joel Feinberg would argue still more emphatically when he writes "protecting the environment now is a matter of elementary prudence, and insofar as we do it for the next generation, already here in the persons of our children, it is a matter of love. But from the perspective of our remote descendents it is basically a matter of justice, of respect for their rights."[16] In his view, we do not even have a *right* to threaten deprivation to future generations of the necessary conditions for life. And these entitlements imply a restriction of freedom on those now living to do as they please. We, in the present, should not exhaust nonrenewable resources, or irrevocably pollute the environment, or intervene in basic life processes without carefully thinking through consequences in advance; or procreate to such an extent that future generations will be left with an unmanageably large number of people.

MORAL BASIS FOR A FUTURES ETHIC

If we do have an obligation to posterity, what is the basis of that moral imperative? Why love humankind of the future? The case cannot be argued in a direct dependency sense, for certainly the present is not directly dependent upon the future (although the inverse of this is true). Expediency cannot be implicated in the defense of a futures ethic. A social-contract hypothesis is also unsatisfactory since it is unnecessary to compromise some of the individual's self-interest and self-love needs for the good of the social order. "Man as his brother's keeper," is also a time-bound imperative that applies to now. It establishes no dependency of the present on the future, no rational self-love grounds for stretching altruism into the distant future.

One possible resolution turns on the issue of whether there are aspects of one's *present* practice of altruism that make a future morality desirable. In other words, a moral obligation to posterity does not base its sanction on enhancing future well-being or avoiding future suffering *per se.* Instead, one's present, personal growth and experience as a truly human being is dependent upon, and is enhanced by, how one acts toward the future. For self-love reasons we should act toward the future so as to most fully *actualize ourselves in the present*. This is the position of social scientist Walter Wagner.[17] Concern for future humans helps us to be more human in the present. This linkage can be the foundation for a futures ethic.

How do we become more human in the present from a concern for the future? In the first sense, a callousness for the future endangers our present idealism and our image of compassion that is a unique characteristic of humanness. It can be shown that compassion and its sentiments are highly adaptive for the human species. Forms of altruism have contributed much to the attainments of truth, justice, and love in the course of human evolution (see Chapter 1). Compassionate sensitivity is instrumental for the good life now as well. But a compassionate humanity cannot restrict itself to decisions and actions which speak only to present conditions for the same reason that one cannot maintain a defensible moral stance if one neglects an obligation toward suffering in distant parts of the globe today. Morality makes no provision for selective exclusions. We cannot pick and choose those areas of moral participation which are to our liking and disregard those that displease us. "I choose to do good to this and these but not to that or those," is offensive to any who practice a truly moral life. So then, just as sincere profession of concern for all of humanity includes the entire household of humans, both our near and our far neighbors, so obligations for future generations must come under this same umbrella of compassion. Proper moral concern is not only for the near neighbor but also for the distant neighbor, both in space *and* in time. Goodness does not allow for omission. If true compassion does not permit selective exclusion, it can then be argued that the exercise of a futuristic compassion leads to a safe and satisfying self-actualization of each of us. Such sensitivity is instrumental for the good life *now*. As Abraham Maslow observed, future concern makes for dynamic and self-actualizing people—mentally healthy and goal-directed.[18]

Theologian Carl E. Braaten suggests how a futures ethic may express itself.[19] Given the exhaustibility of resources and possible irreversible harmful consequences of certain interventions, it is important to think clearly about what justice requires with reference to future generations. We need to ask the question, What is due to coming generations?—not what can we do but rather, what ought we to do? An ethics of the future looks ahead for its clues as to what action to take now. It studies the future to see what in the present is basically destroying the prospects of a just and fulfilling future for all people. This recognition requires not only greater reverence for human life but all life and includes a concern for the nature around us that it, too, be treated justly. Accordingly, another aspect of an ethic for the future must be an ethic of nature. For an ethic of nature is based on the balanced, interrelated, interdependent closed system of nature's life-support processes that have been in operation at least since life began on this planet some three to four billion years ago. An ethic for the future cannot overlook such practical features of existence. The highest calling in these matters may be to understand the human and social ecological systems in which we are centrally involved, to fashion our aspirations and our goals out of this understanding, and then to act so that the quality of the natural world and our own life can move to higher levels.

To adapt a phrase from theologian Reinhold Niebuhr: man's capacity for the control of nature makes a futures ethic possible; man's inclination to misuse the elements of his technology makes the development of an ethic of the future a necessity![20]

VALUES PERTAINING TO INTERGENERATIONAL RESPONSIBILITY

1 The main responsibility of a futures ethic is to pass on to coming generations a world in which there is a reasonable chance of being able to successfully confront the problems they will have been bequeathed by present generations.

2 Traditional ethics is unable to respond effectively to many of the new problems in biology and medicine; therefore, basically new values are needed.

3 Ethical wisdom of the past is not obsolete with reference to the destiny of coming generations.

4 Acting in a manner that responsibly considers the future enhances self-actualization of ourselves in the present.

5 Present generations have no obligations to future generations in regard to setting limits on courses of action.

6 The future is an imponderable; therefore, it is foolish to contemplate intergenerational responsibility.

7 We are bound by ties of justice to real future persons.

8 The lives of future persons ought ideally to be better than our own and certainly no worse.

9 Sacrifices on behalf of the future must be distributed equitably in the present with special regard for those who are the least advantaged.

10 The truly moral person cannot selectively exclude certain persons or certain actions either in place or in time.

REFERENCES

1 James M. Gustafson, "Interdependence and human limitations: reflections by a theologian on the 'energy crisis'," Unpublished paper delivered at the Conference on Ethics and Public Policy, St. Mary's University, Halifax, Nova Scotia (August 1974).

2 Hans Jonas, "Essay one, technology and responsibility: reflections on the new tasks of ethics," in *Philosophical Essays* (Englewood Cliffs: Prentice-Hall, 1974).

3 Sumner B. Twiss, Jr., "Ethical issues in priority-setting for the utilization of genetic technologies," in *Ethical and Scientific Issues Posed by Human Uses of Molecular Genetics*, Marc Lappe and Robert S. Morison (eds.), Vol. 265 (New York: New York Academy of Sciences, 1976), p. 29.

4 Hans Jonas, (in Reference 2), p. 22.

5 Garrett Hardin, "The rational foundation of conservation" *The North American Review* 259 (1974): 16.

6 Carl E. Braaten, "Caring for the future: where ethics and ecology meet," *Zygon* 9, 4 (1974): 311–322.

7   Joseph Fletcher, "Indicators of humanhood: a tentative profile of man," *Hastings Center Report* **2**, 5 (1972): 1–4.
8   Fred L. Polak, "Responsibility for the future," *The Humanist* **33**, 6 (1973): 14–16.
9   Walter C. Wagner, "Futurity morality," *The Futurist* **5**, 5 (1971): 197–199.
10 Martin Golding, cited in Twiss (in Reference 3), p. 38.
11 Gustafson (in Reference 1), p. 4.
12 Ronald M. Green, "Intergenerational distributive justice and environmental responsibility," *Bioscience* **27**, 4 (1977): 260–265.
13 The Abbot of Vallombrosa quoted in Van Rensselaer Potter, "Evolving ethical concepts," *Bioscience* **27** (1977): 251.
14 Sumner B. Twiss, Jr. (in Reference 3), p. 29.
15 Carl E. Braaten (in Reference 5), p. 316.
16 Joel Feinberg, "The rights of animals and unborn generations" in *Philosophy and Environmental Crisis*, William T. Blackstone (ed.), (Athens, University of Georgia Press, 1974), pp. 43–68.
17 Walter C. Wagner (in Reference 9), p. 199.
18 Walter C. Wagner (in Reference 9), p. 199.
19 Carl E. Braaten (in Reference 6), p. 313.
20 David E. Engel, "Elements in a theology of environment," *Zygon* **5**, 3 (1970): 227.

11

AN ETHIC OF NATURE

ETHICAL DIMENSIONS OF THE ECOLOGICAL CRISIS

As with so many of the major problems of society, the precise extent and nature of the environmental crisis is not entirely clear. On the one hand are those who prophesy that humankind is facing global disaster in the near future. Our civilization as we know it will die or be disfigured beyond recognition unless we drastically change our ways. Grim predictions of potential global disaster are so widely broadcast that the present generation of young people have literally been weaned on these dire warnings. On the other hand are those who do have faith in the future. They submit that the human species is too great a biological success to end so abruptly and so soon. A species that can learn from the experiences of its predecessors, and in so doing fashion for itself a world unlike any experienced before, can continue to build new knowledge, achieving thereby still higher levels of attainment. Which view will be correct cannot be determined with certainty, at least not now.

Regardless of one's view, many Americans today are deeply distressed with the condition of both their social and natural environments. A large number of individuals have become apprehensive to the point of feeling threatened in a fundamental way. For example, we do not know how many people this earth can provide for or at what level of existence, but we do know that there is a limit and we may be approaching it. We do not know how much wider the gap can grow between the rich and poor nations before Armageddon, but we do know there is a limit to how much suffering and oppression people can and will tolerate. We do not know the extent of the world's nonrenewable natural resources, but we do know the world is running out of gas. We do not know how much pollution this earth can absorb before it lashes back at its human antagonists, but we do know that the air is bad, sometimes the water may be unsafe to drink, and toxic substances are being let loose in the land (over 100,000 of them, according to a recent EPA report). Thus to many, the environmental crisis goes far beyond the inconveniences and nuisances of modern living—the noise, ugliness, and unpleasantness; it goes to the most fundamental levels of concern about the future of our species on this planet. Our greatest danger is not that humans will become extinct. That is probably quite unlikely barring some unforeseen catastrophe. The extraordinary adaptability of the human organism leads to the conclusion that at the very least some will survive somewhere. The basic fear is that cultural values which make us human may be lost. For example, in our attempts to manufacture the good life, we have deprived ourselves of some fundamentally important aspects of living, such as clean air and water, open natural areas, serenity, individual purpose, and opportunities to perceive beauty.[1] Furthermore, altruistic love and concern for others is difficult to achieve when one's own existence is in peril or is marred by a deteriorating and stifling environment. The basic structure of our relationship to the world seems to be out of order in this our highly technological age.

What is the *right* relationship? A resolution to this question will involve a redefinition of humans' relation to other humans as well as their relationship to nature. Earlier notions of humans opposed to nature or humans as the exploiter of nature will have to be replaced by the more inclusive concept of humans in nature, or humans with nature. Nature, now as never before, depends on us; our activities have become determiners of nature's future (see Chapter 10). So powerful have we become that human activity has become the equal of a geological force in our capacity to work profound changes in the earth's waters and atmosphere. Ecologically, *Homo sapiens* is the dominant life-form on this planet, its most successful species, occupying a greater variety of habitats, over a greater geographic range, than any other species. But it is also we who are the sole cause of the population explosion and the ecological crisis.

In acquiring the present position of dominance, humans have snatched the control of their destiny from the processes of nature to which they were once forced to submit. "Whole landscapes are now occupied by man-dominated fauna and flora."[2] We can climb mountains, eliminate disease, transplant organs, and explore the moon. However, according to biologist Daniel Kozlovsky, this power has placed us on the brink of extinction. Attempts to clean the air and water, recycle cans and bottles, fight power plants and dams and highways are worse than useless in that they merely prolong the agony. "Until there are fundamental changes in the social order," he goes on to state, "accompanied by equally fundamental changes in our view of man and of reality, such measures are stop-gap only."[3] Our current knowledge enables us to do miraculous things, but we are still ignorant about whether accomplishing these things would be in our or our planets' best interests. What is needed is a different base to guide our activities with and in nature—a new philosophical and ethical system.

Dr. Kozlovsky may or may not be right, but his appraisal of our present plight has many followers. We simply cannot reach a future for our kind if we continue in the way we are going now. As to the need for a new ethic, most thoughtful people heartily agree. Today's ecological problems demand a new ethical stance toward the natural environment—a future-oriented ethic which stresses the humanity of persons and community with nature. People who care about the present and the future earth must find ways of creating a "totally new form of human society."[4] Our present plight is not hopeless; we still have a little time left and we can act constructively and effectively in the present crisis.

HUMAN-NATURE RELATIONSHIPS

The relationship between humans and nature and the extent to which it should be controlled plays a central role in any system of ethics. According to ethicist Daniel Callahan, some conception of nature and our relationship to it stands behind every ethical system and specific ethical decisions are derived from this conception.[5] What we do with nature depends on our ideas of the human-nature relationship and an ethical decision will show what persons think nature to be. Callahan identifies three major positions on the matter of relationships, each providing a way for utilizing nature.

In the first—*man apart from nature*—nature is viewed as something to be conquered. The human species has the right to use and manipulate nature for its own purposes. Since nature is dominated by impersonal physical forces which in themselves have no inherent values, the world can be shaped in any fashion deemed desirable. It is our unrestricted right to manipulate nature by the use of whatever power we can bring to bear in the service of our goals. Knowledge of how nature functions gives us power to control it; therefore discovery and acquisition of knowledge are prized virtues. Any ethical problems arising from the use of this power are measured against the ends sought. Humans create all ethical and/or moral norms; accordingly, there are no moral codes or absolute guides other than what persons invent or choose. The application of this ethic results in unbridled manipulation and control of nature and if there are any limitations to this exploitation it is that nature can fight back in the event certain cautions are not followed, but these cautions arise from our lack of knowledge, not from any intrinsic limitation imposed on us by nature. They can, therefore, be overcome by more diligent effort and more knowledge. Knowledge maintains us on top of nature; we are its lord and master.

A second view proposes *man in nature* or *man a part of nature*. As advocates of this view, we feel we are not unique in the sense that unlike any other life form we can claim title to the whole biotic and abiotic realm. Rather, humans are one kind of creature among many kinds, differing not because we have special privileges but in degree only. As the donkey is different from the chicken so we are different in terms of our special adaptations, but this does not bestow on us any higher rank. This image has two forms, a religious and a secular one. In the religious form, nature is seen as part of God's creation to be heeded and cared for as good stewards should. Humans are not its master, but nature has been left in our trust. The early Christian saint, St. Francis of Assisi, is the foremost exemplar of this view when he adumbrated the idea of the equality of natural objects—for example, Brother Ant and Sister Fire. The spiritual autonomy of all parts of nature is substituted for limitless exploitation and rule over creation.

The secular image submits that man and nature are one. Just as humans are worthy of respect and possess intrinsic value, so nature, too, has value in and of itself; it demands our utmost respect. By living in harmony with it, lessons for life can be derived. In this model, nature is the teacher, showing us how to live with it and with ourselves. Passivity and quiet contemplation are central virtues, and ethics is derived by pondering nature's way; that which is most in harmony is the greatest good. The "back to nature" or the Walden Pond concept exemplifies the secular manifestation of this view.

Third, there is the teleological view (from the Greek, teleos, meaning end or final form) which asserts that there is *purpose and logic* to be found in nature. Although nature is not inviolable or sacred or an object to be manipulated, a proper study of nature can provide important insights applicable to human conduct. For example, an understanding of the interrelatedness of nature's many parts can lead to the recognition that monodimensional meddling can have significant negative consequences; or that unlimited growth is folly in a world with finite limits. Since for our very survival humans need to utilize parts of nature, nature requires some controls, but nature provides the guidelines for these interventions. For instance, roads must be built to facilitate movement of people but their construction should make wise use of the natural landscape rather than connecting two geographic points in the most expedient fashion. The major difference between this view and the previous two is that whereas we still must utilize nature and change it, the aim is not to subjugate it nor to simply live with it. In terms of an ethical system derived from this view, humans must create their own ethical norms but nature can provide us some guides for developing the good moral life. Systems of bioethics are examples of human values based on this view of nature (see p. 371).

The present environmental crisis reflects our failure to develop a consistent and adequate view of a human relationship to nature. Until more progress is made than is now observed in the attainment of this goal, attempts at resolution of the crisis will be like the shuffling of the pieces of a puzzle here and there with none of them quite fitting together. This is no doubt what Kozlovsky intended when he stated that efforts to rectify our environmental problems are stop-gap only unless we change our view of who we are and of the reality of our existence as based on nature. If it is true that the relationship between humans and nature predicts ethical decisions and if ethical behavior is to be changed, then we really have no choice for survival but to reorient our perceptions.

ENVIRONMENT AS A MATTER OF ETHICS

The first requirement is to make environmental concerns a matter of ethics rather than economics, legal coercion, or even fear for our survival. This involves extending the same concepts of right and wrong that now apply in theory to human beings to other forms of life and ultimately to the environment itself. Theologian D. S. Jordan writes, "the time will come when civilized men will feel that the rights of all living creatures on earth are as sacred as his own." Biologist Julian Huxley expresses this opinion: "In ethical terms, the golden rule applies to man's relations with nature as well as to relations between human beings."[6] A number of other writers have expressed a similar view. Van Rensselaer Potter, one of the early users of the term bioethics, stated in a book by that title that "we must now face up to the fact that human ethics cannot be separated from a realistic understanding of ecology in the broadest sense. Ethical values cannot be separated from biological facts."[7] Aldo Leopold, one of the great conservationists of this century, iterated in his monumental work *A Sand County Almanac* "an ethic may be regarded as a mode of guidance for meeting ecological situations so new or intricate, or involving such deferred reactions that the path of social expediency is not discernible to the average individual."[8]

One final description by geneticist and humanist Bentley Glass clinches the case for an ethical reorientation:

> I believe that only a religious ethic (toward nature) will serve to protect us, an ethic that regards man as the trustee of nature for the welfare of all people, now and into the remote future.[9]

To return to an earlier reference, the evolution of ethics was conceptualized as an inverted pyramid as shown in Fig. 11.1. (See also Chapter 1, p. 25.)[10] In this model, ethical concepts grew over time to embrace larger and larger groups—from individual family, to tribes, to region, nations, races, and finally humankind. The last stages of this phylogeny—to encompass races and all of humankind—are still gestating and it remains to be seen when this ethical leap forward will be made. But going even beyond that, a new postulate, yet to gain serious attention by policy-makers at least, extends the ethical domain to nonhuman forms of life. It is of interest to note that this attitude has begun to attract followers, at least in regard to higher mammals. Some people today, albeit few, are willing to concede that dogs, horses, deer, and similar animals are partially within the ethical sphere. The movement to prevent cruelty to animals reflects an aspect of this consciousness, and so does the motivation for wild-life conservation. (More generally, though, pragmatic considerations guide wild-life policy such as cropping of excess individuals through controlled hunting.) Some vegetarians are motivated to refrain from eating meat for reasons of genuine concern for animals. But neither spiders nor snails nor plants nor protozoa are included here. Only a few people, such as Albert Schweitzer with his reverence for all life, stand as examples of those who have taken the giant ethical step to encompass *all* forms of life on this planet. A more recent movement exemplified by philosopher Peter Singer in his book *Animal Liberation* is pushing for equal consideration of animal interests.[11] The concept is beginning to receive serious attention from the scholarly community.[12]

The last stage in ethical evolution projects an extension of ethics to the environment itself (see Fig. 11.1). The American naturalist Aldo Leopold, keenly aware of the necessity of this ethical expansion as far back as 1949, wrote the following passage in his oft-reproduced essay "The Land Ethic":

> The extension of ethics to . . . the human environment is, if I read the evidence correctly, an evolutionary possibility and an ecological necessity. . . . Individual thinkers since the days of Ezekiel and Isaiah have asserted that the despoliation of land is not only inexpedient but wrong. Society, however, has not affirmed their belief. I regard the present conservation movement as the embryo of such an affirmation.[13]

Throughout his essay Leopold speaks of "the extension of the social conscience from people to land." Basic to this view is the recognition that an individual's well-being depends on the well-being of his ecological (i.e., life) support system. To have a "valid ethic of nature we must affirm the intrinsic value of every item in creation."[14] As knowledge of our dependent relationship with nature grows, we place value on an ever greater variety of things. For instance, plant life of the ocean becomes valuable when we recognize the key role it plays in rejuvenating the earth's oxygen or the higher value placed on preserving soils and vegetation when we apprehend their ability to absorb air pollutants. In practice this attitude does not require a total ab-

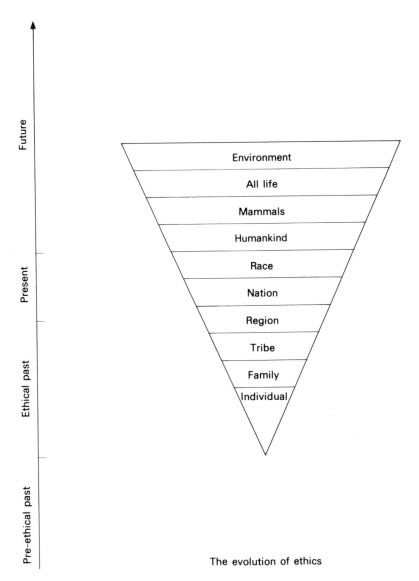

The evolution of ethics

Fig. 11.1 *The evolution of ethics over time to include an ever-widening circle of concern. (From Roderick Nash, Reference 10. Used by permission.)*

stention from the utilization of the resources of nature, for we must still depend on them for food, shelter, clothing, transportation, and recreation. As Murdy writes:

> I may affirm that every species has intrinsic value but I will behave as though I value my own survival and that of my species more highly than the survival of other animals and plants. I may assert that a lettuce plant has intrinsic value, yet I will eat it before it reproduces itself because I value my own nutritional well-being above the survival of the lettuce plant.[15]

By recognizing the value of things as opposed to a strict utilitarian view, sufficient motivation for environmental preservation will be forthcoming.

SOURCE OF AN ENVIRONMENTAL ETHIC

Are environmental values intrinsic or secondary? Should the natural environment be preserved because of its present and future contributions to human welfare or is there some more profound reason for insisting upon its preservation? People of good-will presuppose that nature ought to be preserved, but few have bothered or have been able to articulate reasons in defense of that position.

Do we possess an organic need to preserve? Although the question can be argued both ways, the answer is probably no. Technology could provide us with the mechanism for addressing any imbalance now being wrought in the environment. To assert that it is not doing this now does not imply that with fuller knowledge guided by purpose, technology could not redress our perturbations of nature as well as provide our essential needs. For example, the problem of photosynthesis can theoretically be solved and we may be able to implement an artificial technology for food production more efficient than the present one carried out in vegetative living tissue. Our oxygen needs could be accommodated by planting varieties of fast-growing plants or by generating it from inorganic oxides. Plastic vegetation could satisfy our aesthetic sense as it already does in a number of instances where differentiating the natural from the artificial cannot be easily done. That technology at the present time is unable to provide all of our wants and needs misses the point. The point is that a perfected technology may very well possess the capacity for providing us all of life's necessities, including our aesthetic desires; and technology possesses no need for conservation except perhaps to curb its excesses.

But there is more to the story. Preservation and maintenance of the environment is not a come-see, come-sigh thing; it is not an option whose choice is dictated merely by individual or societal preference. Environmental values are primary and the case can be defended this way. Humans are simultaneously biological organisms and parts of nature, and they are the possessors of individuality, a conscious self-awareness, and an other-awareness. Here is our uniqueness. What needs to be emphasized is that earth, at least that part most interesting to us, was shaped almost exclusively by other living species. The interdependence between us and other life forms is so complete that it accounts for the adaptability and richness of human life. Our evolution has been shaped by this association; our individual life is conditioned by stimuli we receive from nature during our own brief existence. We constantly seek out other living things probably because our species evolved in fellowship with them and we have retained from the evolutionary past a biological need for this partnership.[16] All of us incorporate part of the universe into our very being; we realize our own humanness in our dealings with the environment. If we are to realize the wondrousness of ourselves we must respect other living organisms equally. A sterile environment can only produce sterile souls.

The relationship that links humankind to other living organisms and to the earth generates an overriding need for us to experience as much of nature as we can. It would seem, then, that there is something more basic than mere expediency for constantly seeking to preserve nature. If it is desecrated, we run the real risk of losing some or all of our humanness. The ethical criterion for judging the intrinsic value of a course of action was given us by Leopold in this statement: "A thing is right when it tends to preserve the integrity, stability and beauty of the biotic community. It is wrong when it tends to do otherwise."[17] This condition shapes all other values and is, therefore, morally prescriptive.

In constructing a new ethic to protect the land, Leopold implied also a concomitant change in the philosophy of law. Major changes for the better are not only matters of conscience and ethics but require the formulation of new rules to explicate such problems as pollution, destruction of fragile resources, and the like. Now, in less than a generation after the publication of Leopold's classic essay, the foundations for just such a philosophical change are being laid. The occasion was the publication by lawyer Christopher D. Stone of the book *Should Trees Have Standing?: Toward Legal Rights for Natural Objects*. Based on a Supreme Court decision concerning the proposed development by Disney Enterprises of Mineral King in the Sierra Mountains of California, Stone's thesis is that natural objects should have legal standing in the Court. Although the judgment was against those bringing suit (the Sierra Club) to block the development, the closeness of the decision (4 to 3) as well as the wording of the majority opinion reflected a changing attitude in this country. Do the elements of the environment have rights? Do many of the ethical constraints that govern our actions toward other humans govern our use of the ocean, the sky, the soil? Questions of this sort reflect the new consciousness needed to actualize a quality future.

PRINCIPLE OF RECIPROCITY

As a guide in shaping the new social institutions, humans must recognize that they stand in necessary relationships of interdependence and reciprocity;[18] that is, not only do we need our fellow persons, we also need the other species, animals and plants, *and* the materials of the earth and atmosphere. Human life now depends and will continue to depend upon the proper functioning of the earth's present ecosystem. The day-to-day maintenance of our life-support system relies on the functional interaction of countless interdependent biotic and physiochemical factors. Ecology has shown that no living entity can exist by and for itself; everything is connected to everything else. This concept has been called the *principle of reciprocity*. One form of this principle has been known a long time, appearing in various forms in religious and primitive societies in their dealings with other human beings: "Do unto others as you would have them do unto you." Reciprocity is recognition of mutual obligation. What an ecological ethic must do is to force upon us the recognition that this principle is truly universal; biologist Barry Commoner calls it the first law of ecology. Reciprocity includes not only the *who* but the *what* as well. Not just our next of kin, or those who belong to our tribe, or social class, or nation, not even the human population as a whole, or even future generations, but all living things and the nonliving substances with which we must work—all these are bound together in a variety of bonds of mutual dependency. Everyone's environment merges into everyone else's; the environment does not have state or national boundaries. Continued growth in awareness may lead to the recognition that no event in nature is without some effect on the whole environment of which we are part, and we should value all items in nature. We don't always know how or why a human-made upset may imperil the balance on which all living things, including our own species, depend. But until we do, it behooves us to be careful of all elements of the system and not wantonly destroy any of them. Does it then not follow that the rocks themselves have rights? The water, the landscape, the air? The movement of ocean currents and the activity of soil microbes are as essential to our existence as the oxygen we breathe. We must learn how far the network of reciprocities reach, beyond just plain economic considerations; we must develop a morality of interdependence going far beyond our present commitments. Elliot T. Richardson, U.S. Ambassador-at-Large, perceived this relationship in the following exhortation:

> There was a time when the seas seemed endless and the skies vast enough to swallow any of the mistakes and errors of man. The world used to be big and men could afford to be small. Now the world is small and men must be big.[19]

In the extreme, reciprocity seriously challenges the right to own property. Can someone or some company *own* a piece of the environment and do with it what he/she wishes; can someone buy a mountain, sell a forest, lease an oilfield? Is the environment a commodity to be possessed? In a more practical sense, reciprocity expresses itself in many ways. It may mean not draining marshlands because they play a key role in recharging aquifers (water-bearing strata of rock, sand, or gravel), or not constructing a highway across productive farmland. Reciprocity may mean increasing population densities at certain points to free open space elsewhere (i.e., planned urban development and cluster developments). Reciprocity may mean placing interdependent functions close together; one major variable in our traffic jams is the length of the journey to work because we have encouraged the segregation of work and residence. In this view, human cultural achievements are seen as occurring within the context of interdependences, expanded to include not only the cultural and biological but the physical environment as well.

A final observation concerning the ethical pyramid (Fig. 11.1). The last stage, or even those stages just preceding it, is conceived of primarily in the abstract, at least for the moment. "The extension of the social conscience from people to land" as proposed by Aldo Leopold has not yet occurred nor is it likely to occur in the near future. The higher levels of the ethical pyramid apply to an ideal, not to real present-day behavior, but the higher levels are not to be discounted. Rather, they are to be strived after much like the Biblical admonition: "Be ye therefore perfect even as your Father which is in heaven is perfect." Obviously, at different times and depending upon the circumstances, all of us are still mired in the lower ethical echelons. Although we consistently fail to live up to the higher levels, at least we have the ideal to motivate our actions; at those rare times when we attain the ideal, we are privileged a transcendent experience; we encounter the mountain-top, and another dimension of our humanhood is fulfilled.

TWO CONFLICTING ETHICS: NATURE VERSUS THINGS

Right relationships between humans and the natural world involve not only a new definition of our kinship with nature but our utilization of it as well. Since we must use the resources of the natural world for our subsistence, humans and nature must find sustainable and satisfactory arrangements in packages of different sizes than those presently used. Our appetite for things must somehow be reduced.

One of the most outstanding features of human history has been the shift from biological to cultural evolution. Our ability to solve problems, remember the solutions, and transmit this information directly or indirectly to subsequent generations has developed in humans to a spectacular degree. It has given rise to an innovative kind of heredity, cultural heredity, as distinguished from genetic or biological heredity. The invention of this new heredity has made possible the process of cultural evolution, a process so much faster than biological evolution. By permitting *Homo sapiens* to circumvent or delay many of the ecological limitations that keep natural species in check, cultural evolution has made it possible for our species to reshape the face of the earth. For the first time in earth's evolution, one species can live in almost every kind of habitat found in this world (and now even out of this world for short times at least); it has appropriated about one-fourth of earth's land surface for its own private food production and is covetously grabbing up more; it gobbles up about one percent of all the food energy in the ecosphere, more than 10,000 times its share; it has invaded the air and the sea, and burrowed into the earth in search of raw materials to sustain its activities.

To support their ever-increasing numbers as well as individual appetites, humans have invented thousands of "synthetic organisms," such as automobiles, factories, nuclear power plants, and the like. These synthetic organisms, like living organisms, are open systems. They require an input, have an output, and require a source of energy. They ingest all manner of natural resources and various sources of energy (usually in enormous quantities), then transform these into a great variety of products and by-products, some of which are consumed by the species and some of which are not. Those which are not pile up in the form of environmental junk, more commonly called pollutants, that the species tries to get rid of by depositing somewhere else. The three primary economic processes—extraction, production, and consumption—with their yield of unavoidable by-products (as predicted by the Second Law of Thermodynamics), are frequently in conflict with the natural ecosystem. Thus, natural ecosystems have been replaced by those judged to be of greater worth, namely, artificial ecosystems.

The driving force behind this rapid development, as the recent world-wide events of inflation and shortages impress upon us, is consumption. It is the force that drives production and extraction. Not only is consumption a function of ever-increasing numbers but during the century or so since the scientific-industrial revolution began, the level of consumption has increased conspicuously as members of industrialized societies have become wealthier. As Philip Handler, director of the National Academy of Sciences, observed, world population has been growing at a two percent annual rate while world food production has been increasing at a rate of two and a half percent, but world food demand has risen three percent.[20] Thorstein Veblen, the early twentieth century economist, invented the term *conspicuous consumption* to describe that kind of demand upon products where actual consumption is greater than necessary consumption. During the past several decades, as individual and corporate wealth has continued to increase, consumption required to be conspicuous has increased accordingly. The consequences of the acquisition of wealth by larger numbers, coupled with rapid development of technology, have led to extensive changes in culture; that which in former times was judged to be a luxury now becomes necessity. What Veblen called conspicuous consumption has now been called *galloping consumerism*. Production, aided by technology, has responded to increased per capita consumption and population growth; this response has accelerated both the extraction of raw materials from natural resources and the introduction of garbage into the environment. Consume more, to produce more, to consume more has become the marching orders of our generation. Spend to keep the economy healthy is the incessant message broadcast by our leaders, both public and commercial. An eminent biologist has remarked "growth for growth's sake is the philosophy of the cancer cell." It is within this context that Leopold said, "we will soon be dead by owning too much." In the United States and elsewhere, however, this accelerating consumption is called progress or economic growth. In fact, it is a kind of pernicious, ecological myopia, for as soon as one essential resource has been exhausted or made useless by pollution—perhaps even before this happens—the concept of complex reciprocity (interdependences) warns us that some vital link in the ecosystem and/or the economic system will be used up and the quality of our lives is diminished yet again!

Not so long ago we were getting mainly good news about what we with our machines were doing. Our abundant creativity was capable of transforming almost any aspect of the environment into something useful. Now, though, the news is bad; trends have been set in motion that can carry away our *human* future and lay it in a tomb. We simply cannot reach a good future by the way we are going now. The environment that called us into being, that directed our evolution over countless eons of time, was vastly different, naturally and socially, from the environment to which we are now exposed. Daniel Kozlovsky points out that the organism is most interesting and healthiest when it is exposed to an environment fundamentally in harmony with the one that called it into being.[21] What he means, of course, is that you need the environment you evolved in to be you. Our present competitive and conflictual modes of behavior are making the human environment more and more unreal—i.e. less natural.

A fundamental ecological principle applicable to human activity says that we can make an unlimited amount of anything only with the inevitable, irretrievable loss of something else.[22] Many times this something lost is a something we must have to be healthy and happy. The ingrained attitude of many persons is that we can do anything, and it sometimes seems so; it is important, however, to accept the obvious fact that anything we do has environmental implications, almost all of them disturbing. It may well be that the present energy crisis and the wider ecological crisis are going to become the occasions for an historical and social testing. Can we learn, accept, and then implement with proper policy the central principle that there are limitations to what should and can be done? The United States and other advanced industrialized nations must sooner or later realize the folly of their growth mentality. The earth is simply too small for all the nations of the world to have standards of living like those prevailing in the West.

Unfortunately, the wants and desires of humans appear to be insatiable. It is, therefore, a self-deception to think that restraints upon human action are not going to have to be developed and enforced. There is scant evidence from human history to arouse confidence that leaders or citizens will easily adopt a course that proceeds from other than narrow egoistic motives, a course that will sacrifice for the good of the world community or posterity. Such sacrifice is something that we Americans especially are finding extremely hard to accept since the majority of us are inordinately fond of affluence no matter what effluents may happen to accompany it.[23] A case in point: in October of 1974, the president was talking about an increase in taxes as an income surtax to curb inflation; in January of 1975, he suggested a reduction of income tax to take our economy out of the doldrums; in July of 1975, he proposed a "detente with nature" until our momentary economic difficulties could be overcome. It is time to stop kidding ourselves. Present destructive progress cannot continue, and the current economic philosophy is not only incapable of changing it, it is opposed to changing it. As long as there remains the primary motivation for profit, the situation will remain unstable and can have no other result except continued deterioration of the human environment. The solution to the ecological crisis and, in the broader view, the upgrading of the human condition is not a blind self-indulgence, each one grabbing what he/she can out of the common resources that exist for all.

There are fundamentally two courses that lie before us. Either we can continue the present course of disintegrating development or we can build a new consciousness whose dominant values are far different from present ones. Richard Falk, in his book *This Endangered Planet: Prospects and Proposals for Human Survival*, proposes this plan:

> First, we need to understand the inability of the sovereign state to resolve the endangered-planet crisis; second, we need a model of world order that provides a positive vision of the future and is able to resolve this crisis; third, we need a strategy that will transform human attitudes and institutions so as to make it politically possible to bring a new system of world order into being; fourth, we need specific programs to initiate the process, as with learning to walk—we need to learn to walk into the future.[24]

Several years have passed since this was written in 1972. The transformation of attitudes called for seems to be floundering; if there is any movement at all, it is movement in the reverse direction. If Western civilization fails, it will be because it has been unable to discover a concept which could impart an attitude of responsibility governing our interactions with nature; and at this point in time, it does not seem that we are capable of rendering one.[25]

At least one part of the problem involves priorities that ultimately derive from the values we hold. As these remarks have shown, the majority view in terms of basic values is antiecological. In a comprehensive sense, a shift in our ways of thinking and making decisions is required; this is part of what Aldo Leopold meant by "an extension of the social conscience." The ethic of utility and consumption, as it has developed in America, says that the environment is a commodity whose economic utility determines its goodness. Individual success, usually gauged by the accumulation of wealth, is still the acclaimed virtue and is accounted to be a great moral achievement. But this ethic must be redefined, away from quantitative indices and toward qualitative ones. Only when our basic values direct us toward a new understanding of what constitutes the good life, can the quality of life, including human life, be enriched.

Restraints on our demand, or even reducing our demand for things is seen as the primary necessity in terms of changing value systems. A more desirable ethic would accept the fact that too many of us want too much. Within this ethic would be the necessity of learning to share and to do without. As Daniel Kozlovsky suggests in very harsh terms:

> The American way of life is ecological criminality. From the point of view of ecological ethics, it is a criminal act to own and drive a big automobile, to live in excess of your needs, for by reveling in such luxury and opulence, you are denying other persons what they need for survival as well as bringing about the deterioration of the entire earth ecosystem . . . within this framework the American way of life is a criminal act and anyone who owns more than the necessities of life is an ecological criminal.[26]

This is strong language, but perhaps it may force us to pause for reappraisal of the life-styles we live. The embryonic movement under the title "think small" emphasizes this need for review of our whole perspective of what makes the good life. Ernest Schumacher, an English economist, in the tract *Small is Beautiful* contends that we must develop a life-style designed for permanence, with new modes of production and consumption. The customary Western yardstick of a person's happiness—standard of living—measured in terms of material goods is utterly misleading and must change. Modern economic theory implemented by production-consumption policies will in the final analysis consume itself as demonstrated by the increasing industrial threat to the environment, the growing scarcity of natural resources, and the mounting discontent and ungovernability of populations.[27] Whereas a few years ago many of us thought that saving the environment would require little more than recycling newspapers, collecting soft drink bottles, and passing air-pollution control laws, today it is clear that nothing less than a complete reassessment of our whole life-style—intensive and energy-extravagant—and some rather radical surgery on our wasteful habits are demanded. Bigger and better things means bigger and "better" resource depletion and pollution.

A NEW VALUE SYSTEM

This new value system, whatever form it may take, can contribute to a restructuring of social institutions, technologies, decision-making processes, and attitudes toward environmental resources. Why shouldn't we have an environment to live and work in where we would not have to worry about someone disturbing our peace and quiet, or someone building a nuclear power plant in our community, or putting up another hamburger stand or sleazy bookstore across the street, or dropping a bomb on us, or slowly, insidiously poisoning us to death? Some are beginning to ask the question, do we have a *right* to a livable environment? If human rights are those rights each of us require to live a human life, permitting us to fulfill our capacities as rational and free beings, then might not the right to a decent environment be properly identified as such a human right?[28] If our troubles result from the unlimited application of a single-minded economic philosophy, why not change it? The beginnings of these concerns are just now stirring. Although we as individuals cannot constrain the larger forces that govern our economy (it remains to be seen whether anyone can), we can control ourselves. It is contradictory to moralize against the violence of a society threatening to destroy the natural world and itself and then conduct one's personal affairs in a way that contributes to this very route to the future. In fundamental terms this demands that people who care will live lives that show they care! Good ecological thinking and acting in our personal lives must break the bad habits we have learned from the past. I am not so foolish as to think that not buying a new pair of shoes when I already have sufficient would help resolve the ecological crisis, but it would certainly demonstrate one person's commitment. Further, it is consistent with the self-actualization theme of the previous future ethics discussion (see p. 353). It does seem clear that each of us has the responsibility to change him/herself, to abandon those things which are inconsistent with an ethic of nature. I am here reminded of the short but simple verse of Edward Everett Hale:*

> I am only one—
> But still I am one;
> I cannot do everything
> But I can do something.
> And because I cannot do everything,
> I will not hesitate to do
> The one thing I can do.

If a fundamental solution to the environmental crisis requires the balancing of consumption against the rates of energy flow and materials recycling in the ecosphere, then concerned people must abandon the ecologically destructive life-style of conspicuous consumption. It is as simple as that!

At a higher level, restructuring our social system and redirecting economic growth must be the highest of humankind's aspirations. New and unprecedented changes in value structure, attitudinal make-ups, educational practice, and world views must be postulated. What might these postulates be? What is the good life? What is the good society? Is it a free society? Is it a stable society? What is really harmful and what things are really beneficial? We have to ask ourselves what really matters. Although no clear listings or formulas presently exist, at least none that meet with general acceptance, one could suggest as a starting point some basic human needs, needs which ideally should be met if the good life is to be nurtured. At least three general aspects concerning human needs demand attention. These are:

1 Optimum genetic composition of the population.

2 Optimum individual development.

3 Optimum environment.

---

* John Bartlett, *Familiar Quotations*, Little, Brown and Company, Boston, 1955, p. 624.

The first two in this list will be discussed only briefly here; they more properly relate to a discussion of the social environment. They are included here for completeness only. The first implies certain needs for individuals and others that apply to the population as a whole. For the individual, the optimum may not be the right to reproduce but rather the need of children to be born physically and mentally sound. For the population, the greatest genetic need is to safeguard the breadth of human diversity, which for a million or so odd years of evolution has been basic to our success as a species. There is no single genetic ideal, for in genetic diversity there is population stability.

The second need, optimum individual development, may be achieved through optimum nutrition, optimum health, provision for challenging activities, and growth in an atmosphere of love. As Schumacher writes, the difference between Buddhist and Western philosophies is that the former "tries to maximize human satisfactions by the optimal pattern of productive effort." As one social scientist put it, development begins with people, not with things. The commandment "love thy neighbor as thyself" needs to be expanded to "love thy species as thyself."[29]

As to the third requirement, optimum environment, Van Rensselaer Potter in his book *Bioethics* lists what he considers to be the properties for such an environment:[30]

1. Basic needs; food, shelter, clothing, space, privacy, leisure, education (moral and intellectual).
2. Freedom from toxic chemicals, unnecessary trauma, and preventable disease.
3. A culture having respect for sound ecologic principles.
4. A culture that prepares us for individual adaptive responses.
5. A sense of identity, with individual happiness that understands oscillations between satisfaction and dissatisfaction.
6. Productivity that involves commitment to other members of society.
7. An ongoing search for beauty and order that does not deny the role of individuality and disorder.

It is to be noted that the optimum environment is one that goes beyond the basic elements for sheer survival (e.g., absence of disease). It is one where positive health is achieved; a happy and productive life is encouraged. The thrust of Potter's criteria is quite clear: Human beings can never be free from the forces of nature; survival is not merely a problem in economics or political science. These concepts correlate well with the earlier-mentioned evolutionary principle that submits that for an organism to survive, it must encounter an environment to which it is adapted. If an inappropriate environment is encountered, these adaptations are frustrated and the organism becomes distorted, diseased, or deceased. Furthermore, it is essential that the organism not destroy the environment that it needs. (And here we might heed the lesson of the parasite.) We must fashion, then, a system that allows us to remain adaptive, that provides each human individual with the environment needed for full development while at the same time does not destroy that environment. We must abandon ethical systems that cannot see our species in this evolutionary and ecological context.

We add, then, another principle to a nature ethic: Insofar as possible, we must engage in nondestructive activities and programs. Behavior that is destructive to other humans or to the surface of the earth is ultimately destructive to all. Such a nature ethic would promote an harmonious equilibrium relationship between human needs, desires, and activities and the rest of the world, living and nonliving; it would accept the fact each of us wants too much; it would accept the fact that there are too many of us; it would treat all substances of the earth with respect, to be used carefully and recycled, if used at all; it would comprise a society wherein each individual lived in direct contact with his/her physiological and psychological life-support systems, close to the earth, in contact with nature. It would, in short, provide to each person an opportunity to develop and live a biologically sound philosophy of life, free from the high-pressured economic demands of today; free from the competitive, superficial, insecure social groupings within which most of us now interact.[31]

BIOETHICS

To work toward this new world view, Potter proposes a new discipline which he has called *bioethics*. The derivation here is a dual one to emphasize the two most important ingredients to achieving the new wisdom that is needed: (1) Biological knowledge, and (2) human values. As Potter envisions it, bioethics would attempt to relate our biological nature and realistic knowledge of the biological world to the formulation of policies designed to promote social good. He goes further to state what he considers to be acceptable courses of action based on biological paradigms in what he labels "A Bioethical Creed for Individuals" (see below). Each begins with a statement of belief or value preference (ethic) followed by a commitment to a course of action. Such a code of ethics, as Potter emphasizes, should never be considered finished but undergo continual reexamination and refinement, and new statements should be added:

A Bioethical Creed for Individuals

1. *Belief.* I accept the need for prompt remedial action in a world beset with crisis.

    Commitment. I will work with others to improve the formulation of my beliefs, to evolve additional credos, and to unite in a worldwide movement that will make possible the survival and improved development of the human species in harmony with the natural environment.

2. *Belief.* I accept the fact that the future survival and development of mankind, both culturally and biologically, is strongly conditioned by man's present activities and plans.

    Commitment. I will try to live my own life and to influence the lives of others so as to promote the evolution of a better world for future generations of mankind, and I will try to avoid actions that would jeopardize their future.

3. *Belief.* I accept the uniqueness of each individual and his instinctive need to contribute to the betterment of some larger unit of society in a way that is compatible with the long-range needs of society.

    Commitment. I will try to listen to the reasoned viewpoint of others whether from a minority or a majority, and I will recognize the role of emotional commitment in producing effective action.

4. *Belief.* I accept the inevitability of some human suffering that must result from the natural disorder in biological creatures and in the physical world, but I do not passively accept the suffering that results from man's inhumanity to man.

   Commitment. I will try to face my own problems with dignity and courage, I will try to assist my fellow men when they are afflicted, and I will work toward the goal of eliminating needless suffering among mankind as a whole.

5. *Belief.* I accept the finality of death as a necesary part of life. I affirm my veneration of life, my belief in the brotherhood of man, and my belief that I have an obligation to future generations of man.

   Commitment. I will try to live in a way that will benefit the lives of my fellow men now and in time to come and be remembered favorably by those who survive me.[32]

What is contained here is "bioethics of humility with responsibility."

Potter's ethical code is but an example of what is needed, a vision to help shape present and future values and decisions of people. The important thing is that the ethic recognizes the ties between humankind and the world of nature. Such thinking can foster a morality that insists upon the wise use of the natural world as it is necessary to sustain human life. As a concomitant outcome, the human species can survive and develop further.

For the question, What *ought* the culture do to survive? the answer is not hard to find, as this discussion has shown. For a second and more practical question, What ought we to do to develop such a culture? an answer is far more difficult. A mere contribution of every concerned individual simply doing his/her own thing is not likely to lead to a culture that can survive. Maximizing laissez-faire culture in this dimension is as bankrupt as we saw it to be in matters of medical ethics. Collectively, as a society, we ought to first agree that some things are more important than others and then get on with the task of naming the important things and deciding how to implement them in our culture. Governmental efforts at articulating a national energy policy underscores the difficulties here. The next quarter-century may be one of the most crucial in history. We must either learn how to control ourselves or suffer the consequences from our lack of discipline and foresight. This observation is neither extremist nor hysterical for civilizations before us have succumbed despite vast intellectual and material resources. It seems likely that survival with quality is possible only if the systems of ethics are compatible with the real world, and this will require some painful reorientation in our ways of thinking and behaving. It would, indeed, be surprising if the human species could continue in an acceptable form without major revision of many ancient and diverse beliefs. The Nobel-laureate scientist George Wald once ended a lecture with the observation that it took the planet earth 4.5 billion years to discover that it was 4.5 billion years old. Then he added: "Having got to that point . . . have we got much longer?"

POSTSCRIPTS

Postscript I. This discussion has touched upon only few of the significant ethical questions as they relate to environmental issues. There are many other questions, those of social goals, of personal attitudes and behavior, of setting and enforcing standards, of providing incentives to influence both individual and corporate activities, of education and indoctrination of people to think and act along certain lines, of the extent to which technology should be encouraged as a solution to environmental problems when the ultimate effect may be to cause more problems than it solves, and others. New visions of the future, new social systems, new political structures, new symbols—the development of a new ecological humanism that is worldwide—these are all problems so varied and so vast that their solutions may seem to go far beyond our resources and knowledge. It will not be easy to crystalize thinking on the ethical dimensions of the current ecological crisis.

Beyond that, the major and extremely difficult question remains: How do we move from the philosophical position to a responsible social state? Potter has generated a sequence that may be helpful in effecting this transition. He includes these steps:[33]

1. Environmental damage becomes visible to "average individuals" raising moral indignation;
2. Knowledge of these problems evolves a new discipline—environmental bioethics;
3. Moral indignation demands preventive countermeasures;
4. Moral pressure plus factual information generates bioethical guidelines;
5. These are converted into legal sanctions.

If there is any reason for optimism as we anticipate the future it lies in the observation that beginnings are being made. There is some evidence that the scenario above depicted by Potter is being followed. Colorado voters, in 1974, turned down the offer of hosting the Winter Olympics Games of 1976 on environmental grounds. Citizens in coastal South Carolina rejected a chemical factory, this despite the fact that unemployment was high in the area. Oregon invites vacationers to come but not to say. Petaluma, California was granted legal authority to limit its growth by the Supreme Court in order to preserve its environment. The office of Governor Edmund G. Brown of California issued a committee report which embodies a comprehensive set of policies for orderly growth, development, and maintenance of environmental quality for the whole state. Public polls still support environmental goals. The Opinion Research Corporation of Princeton, New Jersey in the summer of 1975 polled a cross-section of the American public on their attitudes toward environmental issues. The poll showed that despite recession, high unemployment, and rising fuel costs, those interviewed opposed cutting back environmental control programs. Although it is impossible to prove, the impression is felt that at no other time in our history have the people been so far out in front of our political leaders. Many of the general public show a great deal more awareness of the complexity and interdependencies of modern life and receptiveness to new approaches to ordering their lives than do politicians. But still the call for change lies heaviest on the individual. It does seem clear that each of us has the responsibility to change him/herself to abandon those actions that are inconsistent with a natural ethic acceptable to all people and to the earth.

Postscript II. Much effort has been made to search out the historical roots of the present environmental crisis. The reasons motivating this quest are apparent: if modern civilization's attitude toward nature is out of line, in order to prescribe a cure we must know the cause. Historian Lynn White lays special blame on the Judeo-Christian tradition and its heavy influence on thought and practice in Western societies. He contends that modern science and technology, wherever it is found in the world, is based on the Western model. The Western model is conditioned by the scriptural admonition of domination over, not cooperation with, nature. Factors he cites in support of this thesis are the following:

1. Divine creation started everything including time. Linear or nonrepetitive time rather than a cyclical notion of it is a special mark of Western thought. Creation was a series of events culminating in the formation of humans (males first), the reason being that all the prior inclusions found in the physical world were put there to service man. Genesis 1:28 describes the charge given by the Creator to His last and greatest creation: "fill the earth and subdue it and have dominion over the fish of the sea and over the birds of the air and over every living thing." The whole cosmic system will ultimately end in the final day of reckoning or Judgment Day.

2. Man was created in God's image. He was not part of nature as were the other creatures who came into being by divine command; something special went into human creation, including the "breath of life." This clear separation prompted dualistic interpretations of a living world. Whereas we share in common some features with the biological world, humans stand noticeably apart from it—the possessors of the "breath of life," an immortal soul. Christianity thus became the most anthropocentric religion the world had yet to know; humans were set apart from nature and it was God's will that nature be used for man's purposes. This was in marked contrast to ancient paganism which revered nature, even worshiped it—e.g., the sacred groves of the Old Testament.

3. Christianity wrought the destruction of pagan animism (i.e., God in nature view). Whereas Animism required that spirits must be placated before parts of nature could be used lest there be retribution effected on the perpetrator—the cutting down of a tree, the damming of a brook—Christianity made it possible to exploit nature independently of any feelings natural objects may hold. This indifference made possible exploitation without fear.

4. Christianity promoted the development of a natural theology. A study of nature was presumed to lead to a better understanding of God. This became the motivation of all science—"to think God's thoughts after Him." Western science became cast in the mold of Christian theology, that is, knowledge of nature leads to a greater utilization of what the Divine had made available.[34]

In Lynn White's view, human transcendence over nature validating the rightness of mastery over nature, was attributable to Judeo-Christian precepts; consequently, it must bear the major burden of guilt for the present environmental crisis. He goes further by asserting that the way out of our present quandary is to "reject the Christian axiom that nature has no reason for existence save to serve man." White's interpretation was widely publicized and at the time received a good deal of acceptance even by the intellectual community. More recently, though, the view has been challenged as being much too simplistic; furthermore, it has little factual support on its side. An alternative position based on cultural factors was submitted by Lewis Moncrief.[35] Here, although the Judeo-Christian tradition may have been one contributory cause, it by no means was the only one nor was it probably the most important. The anthropologic record informs us that humans have been altering their environment, sometimes drastically, since antiquity. Examples are slash-and-burn agriculture, the fire-driven method of hunting, irrigation and terracing, overgrazing, lumbering to the point of depletion, and the like. The prompting factors here are the desire for a better life; this is a universal wish whether one is rich or poor, religious or atheistic, occupying this time in history or some ancient one.

Also, for the vast period of human existence, the majority of the wealth was concentrated in the hands of the few. However, in the eighteenth and nineteenth centuries things began to change, for two profound revolutions were stirring in the West. (This probably accords the West its position of uniqueness, not the fact that Christianity is its major religion. Furthermore, it may have been pure happenstance that it occurred here at all.)

The first contributing factor was the French revolution which ushered in widespread democratization. Concomitant with liberalization of the political climate was a redistribution and reallocation of natural and human resources. Wealth became accessible to more and more people.

The second element prompting change was the Industrial Revolution. The productive capacity of each worker was increased by several orders of magnitude. The skills of the artisan gave way to production methods of industry. Goods that formerly could not be produced in quantity now could be manufactured on a commercial scale. Wider availability, coupled with a lowering in cost, made these goods available to larger numbers of people. Later integration of these two revolutions—democratic ideals with technological ideas—resulted in a more equitable distribution of material substance and increased the overall wealth of society. It was this joining that set the stage for environmental degradation, for with larger segments demanding more goods and services, despoliation and waste were the predictable outcomes.

America added something to this, too. With the opening of new lands attracting the former landless from Europe as colonizers, the concept of private ownership by the few broke down. Natural resources became the possessions of the citizens. The problem of decision-making became compounded as a result since many landowners now had to be involved. So burdensome has this become that decisive conservation measures many times cannot be taken because of lack of consensus or cooperation.

A second American contribution to our attitudes toward the environment stems from the Westward movement of settlers. As pioneers moved into new lands, they encountered many obstacles—a primitive transportation system, hostile Indians, forests, the competition of wildlife, sod that must be turned for planting. All these had to be changed if the land was to be made desirable and useful. Thus, many of the natural resources that we highly value today were perceived as nuisances rather than assets in the days of the westward expansion.

A summation of all these cultural variables—democracy, technology, the desire for the good life, urbanization, and antagonism toward nature—are probably the factors which have driven us into our present environmental plight. The universal tendency to maximize self-interest has resulted in a complete absence of personal moral direction concerning our treatment of nature. The dogged defense of the democratic tradition accounts for the inability of social institutions to make proper adjustments to relieve the stress. Our abiding faith in technology to solve any and all of our problems precludes a reorientation in our perceptions of what really counts (we believe no evil until the evil is done, if then—Fontaine's Law).

In this second view, our environmental problems do not stem from the religious perceptions held by Westerners. All cultures, but especially Western cultures due to a variety of motivations, have despoiled their environments. Realizing these historical and philosophical trends, we return to our initial proposition: The environmental crisis is an extension of humankind's failure to see itself as an integral part of the global ecosystem!

VALUES PERTAINING TO AN ETHIC OF NATURE

1 All ethics rests on the single premise: The individual is a member of the community of interdependent parts.

2 An ethic of nature enlarges the boundary of the human community to include soils, water, plants, and animals.

3 An ecological ethic requires a critical thoughtfulness about the consequences of our actions and our life-styles.

4 Humans need nature to realize the full potential of their humanhood.

5 People who care about the environment must live lives that show their concern.

6 The solution to the environmental crisis requires new values, new social systems, and new political structures.

7 Human ethics no longer can be separated from biological facts.

8 The environmental crisis is much more profound than the inconveniences of noise, ugliness, and unpleasantness; it touches on matters of our very humanity, our relationship to nature.

9 It is essential for the full development of an organism that it encounter an environment from which it has evolved.

10 Economic gain should not be the ultimate determiner of environmental utilization.

11 The American way of life is a criminal act.

12 Science and technology can be utilized to solve environmental problems.

13 Cries of crisis and impending doom are nothing new; the world has had its doomsayers throughout its history.

14 Attempts to forecast the future have not been singularly successful, hence, the future as an imponderable does not mean that it will destroy all or any part of us, humans will prevail.

15 Every species in the environment has a right to continued survival.

16 All aspects of the environment should have legal standing.

17 Private interests should not have to sacrifice and suffer for the uncertain and unquantifiable concern for ecological values.

18 Our well-being now should take precedence over the well-being of future generations.

19 Resource ownership is morally untenable.

20 Society has the primary obligation of caring for the land.

REFERENCES

1 Daniel G. Kozlovsky, *An Ecological and Evolutionary Ethic*, (Englewood Cliffs: Prentice-Hall, 1974), p. 101.

2 W. H. Murdy, "Anthropocentrism: a modern view," *Science* **187** (1975): 1168–1172.

3 Daniel G. Kozlovsky (in Reference 1), p. x.

4 Donella H. Meadows et al., *The Limits to Growth*, (New York: Universe Books, 1972).

5 Daniel Callahan, "Living with the new biology," *The Center Magazine* **5**, 4 (1972): 4–12.

6 D. S. Jordan and Julian Huxley (quoted in Reference 2), p. 1168.

7 Van Rensselaer Potter, "Evolving ethical concepts," *Bioscience* **27**, 4 (1977): 251–253.

8 Aldo Leopold, *A Sand County Almanac,* (New York: Oxford, 1969).

9 Bentley Glass, "The scientist: trustee for humanity," *Bioscience* **27**, 4 (1977): 277–278.

10 Roderick Nash, "Can government meet environmental needs?" *Transactions of the 36th North American Natural Resources Conference* (Wildlife Management Institute, March 1971).

11 Peter Singer and Tom Regan (eds.), *Animal Rights and Human Obligations*, (Englewood Cliffs: Prentice-Hall, 1976) and Peter Singer, *Animal Liberation* (New York: Random House, 1976).

12 Michael E. Levin, "Animal rights evaluated," *The Humanist* **37**, 4 (1977): 12, 14–15.

13 Aldo Leopold, "The land ethic," in *A Sand County Almanac*, (New York: Oxford, 1969), pp. 201–226.

14 C. Birch (quoted in Reference 2), p. 1169.

15 W. H. Murdy (in Reference 2), p. 1169.

16 René Dubos, "A theology of the earth," (New York: Charles Scribner's and Sons, 1972).

17 Aldo Leopold (in Reference 13), p. 209.

18 Karl H. Hertz, "Ecological planning for metropolitan regions," *Zygon* **5**, 4 (1970): 290–303.

19 Eliot T. Richardson, "Worth repeating," *Conservation News* (Mar. 15, 1977) p. 15.

20 Philip Handler, "On the state of man," *Bioscience* **27**, 7 (1975): 425–432.

21 Daniel G. Kozlovsky (in Reference 1), p. 15.

22 William E. Martin, "Simple concepts of complex ecological problems," *Zygon* **5**, 4 (1970): 330.

23 Daniel G. Kozlovsky (in Reference 1), p. 101.

24 Richard Falk, quoted in "Caring for the future: where ethics and ecology meet," by Carl E. Braaten, *Zygon* **9**, 4 (1974): 318.

25 Joseph Sittler, Reviews, *Zygon* **5**, 4 (1970): 370.

26 Daniel G. Kozlovsky (in Reference 1), p. 102.

27 Ernest R. Schumacher, *Small Is Beautiful*, (New York: Harper & Row, 1973).

28   William T. Blackstone, "Ethics and ecology" in *Philosophy and Environmental Crisis*, Wm. T. Blackstone (ed.), (Athens: University of Georgia Press, 1974).

29   Nicholas Georgescu-Roegen, "The steady state and ecological salvation: a thermodynamic analysis," *Bioscience* **27**, 4 (1977): 266–270.

30   Van Rensselaer Potter, *Bioethics, Bridge to the Future*, (Englewood Cliffs: Prentice-Hall, 1971).

31   Daniel G. Kozlovsky (in Reference 1), pp. 104–105.

32   Van Rensselaer Potter (in Reference 30), p. 196. Used by permission.

33   Van Rensselaer Potter (in Reference 7), p. 252.

34   Lynn White, Jr., "The historical roots of our ecological crisis," *Science* **155** (1967): 1203–1206.

35   Lewis W. Moncrief, "The cultural basis for our environmental crisis," *Science* **170** (1970): 508–512.

BIBLIOGRAPHY

Douglas, William O., *A Wilderness Bill of Rights*, (Boston: Little, Brown, 1965).

Dubos, René, *Reason Awake*, (New York: Columbia University Press, 1970).

Hardin, Garrett, *Exploring New Ethics for Survival—The Voyage of the Spaceship Beagle*, (New York: Viking Press, 1972).

Stone, Christopher D., *Should Trees Have Standing?*, (Los Altos, Calif.: William Kaufmann, 1974).

12

POPULATION AND ETHICAL CONCERNS

POPULATION GROWTH

It now appears that one of the most controversial issues which will be debated in this latter quarter of the twentieth century will be the question of population growth. We know that the world population has reached over 4 billion and cannot be halted far short of 6 billion by the year 2000. According to some recent estimates, the world population is growing by about two and one-half individuals per second—over 200,000 each day; 75 million new faces are added every year. The specter of possible death by famine of as many as 30 million people in the next few years is before us. Today predictions abound that more people will starve to death in the twentieth century than in any previous century in the human history, with the numbers running as high as 500 million by the end of the century.[1] Current inadequate reporting indicates a toll of more than 10,000 such deaths per week.

Many have gone on record to express the position that the growth of human populations is the principal threat to the future of our species. For example, the well-known first Club of Rome study, *The Limits to Growth*, asserted that in a world that is finite, continual growth is simply not possible. Given the current rates of growth, the study projected imminent and inevitable catastrophe within the next 50–100 years if things remain as they are in the demographic, economic, and political sectors. Their findings have stirred considerable controversy in governmental and nongovernmental offices, in both rich and poor nations, and among academics. The adequacy of the data has been challenged and the computer model on which the study was based has been questioned. Critiques have been published and counter-models proposed. But as some would argue, even if *Limits* is only fifty percent right, it still presents a stark picture of the future and must be dealt with realistically now.[2]

Additions in actual numbers to the human population, expressed as a percentage of the base, is higher than at any other time in human history. The present annual growth rate worldwide is 1.64 percent. However, the world is demographically divided in that different sectors are growing at different rates. Figures for 1975 reveal these conditions:

North America—0.6 percent
Western Europe—0.32 percent
Eastern Europe—0.86 percent
South East Asia—1.18 percent
South Asia—2.13 percent
Middle East—2.72 percent
Africa—2.71 percent
Latin America—2.65 percent

Overall, the less developed world is growing between 2 to 3 percent a year. Those areas have built into them the potential for rapid growth most easily understood as population doubling time or tripling time. The following conversion factors are useful for this purpose:

$$\frac{\text{Doubling time}}{\text{(in years)}} = \frac{69}{A} \quad \text{where } A \text{ is percent of growth}$$

$$\text{Tripling time} = \frac{110}{A}$$

Thus, at a growth rate of 2 percent, a population will double in about 35 years, or triple in 55 years. In these terms, areas like Africa and Latin America will double their population size in about 25 years barring any factors that would mitigate this explosive growth.

Those who are alarmed with figures like these can take some comfort in the peaking of the rate of increase of the world's population that is now occurring. The annual rate of increase of 1.64 percent is down from a high of 1.9 percent in 1970. This may be the first time that the growth trend has reversed since the discovery of agriculture 12,000 years ago! But before taking too much solace, it is well to remember that it is the absolute increase in numbers, rather than rate, that really matters. There are more of us now and even though we are having fewer babies, the size of our population continues to grow astronomically. The annual increment is projected to be about 100 million persons by the end of the century. Just to feed the present yearly increases requires nearly 20 million tons of additional grain each year. This is more than the total Canadian wheat crop and about the same as the crops of Argentina, Australia, and Romania taken together. The real issue is not how many people can live on planet earth but how many people can live well.[3]

In the developing countries the benefits of medical and sanitary measures, along with food aid and agricultural technology alleviating the catastrophic effects of famine, have been brought rapidly to the people, especially since World War II. Death rates have gone down sensationally while birth rates have remained at historically high levels. The main difference between the population situation in developed and developing countries is shown by the two graphs (See Fig. 12.1).[4] In the first case, as death rates declined, birth rates declined. It is also significant that the transition to low death rates in the developed countries came after agricultural and industrial development; populations were not exploding at the time of development. In developing countries, the situation is reversed: Development is trying to catch up with a growing population. Grinding poverty, unemployment, underemployment, lack of educational opportunity, and other social services, all the

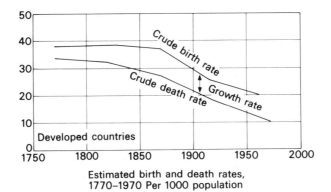

Estimated birth and death rates,
1770–1970 Per 1000 population

Source: United Nations. A concise summary of the World
Population situation in 1970. New York: United
Nations, 1971.

Fig. 12.1 *Population growth rates in the developed and developing countries. In the first, birth and death rates parallel one another while in the second, births outstrip deaths. (Source: United Nations. Adapted from a concise summary of the World Population situation in 1970. New York: United Nations, 1971. See Arthur McCormack, Reference 4. Used with permission.)*

result of larger numbers than can effectively be accommodated within the system, make the task of economic and social development exceedingly difficult. (It has been said in this respect that if America had had modern medicine and sanitary technology available to it in the 1800s, the country would never have developed). The disparate world demographic situation has led some to express concern that Asian populations will overwhelm all others. If present trends continue, Asians will account for two thirds of the world's population by the year 2100. The inexorable swing toward the "havenots" from the present 30:70 ratio to 20:80 or 10:90 in the future conjures up images of massive political and economic instability and world unrest.

There is another feature of western development that commands attention, largely because it bears directly on what will be the response of the developed countries to the plight of their less fortunate neighbors. George Borgstrom writes in *The Food and People Dilemma* that many of the world's present population difficulties can be traced to the "Europeanization of the world," a process that took place between the seventeenth and early twentieth centuries.[5] During that period, an enormous demographic expansion occurred in which European populations multiplied sixfold in three centuries while the total of all other people grew only threefold. The biggest surge occurred between 1850 and 1950. As a result, Europeans swarmed all over the globe, creating colonies and extracting the natural wealth of the newly claimed areas. Mass migrations of Europeans into the colonies, driven partly by population pressures at home, tightened their hold on the "white man's booty." Vast supporting colonies contributed enormous stores of resources for the development of the western economy; population growth in Europe was stimulated and industrial expansion increased. A steady supply of food and raw materials from the colonies, coupled with an expanding work force in the mother country that was turned from agricultural pursuits to factory work, led to a reshaping of the world and its people. To this day, western Europe is a food-deficient land. The encroachments by Europeans into all corners of the globe generated critical imbalances between population and resources, as land, soil, forests, mineral resources, and water were pushed to the limit. Industrialization boomed, world-trade markets were opened, medical technology and hygienic practices were exported to protect and fortify colonizers and those being colonized—all of these factors contributed to an overwhelming increase in the numbers of people. Migrations, many times into areas that were already existing at Malthusian limits, became the inevitable outlet for excessive numbers from the motherland. "For one crucial century in the sequence of history, technology and economics created the unique opportunity to unfold their tricks without taking biology seriously into account," says Borgstrom. Further, the large-scale activities of resource exploitation in the colonies and industrial production at home, separated from one another by many thousands of miles, contributed much to the western world's losing touch with ecological realities. Long-distance hauling occludes the recognition of dependencies. The old saw, "that which cannot be seen cannot be experienced," holds in this situation. It was the massive loads of resources that became important to these expropriators of wealth and not how or what was done to get them. These are key factors in the present population and environmental crisis. But technology, regardless of its sophistication, has not changed our basic dependence on soil, water, and food.

Thus, Europe created huge beachheads around the world for its exclusive survival, with little or no consideration for the world at large. Colonies were taken for granted, part of the "white man's domain." This narrow ethnocentricity led to such fabrications as "manifest destiny" or "only Western man counts." According to this observation, and contrary to what many in the West prefer to believe, we did not pull ourselves up by "our own bootstraps"; we were not solely the product of our ingenuity, motivation, perseverance, diligence, resilience, and hard work. Any nation that does not have the things we have is not necessarily indolent, slovenly, or stupid. Rather, high living standards enjoyed in the West were achieved and continue to be supported in part by a massive exploitation of the world's total resources and a concomitant accumulation of fabulous wealth in the West.

Although it is unfruitful to become preoccupied with the question of who is to blame for the gross inequities extant in the present world, the fact is that some of it is a legacy of practices that have been carried out over a long period of time by Western nations. This raises some questions about moral obligations, a consideration we will return to later.

GLOBAL FOOD INSECURITY

A particular problem directly related to continuing population growth is growing global food insecurity. For a variety of reasons the demand for food by the consumer has begun to outrun the capacity to provide. Where all attention was previously focused on population growth as the sole source of demand on available food stocks, today an equally important source of demand has become apparent and that is affluence. As per capita income increases, purchasing power climbs and with it a demand for higher quality foods, especially foods of animal origin such as meat, eggs, milk, and milk products. Eating meat can be considered an inefficient way of utilizing grain. In the United States it takes three pounds of grain to produce a pound of poultry; 5:1 is the ratio for pork, and 10:1 for beef. In the end, Americans eat eighty percent of all the grain they consume indirectly, first using it for feed and then consuming the meat. On the basis of these data, Americans consume the equivalent of one ton of grain a year while inhabitants of poorer countries consume one fifth as much. Outside our borders, other nations with growing economies but without comparable agriculture have also increased their appetites for animal protein. Hence, sixty percent of North American agricultural sales has been to nations whose people are already rather well fed. At this time, the approximately one billion people of the developed world feed enough grain to their livestock and poultry to provide minimal nutritional requirements to another 2 billion people. Over the last twenty years, the rich minority of the world has doubled its meat consumption. This is, however, not due to eating twice as much meat per capita, although there has been some rise here. Rather, there are twice as many people with the money to buy a higher quality protein-rich diet. The net result is that while world population has been growing at 1.6 percent and agricultural production at 2.5 percent, world demand for food has been increasing at 3 percent per year.[6]

It is to our advantage and the world's as well that the United States grain harvests in the years 1975-1977 have resulted in bumper yields. Overflowing granaries and low grain prices are the mark of this high productivity. But the great increases in food production have not occurred where populations are growing the fastest. Gains in production require modern energy-intensive methods combining irrigation, pesticides, herbicides, fertilizers, genetics, and mechanization. One reason, among several, why poor countries have lagged behind in food production is because their farmers have not had access to appropriate technologies, such as sufficient fertilizers, irrigation, improved seeds, pesticides, storage facilities, and transportation. The world's poor are thus driven to world food markets to supplement their needs. However, they must compete there with richer nations whose own increased demands have forced the price of grain upward. Caught in the price-squeeze of competition in which rising food prices outstrip purchasing power, the poor countries can buy less and less with their precious dollars.* So today, we have the producer nations with surpluses to sell, the affluent consumer nations who have money to buy, and the low income consumer countries that cannot effectively compete in the world food markets. World hunger is sustained by scarcity promoted by the economic system of rich countries. According to some estimates, world agriculture could produce enough to feed up to 30 billion people. What appears to be a food shortage may, in fact, be an uneven world-wide distribution of economic power.[7] These differentials represent an ever-growing number of hungry people. The result is famine in some parts of the world, most notably on the Indian subcontinent and some countries of Africa, Latin America, and South America, and an over-abundance of food in a number of others.

But along with this there is also a less visible crisis emerging, the silent crisis of malnutrition, which is denying close to an estimated billion human beings the "basic right to realize their full genetic potential, their full humanity."[8] It is believed that twenty percent of all the people in developing countries—350 to 450 million people—are undernourished due to insufficient caloric intake; kwashiorkor, a disease brought on by insufficient protein but adequate calories, is found in 1 to 10 percent of preschool age children in less-developed countries; marasmus, a protein plus calorie malnutrition disease, has a frequency of 1.2 to 8 percent in preschool age children in low income countries. The effects of malnutrition are farreaching. During infancy, brain size can be reduced and a permanent deficiency in intelligence can result. Physical size and vigor is diminished. Life span may be shortened. Certain nutritional deficiencies can cause specific diseases, such as blindness caused by lack of Vitamin A or anemia by a shortage of iron (see The Malnourished Mind, Reference 9).

If "nothing will work but food," what is the potential for increasing the world food supply? Optimists assert that the earth can easily support a population several times larger than the present one. The future-oriented Hudson Institute calculates that, based on present technology alone, there is enough arable land, food, and resources to support 15 to 20 billion people with an average per capita income of $20,000.[10] According to some estimates, the number of people who could be fed can be increased tenfold by taking the following measures:

1   Bringing marginal or hitherto unused agricultural land into production. One-half to one-third of the total cultivated land is left fallow or used as meadowland; chemical fertilizers, irrigation in some areas, drainage control in others, could bring this land into production. Reasonable estimates suggest the possibility of about a fifty percent increase in usefully cultivatable areas, worldwide.[11]

2   Shifting from nonessential to essential agricultural production. About ten percent of the agricultural land is used to grow nonfood crops such as cotton, tobacco, rubber, coffee, etc.

---

*   In a number of countries, the debt incurred in international dealings is crippling their capacity to purchase. Already, India's interest payments alone to the United States are greater than the total aid she receives from us. A number of so-called low income countries are unable to pay interest due on previous loans much less take out new loans for the purchase of needed food.

3 Simplifying diets from animal to plant protein; e.g., the wealthy minority of the world feeds as much grain to animals as the rest of the world eats; feedlots accentuate the problem, requiring ten times more grain and seven times more high-protein feed than range cattle (see References 7 and 8).

4 Better insect and pest control. Ten to twenty percent of all crops are destroyed in the field or in storage by pests of various kinds.

5 Increased agricultural technology. Irrigation, pesticides, fertilizers, applied genetics, and mechanization could increase yields in most areas of the world. Agricultural technology is thought to be the major way to increase production (both India and China faced famine in 1973, but China did not fear famine, for the past twenty years water control programs have had top priority there; 35 giant reservoirs have been built, rivers have been broadened, and thousands of wells have been dug. China, with 25 percent of the world's people, owns about eight percent of the world's arable land, yet significant hunger has been eliminated from the country. India, on the other hand, has tapped less than three percent of its water resources.)

UNCERTAINTIES CONCERNING THE POPULATION PROBLEM

And so the population issue, like so many others, presents a confused picture. Although not many will deny the gravity and magnitude of the current food-population crisis, there is no general agreement as to its cause (whether it is political and/or economic rather than biological) or its solution. At least three positions on the population issue can be discerned:

1 The crisis is so grave that catastrophic effects can be expected unless drastic action is taken soon to stop population growth (Malthusian view).[12]

2 Population is an intensifier and multiplier of other social problems; in this view, population is not everything, as in number one, but rather a substantial "something."

3 Population is a nonproblem; the real issue is one of development, that is, how to redistribute income, rectify social injustices, or promote technological change. If these could be fairly accommodated, population will automatically come to equilibrium with carrying capacity (Marxian view).[13]

The Malthusian line emphasizes crisis; it focuses on the possibility of major disasters such as famine, plague, exhaustion of natural resources, and ecological deterioration. Unchecked population growth is seen as a precipitator of these disasters and, hence, is a serious if not insurmountable obstacle to economic growth and national development. Population in distressed regions of the world is simply growing too rapidly for development goals to be realized, and what little gains can be made are quickly consumed by more and more people. Focus on development without serious attention to population control is futile. The words of anthropologist Ashley Montagu characterize this view: "Unless we solve the population problem we solve no others."

Population ethicist, Arthur Dyck, labels this view, "crisis environmentalists" and links names like Paul Erhlich (*The Population Bomb*), the Paddock brothers (*Famine 1975*), and Garrett Hardin ("The Tragedy of the Commons" and other works) and others with it.[14] The key assumption of the crisis environmentalists is that population equals pollution and resource depletion. The insistence here is one of species survival, hence, coercive measures are morally justified as part of a population policy. Economic incentives, both positive and negative, compulsory abortion, triage, and state sanctions for procreation are a few of the coercive measures suggested. This position is probably held by the majority in the West including some in very high offices. Critics of this view charge that it smacks of elitist preoccupation with trying to preserve a separatist position of affluence. By applying the easy label "too many people" to the problem, the deeper ethical issue of "too little willingness on our part to share" can be passed over.

The second view, population as an intensifier of social problems, was the judgment of the Commission on Population Growth and the American Future, sometimes referred to as the Rockefeller Commission. This Commission was appointed by former President Richard Nixon in the early 1970s to study the population problem in the United States. In the words of its final report:

> No substantial benefits will result from the continued growth of our population beyond that made almost unavoidable by the rapid growth of the past. On the contrary, it is our view that population growth of the current magnitude has aggravated many of the nation's problems and made their solution more difficult. The Commission believes that the gradual stabilization of population—bringing births into balance with death— would contribute significantly to the nation's ability to solve its problems, although such problems will not be solved by population stabilization alone. It would, however, enable our society to shift its focus increasingly from quantity to quality.

> The nation has nothing to fear from a gradual approach to population stabilization. We have looked for, and have not found, any convincing economic argument for continued national population growth. The health of our economy does not depend on it, nor does the prosperity of business or the welfare of the average person. In fact, a reduction in the rate of population growth would bring important economic benefits, especially if the nation develops policies to take advantage of the opportunities for social and economic improvement that slower population growth would provide.[15]

The Rockefeller Commission Report is the closest thing to an official U.S. government position and probably represents a compromise between those who favor an aggressive population control policy and those who insist that any population strategy whose ultimate objective is control is not a government prerogative. Robert McNamara, president of the World Bank, showed a preference for this view. In a speech he asserted as a condition for receiving World Bank aid, the need for direct intervention in developing countries to curb "the drag of excessive populations."[16]

The key mechanism for population control suggested by the commission is family planning. The objective of family planning programs is encapsulated in the phrase, "every child, a wanted child"; hence, the aim is to preclude the birth of unwanted children through such measures as easy availability and effective use of contraception, sex education at all levels, and community health services. Abortion in some instances may be used but usually only as a final back-up when other approaches fail.

Because of its heavy reliance on this approach, Dyck refers to this second view as "family planners."[17] He points out that this is pretty much the position of countries around the world. The U.N. Declaration on Populations of 1967 affirms this position:

> The opportunity to decide the number and spacing of children is a basic human right and family planning, by assuring greater opportunity to each person, frees man to attain his individual dignity and reach his full potential.

Two reasons are offered in support of family planning: (1) By assisting couples to have only the children they desire by providing contraceptives and information, human freedom is extended, and (2) family planning enhances the health of individuals, that of mothers through the spacing of children and of children who can be accorded better care.

Family planners do accept the fact that overpopulation may be a problem, as do the Malthusians, but refuse the proposition that coercion is required; rather, people will desire smaller families if the knowledge and the methods for attaining them are made freely available. Two additional reasons for disavowing coercive government policies are these: (1) It is assumed that if there is no serious conflict between individuals and society, that family size will automatically harmonize with societal interests (i.e., the ideal carrying capacity of a particular environment will be realized without resorting to coercive measures); and (2) there is a high priority placed on the value of individual freedom. Malthusians reject both these contentions, insisting, as Garrett Hardin does, that parenthood is a privilege, not a right.[18] In his view, noncooperators will always outbreed cooperators, hence voluntarism is doomed to failure because of the innate self-interest of persons seeking to maximize individual actions. Furthermore, society bears a greater and greater burden of rearing children and sustaining its adult members (e.g., education, health services, etc.); hence, it must maintain a stake in the matter of child-bearing. To be sure, what greater asset can a nation have than a multitude of able-bodied citizens ready to stoke its furnaces, work its mines, run its machinery, harvest its crops, build its cities, maintain its armies, raise its children, produce its art, and provide the vast array of goods and services that make a nation strong? But on the other hand, what greater liability can a nation have than a mass of surplus people, living in hunger and poverty, scratching at tiny patches of land whose crops will not feed them all, swarming into cities where there are not enough jobs, living in huts and dying in the streets, sitting in apathy and discontent, and ever-begetting more children to share their misery? The choice between these extremes to Hardin and others is clear; coercion if need be!

The third view, the Marxian line, purports that population is a function of the socioeconomic system, and problems of numbers of people are primarily problems of such factors as nutrition, distribution, economic development, and/or the political system, but not of scarcity of resources. Many Marxist countries, especially the low income ones, interpret population control as an imperialist plot whose design it is to hold them in subjugation. Instead of population control programs they demand a redistribution of the world's wealth. The Marxist view is essentially the position of the Third World as exemplified at the World Population Conference in Bucharest held in 1974. The message that sounded loud and clear was this: The population-food crisis is not a problem of the less developed countries but of the rich countries who attained and continue to sustain their luxuriant status at the expense of the rest of the world.[19] The hungry nations of the world have a right to reduce their population growth rates the same way that the United States and other industrialized nations have reduced theirs: within the context of social and economic gains. The wealthy are morally obligated to provide assistance to those less fortunate while at the same time they must refrain from intervention in the internal affairs of those countries. This was affirmed later in the year at the Rome Food Conference where the position was adopted that said the entire community of nations must work together to overcome hunger, and the most important single goal is to enable small farm families in the developing countries to become more food productive. In practical terms, the potential solution does not call for fewer babies in the less developed countries but rather less consumption in the developed ones. "Population growth problems are artificially emphasized by the developed countries as an excuse for them to escape from their obligations to the international community."[20] (Also see Global Food Insecurity, p. 383.)

Ecological imbalances and nutritional deficiencies will not be eliminated simply by reducing or halting population growth rates. Dyck characterizes this view as "developmental distributionist." High population growth rates are brought on by illiteracy, high infant mortality rates, extreme and unjust distribution of wealth, inability of governments to provide some form of social security, underemployment and unemployment, and low agricultural production. These, as the causal links, must be addressed first. By distributing societal and individual benefits more equitably, lower fertility will be realized. Family planning programs, without at the same time providing economic security, do not lower birth rates. Having small families only makes sense when it is relatively certain that children will survive to a healthy adulthood and that they will have available to them opportunities for education and future employment. People starve because of governmental policies that are economically inequitable and unjust or because people lack knowledge, and not from lack of food or the potential to produce it. From this perspective, a population policy must be an overall social and economic development policy.

The insistence upon distributive justice is a feature of the Marxian view. Social justice taking the form of land reform, better health care and income distribution, educational opportunities, improved status of women, social security provisions, and the like, all constitute population policies that will lower population growth rates. Couples control their family size when they recognize that they themselves have something at stake. The demographer Philip Hauser expressed it well when he said, "the world has yet to witness a population mired in illiteracy and poverty that has managed to reduce its fertility."[21]

Thus, the population issue has become politicized, and much of the current discussion over global population policies is related directly to these three lines of argumentation. The resolution to the problem is not imminent. As long as it remains a political question with political dimensions, progress toward a world population policy will be stalled. There are, however, some hopeful signs that the glacier is beginning to move. Although many Third World countries take a hard line in their official and public statements, unofficially and out of the public limelight there is a great deal of attention directed to internal control programs. It is not difficult to agree that the earth or any part of it cannot sustain an indefinite number of people. Many are of the opinion that an aggressive population policy is imperative. Attempts at developing concerted energy programs, talk of establishing a World

Food Bank, the implementation of economic assistance programs, intensified efforts to better understand population-development dynamics, declining birth rates in many areas of the globe, the acceptance of family-planning programs in parts of the world that formerly and vigorously resisted them (e.g., Mexico)—these and many more signs indicate, albeit tenuously, that a coordinated global strategy is possible if we but have the will.

POPULATION ETHICS

Because the perceived need to reduce population growth is historically new, there exists no developed political or ethical tradition for dealing with this specific problem. Also, the world, especially that part of the world occupied by us, finds itself facing a moral dilemma: What should be our response to a world in which two-thirds of the inhabitants live in substandard circumstances? Should we retreat into a mood of defeatism or isolationism? Or should we provide whatever assistance we can to help overcome the present crisis and cooperate with others of like interests in the formulation of long-range, coordinated global strategies? What are the dimensions of the population problem and what ethical norms might be brought to bear in responding to these pressing needs?

Excessive population growth raises ethical questions because it threatens existing or desired human values and ideas of what is good. In addition, all or some of the possible solutions to the problem have the potential for creating ethical dilemmas.[22] For example, traditional ethics embodies a concern for human life, including the helpless lives of infants. Consequently, ethics winces at the suggestion that there may be a surplus of people for it intimates the admission that not every human is valuable. Acceptance of this latter judgment carries with it the threat of destroying something of our humanity. Even the declaration that there exists a population problem or excessive population growth is value-laden, for these judgments express the ethical orientation of those who do the defining (see the above discussion on the three positions of the population issue). M. B. Smith asserts that any consideration of explicit population policy necessarily involves us in ethics because we have to assign priorities to competing values, and arrive at accommodations between competing standards.[23] There are many such conflicts in the area of ethics and population control, and very little by way of common agreement has been evidenced, not at this point in time anyway. But we need to start by discussing some of the basic issues. A new dimension of ethics, population ethics, is beginning to attract study.

Individual self determination versus the rights of the greater society

A basic set of problems concerns itself with the rights of individual self-determination versus the rights of society to protect itself from forces or actions which might upset or destroy it or prevent it from carrying out social policy aimed at promoting the common good. The conflict is between the self-fulfillment of persons and groups and the interests of a just social order, and the old premise of the unlimited right to procreation is now being questioned. Procreation is so fundamental a human activity, so wide-ranging in its personal and social impact, that controlling it poses a whole set of ethical issues. In particular, the question is this: How are the prerogatives of the famiiy and of ethnic minorities, as embodied in international accords on human rights, to be adjusted with the equally sanctioned rights of persons to be provided with adequate housing, health care, education, and economic security?[24] Within the American constitutional framework, the right of privacy has consistently been held to extend to activities relating to marriage, procreation, and family relationships. The rights of procreation are set over whatever other laws or administrative procedures may be enacted and have been so affirmed by the courts (see also the discussions on abortion, Chapter 5d). However, the procreative right makes no real provision for duties and responsibilities and those involved are unprepared to resolve rights in conflict. The earlier mentioned U.N. declaration on populations advanced the position that individual freedom to choose must be the guiding principle in achieving personal demographic goals. This is reiterated in the U.N. Declaration on Human Rights which says, "men and women of full age, without any limitation due to race, nationality, or religion, have the right to marry and found a family."[25] This statement encompasses the right to individual freedom and to some degree, justice, but nowhere is a concommitant responsibility expressed.

Having children is part of humanhood

In both the views introduced here, procreation is seen to be so fundamental to human personhood that to interfere in it without consent is to deny that person humanhood. How can this position be defended? Having children is central to our humanity because they are a link to the future. Choosing children is to choose a personal future since they are a means of extending one's own selfhood into the future, of obtaining some kind of personal continuity. There is an intimate relationship between personal identity and one's own children as numerous parent-child associations attest. Having children affirms that the gift of life is good. Children are a source of regeneration and renewal. They are a form of hope and happiness for all persons but especially for those who live in poverty. The saying hope springs eternal applies to these circumstances, too, in that there is hope the future may be better; my children will be more well-off than me. And hope is part of the human experience. But, on the other hand, if procreation is central to our humanity, are there limits to procreative rights? Are persons free to bear as many offspring as they elect or are there larger considerations? This is the central question.

The poor and population control programs

Particular stress is given to ethnic minorities and the other disadvantaged in the developing world. The reason for this is that these groups frequently constitute the poorer segments of a society and are the ones often accused of irresponsible breeding. Consequently, it is on them that the burden of limiting population falls most heavily; it is on them that coercive measures may be more effectively applied. This is contrary to the equality principle of moral philosophy that insists upon fair distribution of goods and burdens among all. Discrimination against a single group or groups for any reason is ethically unacceptable. Similarly, the principle of distributive justice insists that the application of any population policy should fall equally on all—the poor and the affluent—if it is to be ethically acceptable. Population policies must be constructed in such a way that they are just, equalizing both burdens and benefits.

It is within this context that the issue of group genocide is often raised. Family planning programs are frequently viewed this way by nonwhites both in our country and abroad. These policies are seen as aimed at stopping babies rather than stopping poverty.[26] Studies have shown that there is a significant black group in the United States that is suspicious of population-control programs, especially if they include sterilization and if they are administered by nonblacks. The strength-in-numbers argument is counterproposed where it is felt that black (or ethnic) survival and betterment depends on ever-increasing numbers so as to create a larger political power base for bargaining.[27] At least a partial lessening of genocidal overtones might occur if family planning was based on free choice and was coupled with a general improvement of economic conditions and health services.

Population control and the human rights of procreation

The term *human rights* is still another problem when considering the ethcial issue raised above, for the phrase is an umbrella term being accorded different weights in different societies and under different policies. In general, the only way in which the promotion of human rights has been interpreted is a negative interpretation—the prohibition of actions adverse to certain human prerogatives. Rights are taken as a defense against arbitrary government regulations, but no consistent definition of human rights has yet been codified. Human rights remain simply *prima facie* claims of individuals, groups, or states. They are something we might wish for but in reality they may, in some cases, be impractical. For example, by stressing "the rights of parents to have the number of children they want, it (the concept) evades the basic question of population policy which is how to give *society* the number of children they need."[28] In the face of this difficulty, the task is to differentiate an understanding of rights which distinguishes between the inviolable prerogatives of the individual on the one hand and promotion of social progress and a better standard of life for the community on the other. Unfortunately, those discussing the issue do not shed much light on the subject. Reproductive behavior is a declared human right, but the nature of this right or reasons why this particular form of freedom ought to be retained are not effectively validated. We are still left with the task of articulating an understanding of procreative rights vis-à-vis the conflicting interests of individuals set against those of society.

Garrett Hardin submits that "the morality of an act is a function of the state of the system at the time the act is performed."[29] The present needs of posterity determine what is right and good, not previously ordained dictums and edicts. The proposition of Hardin finds application to the population question in what he calls the eleventh commandment, "Thou shalt not exceed the carrying capacity of any environment."[30]* In an uncrowded world, ethical concern about too many people was simply irrelevant, but that is no longer true today. Ours is a crowded world and

---

*	Carrying capacity can be expressed by the equation $C = B:E$, when C is carrying capacity defined as the ability of any land to provide food, water, and shelter to those who live on it. B is the biotic potential of the land, its capacity to produce plants used as food, or shelter, or clothing. E stands for environmental resistance or the limitations that any ecosystem places on B. E may be of natural origin, such as deserts, mountains, or climate, or of human origin like pollution, erosion, resource utilization, and numbers of people. C, carrying capacity, depends on the balance between these two factors.[31]

we need to order our understanding of the morality of procreation to accommodate the new situation. This, contends Hardin, is paramount to any solution of the population crisis and settles the question of rights in matters of family size.

Ethicist A. S. Parkes adds support to Hardin's position by submitting that although basic human rights cannot be successfully challenged, they are necessarily accompanied by obligations. He proposes a Declaration of Obligations, the major points of which are listed.[32] It is an obligation of women and men—

1. not to produce unwanted children;
2. not to produce children because of irresponsibility merely as a by-product of sexual intercourse or because of religious beliefs;
3. to provide the best possible mental and physical environment for children to grow up in.

The relationship between rights and duties is not a new one and several philosophical analyses have relied on this association.[33] Population ethicist Arthur Dyck insists that the free exercise of procreative rights is as fundamental as the right to life.[34] Choosing to have children is a choice to have a genetic continuance into the future. Children, in his view, bestow upon parents a place in the memory of future generations just as our forebears live on in us. Being deprived of the choice of perpetuating the link from the past to the future denies persons a great deal of the meaning of life; we will have lost the most predictable way known to extending our lives. The only population policies that are ethically valid are those that rely upon voluntary decisions of individual couples. Compulsory birth control or any other form of forced population control must, therefore, be judged ethically wrong.

Philosopher Daniel Callahan also places the focus of ethical concern on the freedom of individuals to choose the appropriate reproductive behavior.[35] But he adds a qualifier. Individual freedom must be exercised so that the freedom of others is not diminished. In its first application, parents are obligated to care for the needs and respect the rights of their children. Their decision to have children must include their capability to meet the intellectual, physical, and emotional needs of their offspring. Societally, encroachment on other's freedoms encompasses those hard-to-measure intrusions as physical competition for space, increased food demands, the need for recreational facilities, and the use of other social recourses. What is still required is a determination of that point at which a couple's exercise of privacy and free choice in childbearing impairs a broad set of citizen's interests so that regulation may be justified.

A possible way out of this dilemma is suggested by Jack Parsons. If individual liberty is prized above all other things, then it must be maximized above all other rights. If it is not the *most* desirable but only one of a number of desirable things, then it may be optimized rather than maximized. In practice this requires that the social system be organized so that individual liberty is accorded a value consistent with other rights. The quantification would include the development or preservation of other desirable values such as equality of opportunity, conservation of the environment, or even survival of the species.[36] In the interest of any or all of these, some compromise of individual freedom is necessary so that although individuals may have the right to procreate, that right must be evaluated against other needs of society. If it is judged that unlimited procreation deprives society of other requirements, then the right to procreate may justly be limited.

Christian tradition has a long history of pronouncements when it comes to issues related to population control. Although they have been many and varied, the traditional position is represented by Martin Luther: "Propagation is not in our will and power. . . . Creation is of God alone."[37] The pronatalist position has long been emphasized in the church's position on contraception, abortion, sterilization, and regard for the sexual act. With the presumption that people are made in God's image, being human takes on an added special or sacred significance. To seek to thwart in any way the union of sperm and egg is to violate God's will. If children are gifts from God then He will necessarily provide for them and numbers of them are of no importance. Only recently has the official position of some churches on a few of these issues started to change. However, it does seem clear that reinterpretations by theologians are coming in response to the behavior of laypersons, not the clergy. Since it is the laypeople who must bear the responsibilies of rearing the young, it is they who render the final choice—the church follows practice rather than leads in these matters.

Lastly, ethicist Drew Christiansen has proposed that in order to avoid causing conflicts of rights when population policies are established, programs aimed at curbing growth should either proceed simulatneously with programs of economic development, or follow soon after.[38] If the majority of people are offered no social security and there is only the *hope* that curtailment of procreation will result in economic growth, then the right of procreation cannot be surrendered. There ought to be some reasonable expectations that the rights relinquished promise a bettering of social conditions and provide minimal social security so that one need not rely on his children to provide this service. An approach of this type, although not insisting on the protection of individual rights, seeks to avoid moral conflict between the individual and society since there is an equal exchange between the two parties and participation could be based on persuasion not coercion.

The role of government in population control

These assertions described here, with the exception of Hardin's and Parson's, generally affirm the position that uninvited government intervention into procreative behavior would be wrong. But are there circumstances where an individual right cannot be honored? Is it possible to say that liberty is a vital human good and yet, for the sake of the other goods, that restriction of liberty seems necessary? As a start, we might inquire into the question, What is the proper role of government? A classical argument for the need of a formal and public structure of government is twofold: (1) It is necessary to regulate the exercise of individual liberty, and (2) liberty must exist to promote the common good. In everyday terms, the government's charge is to act in the interest of the people, to protect human rights, and to guarantee justice and equality. From this it can be concluded that governments have the moral right to take those steps necessary to secure a maximization of freedom, justice, and security-survival.[39]

In this context, then, it can be argued that programs aimed at controlling populations are morally acceptable if it can be shown that the population size poses a basic threat to such values as security-survival or freedom and justice. But this is not as easy to demonstrate as it may seem at first. Many in the Third World would argue that the threat is more properly interpreted as a threat to the freedom and comfort of the affluent. As mentioned earlier in this chapter, there is widespread resentment against the wealthy, developed nations exhorting those who do not have as much to do something about their populations. The continuing admonitions by the high income countries of the urgency to control population growth is but an evasion of moral responsibility to the poor whom they have exploited and continue to exploit. The Third World case is strengthened still further by embarrassing revelations that some aid programs are cunningly disguised to help the donors more than the recipients (e.g., aid is given in the form of trade credits redeemable only in the donor country; or only surplus grains make their way into the aid programs thereby reducing storage costs while at the same time keeping prices high; or raw materials from the recipient country are traded for processed ones from the donor, etc.). Furthermore, many countries of the world do not consider their situation hopeless. Given the potential of existing technology, assistance programs can increase local agricultural production, lower population growth rates, improve nutrition and health, and extend life expectancy. Despite all their problems, including substantial population increases, it has been shown that nearly all countries have more food per capita than they did ten years ago. Without the successful aid efforts that have already doubled and tripled production of crops in some countries, many more people would be dying.[40]

The Malthusian proposition raises a second question, Is the threat to freedom and survival worldwide or is it limited to a few Asian countries? Widely publicized photographs of the starving in the Sahel, Ethiopia, and Bangladesh create the impression that the food-population crisis has grown to unmanageable proportions worldwide. However, these are geographically isolated situations and affect only a small fraction of the populations in those countries. Some countries are hostile to family planning and population limitations and recognize that future development is intimately tied to continued population growth. For example, Brazil insists that a doubling of its population is absolutely mandatory for the development of its uninhabited areas, especially the Amazon basin. Australia, Argentina, Canada, Liberia and others, too, share a similar view.

The burden of proof for proposals to limit freedom of choice in procreation behavior must rest with those who make the proposals, but as these examples illustrate, it is not possible to do so with certainty. While everyone might agree that widespread starvation and malnutrition are bad, not everyone will agree that crowding, widespread urbanization, change in dietary habits, or a loss of primitive wilderness areas are equally bad.[41] Too often, our view of what is good for the world is cast exclusively in the Western image; but Westerners occupy only a small part of the total world and comprise a still smaller percentage of the world population.

SOCIETAL RIGHTS OVER INDIVIDUAL RIGHTS

But still, some would argue that since excessive population growth can touch upon crucial elements of social life, society has the right to take those steps necessary to insure the preservation and promotion of the common good. Where rights make a claim on resources, they involve duties and a call for responsible action. Again, Garrett Hardin is a well-known advocate of this view. By separating the rights to bear children from responsibility, population control is impossible. When control of individual family size depends upon voluntarily restricting fertility, the chief appeal is the moral appeal to conscience. However, nonconscience has a selective advantage over conscience. The children of the conscienceless will make up a larger proportion of the population in the next generation than their parents were in this. To produce a runaway process, it is necessary only for the transmission of conscienceless behavior and the attitudes of children often resemble their parents more than they do the population at large. In both the short- and the long-term, population control programs based on voluntarism, reward the selfish. It thus becomes mandatory for survival that the common welfare of society take precedence over freedom of individual citizens and here, we are not without precedent. We do this in times of war when wars are morally acceptable if they are fought for just ends (e.g., conscription of citizenry for service in the military, etc.). Hardin concludes that "the community, which guarantees the survival of children, must have the power to decide how many children shall be born."[42]

LIFEBOAT ETHICS

More recently, he has carried this argument still further by suggesting that the lifeboat is an appropriate metaphor for understanding the relationship between the rich and the poor countries of the world.[43] This view has been given the designation *lifeboat ethics*. In it, Dr. Hardin rejects the popular metaphor of *spaceship earth* for the reason that a spaceship has a captain who commands and a crew that shares the resources of the ship and cooperates in its operation; together, captain and crew function as a single, interdependent unit. None of this holds true with the earth; it is under no central control but rather it is divided into bickering states not ready to give up nationalistic or parochial goals in favor of the worldwide common good. An important ethical consequence is that the demands are made "on common resources, without acknowledging corresponding spaceship responsibilities." This is essentially the position Hardin has held throughout: The separation of the power and the right to act from the responsibility for the action. A more realistic model, he contends, portrays the world as a group of lifeboats:

> Each rich nation amounts to a lifeboat full of comparatively rich people. The poor of the world are in other, much more crowded lifeboats. Continuously, so to speak, the poor fall out of their lifeboats and swim for awhile in the water outside, hoping to be admitted to a rich lifeboat, or in some other way to benefit from the "goodies" on board.[44]

The ethical question posed by Hardin is this: What should the passengers of the rich lifeboat do? This is the central problem of the ethics of a lifeboat.

Hardin goes on to argue that generosity by the rich in well-provisioned lifeboats will only hasten the approach of disaster for all, whether the assistance be in the form of a world food reserve from which those in need can draw or unlimited immigration or food aid to specific countries with no stipulations attached. If all in need are taken on board the life boats of those who are well-off, all will perish; if attempts are made to be selective, an impossible dilemma of who and how to choose is encountered; by adopting a sharing ethic (sending some aid), another tragedy of the commons is invited in that individual interests of those being swamped are still incompatible with collective interests, and the number requiring need will continue unabated, the result being that the ultimate day of reckoning has merely been post-poned. It is a better alternative to allow normal cycles of nature to bring population size to carrying capacity of the environment. Greater future suffering can only be prevented by allowing some suffering now—and that is more moral.

A moral defense of the lifeboat position submitted by Hardin is contained in the aphorism of Joseph Fletcher (the consequentialist ethician): "We should give if it helps but not if it hurts."[45] Charity can only justify itself by the good that it does; in the case of aid to populations in need, it can be justified by the recipients of that aid. A possible response to Fletcher's formula is raised with the ecological question, "And then what?" In terms of population policy, it may appear amicable and moral to feed the starving, but then what? Present ethics is blind to future repercussions for the problem of starving people can only become all the more severe if feeding is all that is done to end suffering. A more responsible ethic demands that the needs of posterity including that of those receiving the aid be given a weighing at least equal to that accorded present generations. Human suffering in the long term can only be reduced or prevented by taking responsible action now. As numerous studies have shown, the United States is not now self-sufficient nor is it likely that we ever will be and so the question is placed: Must we in the West reduce our desire for things so that the world's poor might be better off? It is at least conjectured that a reduction in our demands would result in a world economically better off and more secure.

As might be expected, the life boat thesis, coming from a scientist of Garrett Hardin's stature and influence, has attracted a good deal of attention both in this country and abroad. It has ignited a great deal of controversey, both pro and con, for in effect, lifeboat ethics amounts to a deliberate decision by rich nations to allow others, judged to be beyond help, to die. This proposition is becoming the underly-ing issue before contemporary civilization—the attitudes of the rich toward the poor. Many predict that depending on the response of the affluent of the world, the stage can be set for what could become the costliest showdown in history. Econo-mist Robert Heilbronner (*An Inquiry Into the Human Prospect*) and others as well are of the opinion that poor countries will align themselves into power blocks to the detriment of the entire world unless they receive a larger share of the world's resources. Lifeboat ethics and the related concept of triage are congruent in that a decision is made to allow certain populations to die. In the first, natural cycles accommodate this end, a sort of benign neglect on a population-wide scale where the decision not to help allows nature to take its course. Triage is a deliberate verdict in which whole populations are marked for extermination as a matter of calculated judgment—a form of passive euthanasia practiced on an entire population.

Triage is a term borrowed from medicine (especially wartime medicine) and involves the allocation of resources when there are not enough for all. Triage divides the wounded into three groups: Those with superficial wounds where minimum care is all that is required (the walking wounded); the seriously wounded where maxi-mum attention will result in a large proportion of survivals; and the fatally wounded where no amount of care will sustain life. Medically, the first group are treated immediately or they are set aside for later care when the immediate stress on avail-able resources has passed. The third group are at most administered pain killers and set aside to die. The middle group can then receive maximum attention of the medical staff and facilities with the consequence being higher rates of survivorship. Applying triage to population policy, those doing the judging are those nations that have resources over and above their needs but the resources are limited so that not all can share. Decisions as to the allocation of these surplus resources focus on the first and second groups, but especially the second. In this group are countries which have the wherewithal for long-term recovery through such indicators as agricultural potential, economic reform, population-control policies, and the like. Those in the hopeless third group are judged to be without redeeming value: Sheer human numbers simply outweigh any possibilities of success; this group is to be written off as nonsalvageable.

Taken at first reading, this seems like the reasonable thing to do, especially if your household is well-provisioned and others are begging for help. Lord Ritchie-Calder, English scientist and humanitarian, recalls the response of a contemporary to Parson Malthus who labeled the Malthusian proposition "a cushion under the conscience of the upper classes."[46] Speaking out against the poor laws of his time, Malthus pointed out that if you did anything to improve the conditions of the poor, they would just have more children and, these "poor things" would only die of hunger. The easy acceptance of triage as a population policy can "put a cushion under the conscience" of the well-to-do. Looking at the problem intellectually and objectively, without putting names or faces on the suffering, does not prick the conscience nor does it cause much unease. By defining a group as hopeless, it is not so morally obnoxious since we, the definers, had nothing to do with the group's plight. The western business sense, of not sending good money after bad, further validates this position. But we easily forget that "population is people";[47] they are living, breathing, suffering human beings.

So to some ethicists, a policy of triage is ethically abhorrent. And, in fact, it is a form of genocide. The torments of those suffering famine cannot be so easily ignored or dismissed simply by defining their condition as hopeless. The problem can and must be dealt with and recent bumper harvests of grain in the United States have indicated that our resources are not so much in short-supply that life and death rationing is at all called for—certainly not at this time. Before the easy and objective decisions are made about who is expendable, or which are ecologically unworthy, or where are those who are to be abandoned to starvation, ethicists would insist that the facts first be examined.

And so a first question—how valid is the lifeboat model? Several of Hardin's propositions need examining. Daniel Callahan poses these rejoinders:[48]

1. *Is ours a self-sufficient lifeboat?*

   Hardin's lifeboats rarely interact with one another, each drifting about as separate and sometimes self-contained units. In the real world, however, there is a great deal of commerce between nations and the present oil situation forcibly brings to our attention that nations of the world do not exist in isolation. The United States now imports over twenty percent of its energy, including almost fifty percent of its oil supplies with that proportion steadily growing. Because of interlocking dependencies, calamities, too, will be felt sharply in all areas, not just in a few have-nots. We are highly dependent upon natural resources from other countries, as indicated in Fig. 12.2, and depend upon world markets as customers for our products as well. An unequal disparity in the balance of trade with other nations resulting in payment deficits seriously affects the economic health of our own country as the recent devaluation of the American dollar on the world exchange has demonstrated. It is fast becoming apparent that the living standards of the rich nations are to a very large degree dependent upon whole-world interactions, including those with the poor nations. The U.S. is not now self-sufficient nor is it likely that we ever will be again unless we collectively and drastically reduce our standard of living. To what extent, then, is the "great American dream" to be perpetuated? Can the U.S. containing six percent of the world's people continue to consume thirty to forty percent of the world's resources? Viewed in these terms, it does not appear that ours is a self-sufficient lifeboat nor, for that matter, are any of the other Western industrialized high-income countries who are in a position to provide aid.

2. *Who is to blame for the condition of the less-developed nations?*

Is the condition due to their listless motivation to improve themselves, or to their irresponsible procreation; or to inept government officials who care little about controlling their own population size? (It has been said in this regard that American population policy-makers are more concerned about population size in many foreign nations than are the rulers of those countries.) In refutation, more recent demographic studies indicate that population growth is a multifaceted problem; cultural, economic, political and religious factors all play a part. The most important factor in reducing family size, according to these new observations, is motivation based on a more secure life in an economically developing country. Where socioeconomic gains are experienced by a substantial majority who are usually situated at the bottom of the economic ladder, people are motivated to reduce their birth rates. Strategies aimed at bringing about improvement in the welfare and the security of the entire population appear to be significant factors in reducing population growth.[49] (See also, "Europeanization of the World" discussed on p. 382 as a factor for population-resource imbalances.)

3. *Is the capacity of poor lifeboats expandable?*

Carrying capacity of the environment is expandable, within limits. Human cultural evolution which converted our nomadic hunter–food-gathering ancestors to domesticators and builders of civilization was accomplished by increasing carrying capacity, especially the biotic potential. Irrigation of soils, seed hybrids, fertilizers, pesticides, extraction and utilization of lowgrade mineral ores, economically efficient production of goods, these and many more have expanded the capacity of the land to support people. Although there is a limit to what can be done, it does appear that the world has not yet reached maximum development either of new resources or the reclamation of old (see, for example, p. 384).

4. *Are people in underdeveloped countries swimming and on the verge of drowning or are they in leaky, inadequately equipped, and poorly provisioned lifeboats which can be repaired?*

If the latter is the case, we can without in the least endangering ourselves, help them plug the leaks in their boats, and give them information for enlarging their boats. This is a much better use of our resources than repelling "boarders." Philosopher Paul Kurtz suggests the following program for "plugging up the leaks":[50]

a) food shipments to keep our fellow humans from starving;
b) large-scale technological efforts to increase food production by fertilizers, technical aid, and economic development;
c) massive programs of population control, especially in undeveloped areas;
d) unremitting efforts to increase the level of education and literacy in the world and to motivate responsible self-help.

U.S. Dependence on Imports of Principal Industrial Raw Materials with Projections to 2000

Raw Material	1950	1970	1985	2000
	(percent imported)			
Aluminum	64	85	96	98
Chromium	n.a.	100	100	100
Copper	31	0	34	56
Iron	8	30	55	67
Lead	39	31	62	67
Manganese	88	95	100	100
Nickel	94	90	88	89
Phosphorus	8	0	0	2
Potassium	14	42	47	61
Sulfur	2	0	28	52
Tin	77	n.a.	100	100
Tungsten	n.a.	50	87	97
Zinc	38	59	72	84

Industrialized nations are becoming increasingly dependent on developing countries to supply them with raw materials. U.S. reliance on imports of the 13 basic raw materials required by an industrial economy has grown steadily since 1950. By the end of this century the U.S. will be heavily dependent on foreign sources for its supply of all of the 13 raw materials but phosphorus.

Data Source: U.S. Department of the Interior

Fig. 12.2 *From George H. Kieffer,* Biology and Human Affairs, *Champaign, Ill.: Stipes Publishing, 1977.*

Daniel Callahan submits the following positive alternative to the grim predictions of lifeboat ethics: Because the United States is rich, it can give significantly more food aid than it is presently giving—we have by no means reached the limit;* the United States could reduce its disproportionate demand on the world's resources; the United States should be aware that there is no clear evidence that any poor country is hopeless and is to be written off—a responsible moral position insists that we act as if every country can be saved; and we must recognize that there can be no moral justification for deliberately allowing others to starve so that some either living or yet unborn can enjoy a higher quality of life. The facts are that enough food is now being produced in the world to feed its population adequately. According to projections made by the United Nations to the year 1985, population worldwide will grow 2.0 percent while food production will increase 2.7 percent.[53] That people are malnourished is due to political and economic factors (see p. 388).

Presuming the lifeboat model became practiced policy, a still deeper moral question is raised: What happens to those who are fortunate enough to survive while masses around them die? Stated another way, how do we in the provisioned lifeboats survive survival? An earlier discussion raised the proposition that my brothers and sisters are not only those within the borders of the United States, they are either everyone or no one (see p. 353). Thus, if sharing now results in the eventual ruin of all, so be it. It is better to die a ruined human being rather than survive a rescued beast. Norman Cousins, former editor of *Saturday Review* now at UCLA, writes in support of this position stating that the principal danger of the Hardin approach is to the West itself, not to those who suffer want because of the decision to abandon.[54] *Hardinism*, Cousins' term, can infect the moral consciousness, for once it is discovered how easy it is to let large numbers of Asians or Africans starve, it is a small step to be insensitive about those in need here at home. Desensitization to others is already the greatest curse in the world today, and it begins by calibrating people—some are judged to be better than others. He concludes:

> We can't ignore outstretched hands without destroying that which is most significant in the American character—a sense of vital identification with human beings wherever they are. Regarding life as the highest value is more important to the future of America than anything we make or sell.[55]

Agricultural expert Alan Berg criticizes the lifeboat model on several grounds.[56] In the first place short, catchy phrases tend to give people the comfortable feeling of having grasped the whole picture when in reality the issues are much more complex. Oversimplification diverts attention from the consequential aspects of the problem.

---

* Robert S. McNamara, president of the World Bank, describes present aid efforts by the developed nations of 0.7 percent of their GNP as "disgracefully inadequate."[51] This is especially incriminating when the pittance for aid is compared to the whopping 6 percent of the gross world product going to the military. Military expenditures of the countries which provide aid to underdeveloped nations are estimated to be 25 times greater than the official development assistance they provide and only 10 percent of world military expenditures could increase the total of fixed investment of developing countries by 33 percent according to the Stockholm International Peace Research Institute.[52]

The problem will not go away simply because it has been given a name. Further, the model distorts reality; countries are neither hopeless nor are they drowning. But most tragic of all, it may encourage citizens as well as governments, already numb or lethargic to the world's population-food crisis, to become even more so. And here, he concurs with Norman Cousins: What are needed are articles to inflame public opinion to the point where what can be done will be done and the certainty not to put a "cushion under the public conscience." These words summarize his judgment of the situation, "given the penalties for delaying a major attack on the food-population problem, fixation on labels is a luxury the world cannot afford."

The effect of life boat thinking on government policies is illustrated by the testimony of Professor Garrett Hardin before a House subcommittee on population growth when he said, "Progress in lowering the rate of increase every year should be the essential condition for receiving food." Professor Wayne Davis (University of Kentucky) at the same hearing testified, "When people have nothing, they starve. When starving people are fed, they reproduce—and they reproduce at the maximum possible rate." New data suggest that people do not necessarily "convert extra food into babies" but into longer lives.[57] The withholding of food will increase death rates but it will not lower birth rates for in order for a few to survive, many must be produced. The Hardin testimony raises the ethical question: Is it right for the government of a developed country to make the establishment of a population-control program in a developing nation a condition for receiving aid? According to Callahan, this would be extremely difficult to justify on ethical grounds.[58] At the very least, it would constitute an interference in a nation's right to self-determination. But even more seriously, it would be a direct exploitation of one nation's poverty in the interests of another nation's concept of what is good for that nation; and that would be unjust since value preference may vary. Finally, a failure to provide needed food aid when that aid could be given without great cost to the donor nation would be a fundamental violation of the right to life. Those already alive and in need of food have a right to survival. To willfully allow them to die or to deprive them of the necessities of life for the reason of saving more lives in some future time cannot be justified in the name of a greater good over evil. If these arguments are convincing, Callahan submits that an enlightened government policy would take cognizance of the sovereign right of states to determine domestic policies, while at the same time providing the necessary aid to help overcome the barriers to economic development, to increase food production, and to assist in programs of population control.

REDUCTION OF POPULATION GROWTH

In almost all discussions of the world's population, it is quite clear that growth must be brought into check. The questions which cause conflict are these: When (how soon must population size be contained without endangering the earth's carrying capacity) and how should it be done? Much study has been devoted to the first of these. In general it has been concluded that disaster is not imminent; the world still has time, albeit it may be short, to respond. Within the next ten to twenty years is a reasonable projection and, as mentioned earlier, there are signs that world population growth is slowing down some, from 1.9 percent in 1970 to 1.6 percent in 1975.

Regarding the second question, the five classical courses of action designed to reduce fertility are these:

1 Persuade (e.g., education and public information).
2 Manipulation services (e.g., making family planning services available, ready access to contraceptives).
3 Change incentive programs (e.g., positive and negative incentive programs).
4 Transform social institutions (e.g., effective social security programs, increase literacy, upgrade the status of females).
5 Coercion.

Each of these raises its own set of ethical issues, especially those methods related to incentive programs and compulsion. Positive incentive programs take the form of direct payments of money, goods, or services to cooperating citizens offered by the government in return for limiting births, usually to some specified number. Negative incentive programs impute tax or welfare penalties on noncomplying families or on those exceeding a stated number. Both types are morally problematic.

In principle, positive incentive programs are designed as noncoercive; they are to give families a choice they did not previously have. Furthermore, they theoretically allow couples to procreate and thus to exercise some degree of individual freedom; but within limits. In practice, though, the programs may covertly be coercive, at least to the poor. The material needs of this group often make the immediate inducements of short-term gain appear attractive. But the poor have less choice than the rich about accepting or rejecting the incentive, and the question of distributive justice is raised. The motivation for participation was aptly described by Shakespeare: "My poverty but not my will consents" (Romeo and Juliet, V.i.) Positive incentive programs are a form of exploitation of poverty. The principle of distributive justice proposes that both burdens and benefits be equally distributed among all social classes. (In a recent study of male sterilization programs in India, it was determined that over 62 percent of those undergoing the procedure did so for the cash payment offered and only 2 percent elected the operation to control the number of children they might father.) Callahan contends that positive incentive programs may be ethically acceptable if: (1) They are the lesser of two evils (i.e., it can be shown that burgeoning population really threatens survival); (2) They provide other benefits besides a single monetary payment (e.g., provisions for old-age security); and (3) They minimize the pressure of covert coercion by keeping the payments small.[59]

Negative incentive programs have come in for special criticism and a number of objections to such programs have been raised. Negative incentive programs are directly coercive in that they blatantly deprive people of free choice. Other arguments against them are (1) the effects may be detrimental to the children as well as to the parents violating the demands of justice; (2) the penalties would be more stressful to the poor than the rich; and (3) the social consequences could be undesirable (e.g., the health of the family might worsen, children would lose needed social and welfare benefits, enforcement would require an invasion of one's privacy, and an unjust economic or political order might be perpetuated). The problem of punishing offending parents is especially serious since it is the innocent children who frequently suffer most. Fines and jail sentences work a hardship on the children as well as parents even if society made provisions for the children's care. Because any penalty scheme raises so many serious ethical questions, Callahan argues that these programs should be implemented only if it can be shown that they will increase the "balance of good over evil" and in many instances one would be hard-pressed to do so.

Would it be right for a government to institute programs in the fifth category of control—coercion—for the sake of future generations? Those opposed claim that compulsion, like incentive programs, discriminate against the poor. Restricting the very poor to two or three children would render their lives much less joyous, less hopeful and more precarious (i.e., reduction in the number of children could result in both a loss of a potential laborer and the old-age security function which children provide). Population ethicist, Arthur Dyck contends that compulsion can be ethically justified only as a last resort, where the threat to security-survival is to those now living (not future generations), where all alternatives have been sincerely tried and failed, and where society combines its population policies with effective efforts to remove gross inequalities in the society.[60] Even accepting these criteria, not every compulsory measure can be justified, for example, the required abortion of illegitimate fetuses can never be acceptable according to Dyck.

India's experience in 1976 with negative programs and legal compulsion can serve as an historical lesson of what happens when ordinary people are deprived of these very basic behaviors. In July of that year, Maharashtra state passed legislation which required that men and women of child-bearing age must be sterilized (at least one of the couple) within 180 days of the birth of their third child.[61] Prison terms of up to two years were threatened for noncompliance. An exemption was permitted to those couples who would use contraceptives (usually only members of the literate middle and upper classes can afford them), and/or would willingly accept abortion in place of sterilization. Similar legislation was considered by a number of other Indian states. At the national level according to governmental decree, every government employee must ensure that he will not have more than three children. Noncompliers will lose such social services as free-outpatient health care and hospitalization, access to government housing, the denial of vacation pay, housing loans, and other benefits. Families with more than two children were not eligible to apply for government jobs. Mrs. Indira Ghandi justified these policies, asserting that:

> some personal rights have to be kept in abeyance for the human right of the nation, the right to live, the right to progress.[62]

This is a statement of the traditional ethical notion that rights may not be denied but their exercise can be curbed when other rights conflict with them (see Parsons, p. 392).

As is well-known, these policies were greeted with widespread popular dissention. In one riot, fifty people were killed. In national elections, held in early 1977, the Ghandi government was overthrown and these laws were abolished. Mrs. Gandhi's firm position on compulsory population control is generally attributed to be the reason for her defeat. Compulsory sterilization was judged to be so serious an affront to human dignity, that a stance in defense of it cost at least one government its continuance in office. What India's population policy will be in the face of this rejection of compulsion remains to be determined.

Returning to the five classical methods of attaining population stabilization, the first, persuasion relying upon voluntary participation, was discussed earlier in this chapter (see pp. 387, 395) and, at least according to biologist Garrett Hardin, was judged to be ineffective. Furthermore, since voluntary programs result in advantages to some people and disadvantages to other people, it is extremely difficult to establish a policy that would have widespread acceptance. To be accepted, a policy of voluntarism must be universally perceived as being reasonably equitable. No person likes to feel as though he/she is sacrificing while some other person, or group, is taking advantage of the sacrificing.

The second method which proposes the manipulation of services with special emphasis on the availability of family planning was described on page 386 ff. It is this approach that is receiving the greatest attention worldwide and a number of governments which formerly and vigorously resisted family planning programs, are now their enthusiastic endorsers (e.g., Mexico and the Philipines). The fourth policy, the transformation of social institutions by programs such as government financed social security, general education for all social classes, upgrading of the status of females, and providing jobs for all who are able to work runs into the obstacle of cost. Presumably huge sums of money will be required to effect these enormous changes in the social structures of the LIC's (low income countries) and the question of the source of these moneys remains largely unanswered. (Witness the present consternation at the highest government levels over the instability of the U.S. social security system and one might better appreciate the immensity of the task.) Are there then population policies that are more beneficial than harmful, which may not involve injustices or serious threats to human freedom and which can be realistically implemented? Fortunately, the answer is yes. Table 12.1, p. 406, is a selection of scenarios of human rights arranged around different population control programs.[63] For purposes here, these are presented to clarify the relative importance of values under certain conditions and will be discussed no further.

Dan Callahan lists some general ethical principles to judge the validity of population policies:

1. Individuals have the right to freedom-of-procreation choice and the obligation to respect the freedom of others.

2. Governments have the right to take those steps necessary to secure a maximization of freedom, justice, and security consistent with survival.

3. In cases of conflict, one is obliged to act to increase the balance of good over evil.

The courses of action, listing them in rank order of preference from most preferable to least preferable, are these:

1. Primacy is given to freedom of choice. The government is obligated to implement this freedom through such programs as voluntary family planning, educational programs, access to effective contraceptives, etc.

2. If voluntary programs can be *proven* to be ineffective and have been sincerely tried, then the government may go beyond family planning into *posi-*

tive incentive programs and manipulation of social structures (e.g., status of women). If these are *proven* to be ineffective, then the government has discharged its moral responsibility and can then move into . . .

3. Quasi-coercive programs (negative incentive programs), but only as a last resort. Provision must be made to allow for rapid reversibility if conditions change.[64]

The major weaknesses with present programs are inadequate financing, poor administration, poor data on which to base programs, and little real effort at education. (In the year 1975, the United States spent thirty percent of its budget on military expenditures and 0.1 percent on population activities according to Margaret Mead) Our country is thirteenth among eighteen donor nations in terms of percentage of GNP given to aid poor countries (see also Reference 51).

Are there alternatives to compulsion or incentive programs that do not violate individual freedom or perpetrate injustices? As has been stated on a number of occasions in this chapter, there is a convincing body of evidence that shows better living standards and lower population growth are complementary. Good socioeconomic conditions motivate couples to have fewer children. These conditions are parental confidence about the future, an improved status for females, and literacy. They require low infant mortality rates, easily available health care, increased employment opportunities and income, and an adequate diet above subsistence levels.[65] When these conditions are met, birth rates fall rapidly, sometimes even before the availability of birth-control technology. Healthy families with low mortality rates depend less and less on large families for security. Lester Brown has said "high birth rates continue for the obvious reason that families living without adequate employment, education, and health care have little security for the future except for reliance on their children." Translated into practice, this means that the demographic transition—where births and deaths are approximately equal at a low level—can be achieved much sooner and at lower cost than was formerly thought. Historically, and as based on the Western model, the demographic transition was brought about through industrialization and economic growth and required some 150 years. As circumstances now stand, the Western model is nonapplicable to the majority of the developing world for a number of reasons. Most especially, we cannot wait that long for the slow and gradual change to occur, and second, there is serious doubt that the world can afford to industrialize since the process involves natural resources, energy, factories, pollution, and markets.

If the most important reason for reducing personal family size is a secure life, aid programs should be implemented that are a balanced mix of technological, social, and economic changes which reduce or eliminate social inequities. It is not necessary that the GNP be very high either. It is essential that social improvements be spread across the entire population but especially those situated in the lower economic categories. Aid designed to help the poorest people of the poor countries (the "lower 40 percent"), encouraging necessary institutional and social reforms, and assistance for development of their own resources and initiatives have the greatest chance of achieving worldwide population equilibrium. Not GNP but GSP, "Gross Social Product", the amount of real welfare in terms of actual income per capita seems to hold the greatest promise for achieving the desired demographic ends.[66] As

Table 12.1
Alternative Policies, Values, and Rights

Policy	Population growth	Controlled technology	Developmental: synergy of justice with population control	Voluntary family planning	Beyond family planning: incentives and disincentives	Beyond family planning: coercive
Measures	Incentives for large families	Nonspecialized community health care with family planning	Women in work force, health care, education, old-age benefits, and family planning	Contraception; women's rights; abortion on demand	Tax benefits withdrawn from families; tax and other disincentives	Licensing: compulsory sterilization-abortion for violations
Peremptory value	Survival and dominance of group or nation-wide	Realization in community	Justice and human dignity	Personal freedom and responsibility	Prevent disaster without affront to human rights	Survival of species at high level of well-being
Relative value	Justice, global survival; individual and outgroup freedom	Technological and organizational expansion	Survival and degree of individual freedom	Survival; justice (in consequences for society)	Justice; freedom to choose alternate social states	Individual and familial pro-creative rights; justice
Concept of right	Self-interest	Social relation	Intrinsic to human nature	Defense for human self-determination	Flexible margins of social control	Fiction of society
Familial right	Procreate without specific limits	Procreate within limits	Procreate within limits	Choice of number and spacing of children	Procreate within limits	Legal privilege

Social right	Security based on growth for group alone	Economic security, health care limited by convivial technology	Economic security and health care for all	Information and means of control; only aids to freedom	Granted only to allotted children	High standard for survivors
Risk	Leads to uncontrollable problem; global imbalance and injustice	Risks certainty of control; entails decline for developed nations	Ineffective due to time lag; both population control, and social justice	Risk survival at high level; risk minimum standard for poor	Subtle but effective erosion of freedom; injustice to poor	No risk in the population area; risk loss of free society and value of justice

From Christiansen et al., "Moral claims, human rights, and population policies," *Theological Studies* 35 (1974): 86–87. Used by permission.

Table 12.2

		South Korea	Brazil
Population growth rates	1958	3%	3%
	1964	2.7%	2.9%
	1971	2%	2.8%
Income per capita (1971)		$280	$395
GNP growth rates in the 1960s		9%	6%
Ratio of income, richest 20% to poorest 20% (1970)		5 to 1	25 to 1
Literacy (1970)		71%	61%
Infant deaths per 1,000 births (1970)		41	94
Unemployment		Negligible	Serious
Effective land reform		Yes	No
Family planning program		Yes	No

William Rich, "Smaller Families through Social and Economic Progress" (Monograph No. 7; Washington, D.C.: Overseas Development Council, 1973). From Peter J. Henriot, "Global population in perspective; implications for U.S. policy response," *Theological Studies* 35 (1974): 55. Used by permission.

is shown in Table 12.2, strategies aimed at improving the welfare of the entire nation appear to be more efficacious in reducing population growth rate.

Population polices of this kind have still another advantage. Numerous criticisms by Third-World people are voiced against the single-dimensional programs which emphasize only food aid and ignore the feelings, values, and aspirations of those receiving the aid. Margaret Mead, among others, underscores the necessity of population-control programs to consider the existing cultures who are the aid recipients. Frequently, they are disruptive and potentially harmful to those cultures. It is for this reason that many programs are so vigorously resisted.[67] By addressing the program to local circumstances and relying upon the voluntary decision of individual couples, the requisite behavior is more likely induced and it is at the same time ethical.

The United States is in an extremely influential position to determine the direction of global-population policy for several reasons: our country is the major donor of aid and family-planning programs; it is the source of numerous private research, training, and service organizations. This position requires that the United States carry out this role responsibly. To do so, the United States should:

1 Adopt a domestic population policy. At present we have no official policy or population goals. This places us in the embarrassing position of asking others to do what we ourselves have not yet done. This policy should make provision for migrations, urbanizations, and age structures, integrated with an encompassing social policy of human development, distributive justice, ecological responsibility, provisions for health care, etc.

2 Focus its aid on comprehensive programs of development aimed at improving the total welfare of the recipient nations.

3 Turn serious attention to curbing its wasteful patterns of consumption. By experiencing even a little want, we may appreciate the lot of the majority in the rest of the world.

We are, whether we like it or not, interconnected parts of the world society and ecosystem. The sooner we face this overwhelming reality, the sooner we can go about solving our problems including those related to effective population programs.

VALUES PERTAINING TO POPULATION ETHICS

1   Life is the highest value, thus every human life is valuable.

2   The right of individual self-determination includes the right to procreate.

3   Individuals (and governments) have the obligation to respect the freedom of others.

4   Society has the right to protect itself from forces or actions which might upset or destroy it or prevent it from carrying out social policy aimed at promoting the common good.

5   In cases of conflicting claims, one is obliged to act so as to increase the balance of good over evil.

6   Discrimination against a single group or groups for any reason is ethically unacceptable.

7   Parenthood is a privilege, not a right.

8   The affluent of the world have a moral obligation to respond to the needs of those less well-off.

9   Responding to the needs of a suffering world endangers the entire world.

10 Consumption pattern of affluent societies is overly wasteful, depriving thereby the less-affluent of necessary resources.

11 Disregarding the needs of the suffering destroys some part of a person's humanity.

12 Population-control programs which are coercive are an ethical affront to human dignity.

13 It is ethically questionable to couple aid to a foreign country with external demands such as an effective population-control policy.

14 Incentive programs are unjust since they tend to exploit poverty.

15 It may be necessary to give up a little freedom in one area to gain greater freedom in others.

16 Sterilization programs without adequate social-security policies irretrievably threaten the future welfare of those sterilized.

17 "Thou shalt not exceed the carrying capacity of any environment."

18 The morality of an act is a function of the state of the system at the time the act is performed.

19 Economic injustice, not lack of food, accounts for much of the suffering in the world today.

20 If a population policy is to be ethically acceptable, it must rely upon voluntary decisions of individual couples.

21 Children are one means of extending personal selfhood into the future.

22 It is ethically unfair to require couples to reduce their fertility without providing them real long-term benefits.

23 Employing aphorisms to depict world problems frequently hinders effective efforts aimed at correcting them (e.g., "cushions to conscience").

24 Providing contraceptives and family-planning information is quite properly viewed as an extension of human freedom.

25 Since overpopulation is the direct cause of pollution, environmental decay, and resource depletion, and if unchecked will result in cataclysmic disaster for the whole species, any population policy, including coercion, is acceptable.

REFERENCES

1 Philip Handler, "On the state of man", *Bioscience* 25, 7 (1975): 425–432.

2 Peter J. Henriot, "Global population in perspective: implications for U.S. policy repsonse," *Theological Studies* 35 (1974): 50.

3 Nathan Keyfitz, "World resources and the middle class," *ZPG National Reporter* 8, 8 (1976): 4–5.

4 Arthur McCormack, "The population explosion: a theologian's concern?" *Theological Studies* 35 (1974): 8.

5 George Borgstrom, *The Food and People Dilemma* (North Scituate, Mass: Duxbury, 1973).

6 Philip Handler (in Reference 1), p. 425.

7 Francis Moore Lappé, "More food means more hunger," *The Futurist* 11, 2 (1977): 90–93.

8 Lester Brown and Erik P. Eckholm, "Let them eat bread," *The Humanist* 34, 6 (1974): 6–10.

9 Elie A. Shneour, *The Malnourished Mind* (Garden City: Anchor, 1975).

10 B. Bruce-Briggs, "Against the neo-Malthusians," *Commentary* (July, 1974): 25–29.

11 Philip Handler (in Reference 1), p. 429.

12 Peter J. Henriot (in Reference 2), p. 51.

13 Peter J. Henriot (in Reference 2), p. 51.

14 Arthur J. Dyck, "Alternative views of moral priorities in population policy," *Bioscience* 27, 4 (1977): 272–276.

15 "Themes and highlights of the final report of the Commission on Population Growth and the American Future," *Zero Population Growth*, 4080 Fabian Way, Palo Alto, Calif. 94303

16 Robert McNamara, cited in "Moral claims, human rights and population policies," by Drew Christiansen, Ronald Garrett, David Hollenbock, Charles Powers, Margaret Farley, *Theological Studies* 35 (1974): p. 90.

17 Arthur J. Dyck (in Reference 14), p. 273.

18 Garrett Hardin, "Parenthood: right or privilege?" *Science* 169 (1970): 427.

19 Donald Warwick, "The moral message of Bucharest," *The Hastings Center Report* 4, 6 (1974): 8 and 9.

20 Donald Warwick, (in Reference 19), p. 9.

21 Philip Hauser, cited in "Bullying birth control," by Donald Warwick, *Commonweal* (September 12, 1975): p. 393.

22 Daniel Callahan, "Ethics and population limitation," *Science* **175** (1972): 487–494.
23 M. Brewster Smith, "Ethical implications of population politics: a psychologist's view," *American Psychology* **27**, 1 (1972): 11–15.
24 Drew Christiansen (in Reference 16), p. 85.
25 A. S. Parkes, "The right to reproduce in an overcrowded world," in *Biology and Ethics*, F. J. Ebling (ed.) (London: Academic Press, 1969).
26 James E. Allen, "An appearance of genocide: a review of governmental family-planning program policies," *Perspectives in Biology and Medicine* **20**, 2 (1977): 300–306.
27 James E. Allen (in Reference 26), p. 300.
28 Arthur J. Dyck, "Procreative rights and population policy," *Hastings Center Studies* **1**, 1 (1973): 74–82.
29 Garrett Hardin, "Carrying capacity as an ethical concept," *Soundings* **59**, 1 (1976): 120–137.
30 Garrett Hardin, (in Reference 29), p. 134.
31 Lord Ritchie-Calder, "Triage = genocide," *Center Report* **8**, 3 (1975): 18–20.
32 A. S. Parkes (in Reference 25), p. 92.
33 Ruth Macklin, "Moral concerns and appeals to rights," *Hastings Center Report* **6**, 5 (1976): 31–38, and Arthur J. Dyck, "Population policies and ethical acceptability," in *The Great American Population Debate*, Daniel Callahan (ed.), (Garden City: Doubleday, 1971), p. 362.
34 Arthur J. Dyck, "Population policies and ethical acceptability," in *The Great American Population Debate*, Daniel Callahan (ed.), (Garden City: Doubleday, 1971), pp. 351–377.
35 Daniel Callahan (in Reference 22), 490.
36 "Legal analysis and population control: the problem of coercion," *Harvard Law Review* **84** (1971): 1856–1911.
37 John H. Scanzoni, "Rethinking Christian perspectives on family planning and population control," *Journal of the American Scientific Affiliation*, Supplement 1 (1976), pp. 2–8.
38 Drew Christiansen, "Ethics and compulsory population control," *Hastings Center Report* **7**, 1 (1977): 30–33.
39 Daniel Callahan (in Reference 22), p. 490.
40 Alan Berg, "To save the world from lifeboats," *Natural History* **84**, 6 (1975): 4, 6.
41 Daniel Callahan (in Reference 22), p. 489.
42 Garrett Hardin, *Exploring New Ethics for Survival* (New York: Viking, 1972).
43 Garrett Hardin, "Living on a lifeboat," *Bioscience* **24**, 10 (1974): 561–568.
44 Garrett Hardin (in Reference 43), p. 561.
45 Garrett Hardin (in Reference 29), p. 31.
46 Lord Ritchie-Calder (in Reference 31), p. 18.
47 Donald Warwick (in Reference 19), p. 9.
48 Daniel Callahan, "Doing well by doing good," *Hastings Center Report* **4**, 6 (1974): 1–4.
49 Peter J. Henriot (in Reference 2), p. 54–55.
50 Paul Kurtz, "Interdependence: oil, food, population," *The Humanist* **35**, 2 (1975): 20.
51 Robert S. McNamara, "A pittance for international aid," *Bulletin of Atomic Scientists* **33**:9 (1977): 36–38.
52 Arthur Steiner, "The enormity of the arms race," *Bulletin of Atomic Scientists* **33**, 8 (1977): 63–64.
53 William W. Murdock and Allan Oaten, "Population and food: metaphors and reality," *Bioscience* **25**, 9 (1975): 561–567.

54 Norman Cousins, "Of life and lifeboats," *Saturday Review* (March 8, 1975), p. 4.
55 Norman Cousins (in Reference 54), p. 4.
56 Alan Berg, (in Reference 40).
57 William Murdock and Allen Oaten (in Reference 50), p. 563.
58 Daniel Callahan (in Reference 22), p. 492.
59 Daniel Callahan (in Reference 22), p. 491.
60 Arthur J. Dyck (in Reference 28), p. 78.
61 Drew Christiansen (in Reference 38), p. 30.
62 Indira Ghandi (cited in Reference 38), p. 30.
63 Christiansen et al (in Reference 16), pp. 86–87.
64 Daniel Callahan (in Reference 22), p. 493.
65 William Murdock and Allen Oaten (in Reference 53), p. 564.
66 Arthur McCormack, (in Reference 4), p. 11.
67 Margaret Mead (in Reference 19), p. 9.

BIBLIOGRAPHY

Berelson, Bernard, "Beyond family planning," *Science* **163** (1969): 533–543.
Davis, Kingsley, "Population policy: will current programs succeed?" *Science* **158** (1967): 730–739.
Ehrlich, Paul, *The Population Bomb* (New York: Ballantine, 1968).
Hardin, Garrett, "The tragedy of the commons," *Science* **162** (1968): 1243–1248.
Meadows, Donella H., *The Limits to Growth* (New York: Universe Books, 1972).
United States Commission on Population Growth and the American Future, *Commission Research Reports*, 8 volumes, (Washington, D.C.: U.S. Government Printing Office, 1972).
  Vol. 1: *Demographic and Social Aspects of Population Growth*, Charles F. Westoff and Robert Parke, Jr. (eds.)
  Vol. 2: *Economic Aspects of Population Change*, Elliot R. Morse and Ritchie H. Reed (eds.)
  Vol. 3: *Population, Resources and Environment*, Ronald G. Ridker (ed.)
  Vol. 4: *Governance and Population: The Governmental Implications of Population Change*, A. E. Keir Nash (ed.)
  Vol. 5: *Population, Distribution and Policy*, Sarah Mills Magie (ed.)
  Vol. 6: *Aspects of Population Growth Policy*, Robert Parke, Jr., and Charles F. Westoff (eds.)
  Vol. 7: *Statements at Public Hearings of the Commission on Population Growth and the American Future*
  Vol. 8: Index
United States Commission on Population Growth and the American Future: *Population and the American Future* (New York: New American Library, 1972). Paperback edition of the above.
Veatch, Robert M. (ed.), *Population Policy and Ethics, the American Experience* (New York: Irvington Publishers, 1977).

13

SCIENCE AND SOCIETY

WHO SHOULD CONTROL?

Problem areas in science

Science has become a social issue. The immediate reason for this judgment is that over the past few years revolutionary changes have occurred in the relationships of science to society. A comparison of present-day scientific activities with those from its "heroic age" indicates that science is in a vastly more powerful position to influence this world's events than at any other time in history. The emergence of science, especially since World War II, has brought a flow of blessings that in the recent past bedazzled the public, but now that same public is not so easily enamored. Its increasing potential for unleashing deleterious social consequences has caused in part what has been described as a "crisis of confidence in science."[1]

Science is being challenged on two fronts: The moral and the materialistic. Classified defense research has been virtually banned from academia as it is branded as immoral; many medical innovations not only relieve human suffering but are seen to yield an overgrowth in human numbers; industrial technology, feeding as it must on science, is being viewed as a despoiler of the environment. As more becomes known about some very fundamental processes, including those in biology, the question is raised as to whether knowledge of certain kinds is dangerous or undesirable. Is ignorance sometimes better than understanding? Is the relatively simple life to be preferred over the one encumbered with massive technology and continuous change motivated by scientific innovation? Should the search for new knowledge in some areas be suppressed? The debate over scientific research in its political and social setting continues unabated.

A second phenomenon characterizes science today. As problems become solved, new questions are raised—as has always happened—but the new questions are further out; they recede like an everexpanding frontier. To solve these questions requires more intensive specialization, more team work, more sophisticated equipment to catch hold of a small bit of that moving frontier. As the easier discoveries are made, those remaining require greater and greater ingenuity and resources. So as time goes on, what we are caught up in is a circumstance where there must be more money, more specialization, more coordination of research, more administrative superstructure, and more political maneuvering both within the scientific community and between science and society.[2] Thus, science generates its own momentum to become even larger. In this ethos of gigantism, science runs the real risk, if it has not already happened, of becoming impersonal and then knowledge becomes detached from the knower. Whereas in former times, scientists and other learned persons pondered many hours over the scientific, philosophical, and social implications of their discoveries, today this concern over relationships has changed. Perhaps Alvin Toffler, author of *Future Shock* is right: We are too busy; we do not stop to reflect anymore.

Modern science has become, in many cases, a way to make a comfortable living.[3] Publications are the essential stepping-stones to bureaucratic preferment, which in most cases entitles the author of research to the material security of official patronage (i.e., the granting agencies). Science in our day, according to legal scholar Harvey Wheeler, has abandoned the image of the highly motivated and concerned amateur investigator in favor of mass bureaucracy. Classical science used to be charismatic and heroic; contemporary science is routinized, frequently boring, and generally not much concerned with values, preferring to dismiss such concerns with the off-hand judgment that science is "morally neutral."[4] Little wonder that laypersons viewing modern science exhibit a certain amount of unease with science itself. A recent National Science Foundation (NSF) poll of 2200 adults representing a cross section of American opinion, rated "new basic knowledge about man and nature" at the bottom of a list of national priorities. The state of the economy, tax policy, the delivery of health care, crime prevention, and pollution control ranked above the need for new knowledge about nature. More frequently, it is the question of where all the dollars are going that excites legislators and the public, and self-appointed watch-dogs of the public coffers like Senator William Proxmire (D-Wisc.) are not hesitant to publicize perceived abuses (e.g., the "golden-fleece" award, bestowed monthly, sometimes with public fanfare, to that government-financed activity which is thought to be wasteful of public money). It is well to insist that there are still within the sciences many who remain highly committed to its noble goal—that is, the search for objective knowledge—who consider the practice of science a calling as it once was. There still are those who toil away in modest laboratories, often with makeshift equipment, with little or no outside research support, searching the unknown. It is, though, not this practice of science that characterizes much of what attracts attention today.

It is of more than passing interest to note that because of its very bigness some are beginning to speculate that scientific research may fast be approaching the point of diminishing returns.[5] There may well be an absolute limit to knowledge, imposing an intrinsic limit to scientific growth. It comes as no surprise to anyone in the least familiar with the conditions in science that its apogee has been reached and we are now in a period of recession. Although there are discoveries still to be made, they will probably not be of the truly creative kind. Rather, they rest on or derive from previously established innovative breakthroughs. Even the discoveries in molecular biology, our most rapidly advancing biological subdiscipline, are said by some to be nothing more than applied physics.[6] According to this rationale, contemporary science is now in a developmental phase in which the technological implications of the visions of former giants are being exploited and systematized by the lesser among us. (But this is a topic in itself and this is not the place to debate the merits of that hypothesis.) Some have carried the arguments of limits to the extreme, contending that in an absolute sense, there may be just so many natural phenomena in the universe to be discovered. Economist Frank Boulding once remarked that only about another 500 years will be required to uncover this remaining knowledge.

To return to the world of the here and now, it has been asserted that bigness breeds bureaucracy, intentionally or not. If you have the first, the second is automatic. They are inseparable. As science becomes both richer and larger, it calls for the application of business management methods. F. T. Cole editorialized in *New Scientist*, "In the large laboratories, the management of people and resources is as important as in a large business enterprise." But bureaucracy has within it fundamental defects, some or all of which could contribute to its demise. For one, bureaucracy tends toward the status quo, whereas science thrives on creativity. The status-quo syndrome is perpetuated this way: Scientific leadership tends to become the monopoly of the scientific establishment under the control of older persons who gradually turned their careers from doing science to the administration of it. Creativity and scientific productivity, it has been argued, is a young person's game. (It has been said that the majority of major scientific breakthroughs are made by persons under age 35.) As funds for research diminish, decline in support for university science naturally follows since most science is done in universities.* As science budgets are reduced, the younger, nontenured scientists suffer the first blows of the axe. The older, tenured scientists remain—youth and genius give way to age and sterility. Because virtually few young scientists can obtain new tenured positions, the feeder-system is shut off. A mediocratizing sets in (what we see now is that the American research enterprise has entered a depression) both in terms of money for support and for talented minds, from which recovery is by no means yet in sight.[7]

Science's competitive nature has yet another effect. Bright young researchers who do obtain positions find competition severe. Untenured faculty are under enormous pressure to publish in order to win grants and promotion to security. They may be forced to be less scrupulous in their methods and cheating in the reporting of scientific "discoveries" has come to the attention of the public. Probably the most celebrated recent case is that of the young researcher, William T. Summerlin, at the Sloan-Kettering Cancer Center. He deliberately falsified the results of his experiments by using a felt-tipped pen to indicate successful tissue transplants in some experimental mice. His experiments were widely reported at the time to demonstrate a breakthrough in transplantation techniques.[8] Another was the faking of research by a bright Harvard student, Steven Rosenfeld, who shook the biological world with his reported isolation of the immuno-transfer factor. Although the number of revealed fabrications are very small in comparison to the amount of science done, the number of shoddy and unrepeatable publications is increasing at an alarming

---

*   The National Science Board, the governing body of the National Science Foundation (NSF), reported that the support for basic research in constant dollars declined by 13 percent between 1968 and 1974 and that the expenditure per active scientist was down a sharp 30 percent over the same period.

rate. Dr. Richard W. Roberts, Director of the National Bureau of Standards, cited estimates that 50 percent of data reported in scientific literature is unusable.[9] Instances like these have led to accusation by science watchers that there are symptoms of a "widespread sickness in science."[10] Dr. Ernest Borek, in an editorial, asks about "the twilight of integrity."[11]

Still another problem-area deals with the matter of funding for research. As overall research funding declines, individual scientists are forced to scramble for research contracts and foundation grants in order to keep their laboratories going; survival may not depend on the merits of the research or the motivation of the researcher. Scientists frequently must conform to the desires of administrators of foundations, of corporations, and of government agencies. The research contract system has within it the implicit potential for corruption. The potential for the coopting of the scientific enterprise is inherent in such a system, for the old saying "he who pays the piper calls the tune" is as applicable here as anywhere else. Why, after all, do governments, companies, and societies support science? A scientist thinks of a grant as a means to carry on his/her research; a business tends to regard research as a means to obtain a payoff. The payoff certainly can take many forms depending upon the sponsoring agency: Warmongering, company profits, political ambitions, prestige, economic growth, or practical needs. What is disturbing to some is that the government is placing emphasis on directed research through the mechanism of contracts. Here the government decides what problem areas are most in need of further research and solicits the scientific community for proposals. For example, the key words to success in searching out funding sources today are cancer and energy, and the scientific community is eager to accept funds on these terms (it has been said, "where money beckons, scientists are wont to stray"). Here we have the specter of government hiring scientists to solve specific problems that are very practical or of the applied variety. In the short-term, this may be all right, but in the long range, the style in which science is practiced will be affected.

> It is inherent in the nature of science that we never know exactly what it is that we are looking for, or even where to look for it. So it is absurd to maintain that we can determine, *a priori*, the most efficient way to find it.[12]

Mission-oriented research can stifle creativity so essential for discovery. And in this regard someone has said, if targeted research had been the policy in the 1950s, polio would never have been solved. We would have instead of two effective vaccines today, more efficient iron lungs (probably portable) and whirlpools.[13] To loosen the strings of the paymasters, the entrepreneur of science must be skilled in public relations and grantsmanship, must be willing to compromise, and must learn to package results to suit client's preferences. Science does reflect the social forces which surround it and if the contemporary scientist is to live and work in that world, his/her research field must reflect that world. But society may well write the rules to be followed.

The cost of modern science

Among the most pressing social and political concerns of modern science is its cost; it is not cheap, and it costs more and more to learn less and less. The amounts of money involved in science are astronomical. There is a restriction to the total investment any given society can devote to the support of science. A few dollar figures vividly illustrate that there may well be fiscal limits to scientific growth. For the fiscal year 1975, total expenditures for research and development in the United States were estimated to be $34.3 billion, seven percent above the $32 billion for 1974. It represents 2.3 percent of the Gross National Product. Of that amount, the federal government funded about 54 percent.[14] Although it is difficult to establish where the breaking point may be, those who have looked into these matters estimate that even in the wealthiest of countries, not more than two or three percent of the GNP can be diverted for this purpose. It has been suggested that the two-to-three-percent breaking point has already been reached in both the United States and Russia. Being forced to spend more for less, sooner or later someone must evaluate what the proposed expenditures will yield in terms of payoff. Because of this inverse relationship, it would seem that modern science faces a limit beyond which further progress is feasible. This of course, raises that most difficult question and also bears on the issue of control: Where does the margin lie beyond which the new knowledge will not be worth the money required to acquire it? How much money should be allocated to the fulfillment of curiosity (i.e., basic research), and how much in the pursuit of hard returns? Should we expect only quick payoffs or make provisions for longer term benefits? Taxpayers and public policy makers as well as scientists do have a stake in all of this.

It is fast becoming a fact of life that science has become so expensive that its support can be justified only on the basis of the benefits that derive from it. The last few years have witnessed a serious challenge from the public requesting an accounting for the dollars spent. A *New York Times* editorial in 1967 said the following about the National Acceleration Laboratory proposal (it has since been built at Batavia, Illinois):

> But there is an even more basic objection to any commitments or expenditures for this expensive research tool at this time. The objection is simply the irrelevance of a 250 billion electron volt accelerator to any real, present national problem. . . . It is a distortion of the national priorities to commit many millions now to this interesting but unnecessary scientific luxury.

More recently, other serious challenges to the federal science budget have been leveled. The previously mentioned behavior of Senator William Proxmire (D-Wis.) and Congressman Robert Bauman (R-Md.) inveighing against federal funding of "damn fool" projects cannot be taken lightly. (Representative Bauman has joined the fray by initiating a "Mickey Mouse of the Year Award" for the federally funded research he judges to be the most inane.) The language of the House draft appropriating NSF funds for 1976 emphasizes that federally supported research is under the gun.

> In recent months particular activities of the Foundation have been questioned. Members of Congress, representatives of the press, and countless American taxpayers have been openly critical of the uses of tax revenues to finance seemingly frivolous and irrelevant scientific research projects.

This wave of resentment peaked with the Bauman amendment, an amendment added on the floor of the House to the National Science Foundation appropriations bill by the congressman. On April 9, 1975, the House voted (212 to 199) that Congress should have a veto power over any and all of the 14,000 grants which the National Science Foundation awards every year. The Senate, at the urgings of Senator Robert Kennedy (D-Mass.), refused the amendment and it was dropped from the final budget bill. Even so, the action had an impact. It was a less than subtle message that some people in government charged with guarding the public purse strings were in a mood to crack down.

The point of this discussion on limits and high cost of science is that the continued growth of science will increasingly come under public scrutiny and calls for its regulation will be emphatic. To Harvey Wheeler, this is good for two reasons: It prevents potential evil from crippling the system from within, and it insures the continued vitality of science by forcing its continuous evaluation. However anathema to scientists the prospect of regulation may be, it seems almost axiomatic that the public regulation issue be raised since science subsists almost entirely on public funds. There is small likelihood that the public will want to continue to pay the price in support of untrammeled scientific research without having some voice in the spending of those dollars.

Furthermore, the massive American scientific enterprise, costing millions of dollars in public funds annually, can no longer justify its continued existence because it is a privileged scholarly enterprise of cultural value. The mass successes of science and its technologies have made it an indispensible part of our culture. Because we can't do without it, like water and air and other essentials of life, it must enter into public governance and public domain.[15] Scientists cannot expect generous public support much longer without explicit responsibility and accountability to the public. And here we have a parallel between science and medicine; the newer conceptions of health care delivery view medical care as a social service and ought, therefore, to come under public control. So, too, with science. But as the medical enterprise resists public intervention so many in the sciences oppose outside interference.

Wheeler is quick to point out that there is probably no other profession that is almost wholly supported out of public funds, while at the same time is almost completely free from public regulations. This situation could be at least tolerated if, first, the demand on the public treasury was not so great, and second, if science was still harmless. But those utopian conditions have ceased to be. For example, the lag between basic discoveries and their social consequences has disappeared in many instances. Scientific breakthroughs, especially in matters touching directly upon the human condition, can coincide with immediate social consequences, for good or evil. (For example, reproductive technology and social dislocations; green revolutions in agriculture and social revolutions; gene-splicing and the potential for unleashing massive epidemics.) The lag time between science and technology becomes shorter and shorter and, in some cases, nonexistent. This demands that a level of control must be inserted before the research is done, not after the fact when shattered pieces must be reassembled. Science is knowledge, but it is not wisdom. As Robert Heilbronner stated in *The Future as History*:[16]

> Advances in science and technology have rewritten the terms and conditions of the human contract with no more warning than the morning's headlines.

The question to be resolved is how to permit scientific activity to remain free while regulating its costs and its technological applications. No one has figured this out yet, but recent events in Washington predict that efforts will be exerted.

The morality of science

Before taking on the question of control, there is another factor that has been implicated in the contemporary adversary relationship between science and the public. It is believed by some nonscientists and scientists alike that the activities of science are value-free. Science is morally neutral. After all, equations do not explode and almost any technology can be used *either* for evil or for good. However, the moral and ethical neutrality of science has been seriously challenged from a variety of sources, both from within and without its establishment. Facts themselves may ultimately be value-free, but the enterprise that discovers them is not. Facts will continue to be a reflection of humans and their culture. Two British scientists, Steven and Hilary Rose, contend that scientists are responsible for the misuse of their findings.[17] They maintain that most of the contemporary scientific research is conceived for specific ends and is linked to the views of those who provide the support. They decry for example, the great outlay of funds that goes for the support of those areas broadly defined as military or for economic gain. Thus, the social and political environments specify the direction of research and no research can be separated from its environment.

Knowledge sought will continue to be a reflection of the society that encourages and supports it. Therefore, it is a delusion to think that science can be separated into socially acceptable and unacceptable parts. Modern science is a composite activity in which a discovery in one part frequently influences discoveries in other, often unrelated areas (e.g., the study of plant growth hormones led to the development of chemical herbicides which were used as defoliation agents in the Vietnamese war). It is no easy thing to separate one aspect of the scientific enterprise from another. What appears to be sometimes morally neutral in and by itself can have significant repercussions when associated with scientific activity in other fields. The important point is not that science in the abstract is amoral, but rather that the scientist in the flesh cannot escape the problem of value judgments in his or her own behavior. The products of scientific endeavor are of enormous importance to the welfare of humanity.[18] This is especially so when one considers the very tiny step from the discoveries of science to their implementation by technology. (The story is told that Albert Einstein, upon learning of the first nuclear explosion, exclaimed, "I wish I had become a blacksmith.")

Philosopher Hans Jonas analyzes the accountability of science as an agent for social action.[19] He contends that freedom of inquiry may be granted as long as it raises no moral problems, that is, when pure theory does not intervene in the practical affairs of society. Knowledge can be considered a private good to the knowers—a state of the mind—only if it does no harm to the good of others, and if it seeks only to comprehend but not to change the state of things. However, he argues, "knowledge for its own sake" for the most part has ceased to be. With the beginning of the modern age (that is, from the nineteenth century onward), the historical separation between theory and implementation has been irrevocably altered. Science has shifted its wares to practical applications. When this happened, science became subject to a moral judgment for whatever has an impact on the real world, hence the welfare of others is of moral concern. As soon as there is power and its use, morality is involved and science has provided power. No longer is the question one of good or bad science but of good or ill *effects* of science. Since, according to Jonas, no branch of science remains whose discoveries are devoid of some technological applications (and technology, the child of science, has its dark sides), then science cannot alibi itself out by claiming moral immunity. Taking credit for the benefits means also taking responsibility for the dangers.

Theodore Roszak, among the sharpest critics of modern science, carries the morality argument still further when he accuses the scientific community of complicity in the destruction of nature. Although it was profiteering industrialists and short-sighted developers, who in the first case wasted and desecrated nature, Roszak insists that it was science which provided that image of the natural world which invited its rape. "Science has been the only natural philosophy the Western world has known since the age of Newton." What he is saying is that science not only tells us how nature works but how it is to be used as well. Again to quote: "Before the earth could become an industrial garbage can, it had first to become a research laboratory."[20]

A possible resolution to all this is that the humanist must be drawn in whenever science undertakes a set of moral experiments (e.g., gene-splicing, behavior modification, etc.) for although new scientific knowledge can broaden our understanding of the natural world, by themselves scientists should not make these choices. We must be continuously reminded that values determine which choices *ought* to be made, not facts standing alone. The choices that lie before us in these matters must be judged against the single criterion: That which improves and preserves human life is good. Increasingly, we must try to separate the good from the bad and then work toward the good, bearing in mind that social and political choices about the uses and priorities of science will be only as wise as those making the decisions. The argument that productive research has no necessary relationship to social health and human freedom must be judged as unacceptable. Dr. James Shapiro, a promising, bright Harvard biophysicist, saw clearly this relationship and put his case this way as he renounced a potentially brilliant career in biology (Shapiro, as a member of a research team under Jonathan Beckwith, isolated the first naked gene at Harvard in 1969):

> In and of itself our work is morally neutral; it can lead either to benefits or dangers to mankind. But we are working in the United States in the year 1969. The basic control over scientific work and its further development is in the hands of a few people at the head of large private institutions and at the top of government bureaucracies. These people have consistently exploited science for harmful purposes in order to increase their own power . . . what we are advocating is that scientists, together with other people, should actively work for [radical political] changes in this country. . . . If our arguments mean that "the progress of science" itself may be interrupted, that is an unfortunate consequence we will have to accept.[21]

If science does not realize that it has been experimenting with morality all along and that ethical neutrality is no longer a permissible moral stance, freedom to do scientific research may be legislated out of existence to the detriment of both science and society.

A restatement of the problem

A new report titled, "The State of Academic Science: the Universities in the Nation's Research Effort" identifies the dampened state of scientific endeavor in the United States.[22] Several significant problems underlie the adverse trend in American university science. These are the weakening financial position of the universities resulting in part from a decline in federal support, a downward trend in graduate enrollments, an aging faculty entrenched by virtue of tenure, deteroriating scientific equipment, tensions between scientists and university administrators over financial support, and demands from federal and state authorities for extensive accounting and compliance with regulatory laws. More serious trouble probably lies ahead and the gap between the prestigious institutions and their smaller counterparts will probably grow. This could result in a drastic decline in the number of serious research institutions. The final statement of the report succinctly summarizes the condition of university science today: "The era of rapid growth is over. Innovations now must be by substitution rather than by expansion."

The sketch of the besieged state of science drawn here is fragmentary and has necessarily omitted much supporting detail. A recapitulation of the points made are:

1 Modern science has grown excessively large resulting in a loss of personal commitment and concern by its practitioners; its support requires enormous outlays of public funds; it encourages bureaucracy which creates conditions for cheating, mediocrity, and counterproductivity.

2 The compression of time between the physical and social effects and scientific advances provides little opportunity to evaluate the social consequences of proposed science.

3 There is a concern among the lay public and its representatives in government with the activities of scientists, and a call for control is being made at many levels of society.

4 Science cannot claim moral neutrality.

To deal with each of these, new social inventions are desirable and in fact are demanded if science and scientists are to maintain a responsible position in society and participate in securing a better future.

Control strategies

Can science—biological science—respond to the challenge? Are there larger social obligations of science and scientists? Does science have anything of value to contribute to the preservation of democracy? By what mechanism should the course of scientific research be directed? How does one secure the "consent of the governed"? Do scientists have a role to play not only in matters scientific but also in participating themselves in debate on sensitive social issues? Can there be an effective partnership between the federal government, private industry, society, and the scientists? The real issue reduces to this: On one side are those who insist that unrestrained scientific research is hazardous and must be brought to bridle, while the opposition views as pure folly efforts to control science in any way. In the matter of control, several alternatives are possible.

Self-regulation

The first considers self-regulation, a frequently resorted to procedure when outside pressures threaten. As a specific case in point, the recent work in gene manipulation using restriction enzymes exemplifies some of the difficulties encountered with self-control. Recall that the new techniques make possible limited gene insertion, posing thereby a real danger to human life if biologists succeed in creating new and/or potentially lethal organisms which might escape the laboratory and infect human beings. This danger is especially acute because the geneticist's experimental organism of choice, the bacterium *E. coli*, naturally inhabits the human intestine. Without recounting the entire course of events that transpired from the first call of alarm in 1973 by a group of scientists, some recapitulation is instructive. (See Chapter 4 for a more thorough discussion.)

Professor Paul Berg of Stanford, a scientist active in this type of research, became a leading voice calling public attention to the danger of recombinant DNA research. Very early (1973), he and several others doing similar experiments suggested careful consideration be given to further recombinant research until such time as appropriate safeguards could be developed and agreed upon. They also recommended to the National Academy of Science, (NAS), that it undertake a study of the matter. The NAS thereupon appointed an ad hoc committee, composed of U.S. scientists under the leadership of Professor Berg, called the Committee on Recombinant DNA Molecules. In the summer of 1974, the committee urged a moratorium on DNA research until the whole situation, including potential hazards, could be studied. An international meeting was subsequently convened at Asilomar, California, February 24–27, 1975, to which 150 scientists from various laboratories around the world were invited. Extensive debate at Asilomar led to a lifting of the ban, the moratorium being replaced with a stringent set of safety conditions which in some instances continued the prohibition on certain kinds of recombinant work. Like the moratorium that preceded it, the conference decision had the power of moral censure only. As far as is known, all scientists working in the area voluntarily participated in these restraints. Throughout the Asilomar conference, the admonition was repeated over and over again that if scientists themselves failed to regulate their activities, the government would. Dr. Sid Brenner of the British Medical Research Council summed it up this way:

> The issue that I believe is central is a political issue. It is this: we live at a time where I think there is a great anti-science attitude developing in society, well developed in some societies, and developing in government, and this is something we have to take into consideration. . . . Who really believes that natural science will increase your GNP? Maybe this is the end of this era. It is very hard to tell in history where you really are. . . . I think people have got to realize there is no easy way out of this situation: we have not only to say we are going to act but we must be seen to be acting.

During 1975, the National Institutes of Health (NIH) Advisory Committee developed guidelines for regulating these researches. After several meetings where they were open for review (and attended mostly by scientists), guidelines were formalized that represented the official position of the government regulating all federally funded recombinant research. One oft-repeated criticism of the NIH guidelines was that they were developed by scientists for scientists.

It is not surprising that this try at self-policing had a galvanic effect on biologists and politicians. What the whole affair has highlighted is precisely the issue that some have politely questioned in times past, namely, can humankind's well-being be entrusted to the integrity, carefulness, and self-restraint of individual scientists who are themselves competing against each other to see who will be first to make the breakthroughs that lead to prestige? In other words, can a vested interest group both encourage and police its activities simultaneously?

The position favoring independence is argued as follows: Pure or basic research must not and indeed cannot be limited. You cannot tell scientists what to think! Efforts to control the development of knowledge are an inherent infringement upon the freedom of inquiry this nation has always valued so highly. (The vision of Lysenkoism in the Soviet Union is frequently invoked.*) Self-regulation taking the form of codes of acceptable and forbidden areas threatens the very foundations of science. However, as this discussion has attempted to show, the older dictum—basic science must remain free while society must decide what to do about the consequences of scientific discoveries—no longer applies in view of the short-lag time between discovery and social ramifications. In the case of the recombinant work, the accidental creation of a lethal organism escaped from the confines of the laboratory would provide society no chance at all to regulate the consequences of the invention. Questions of the following sort pose very serious difficulties when the proposition of self-policing is projected:

1 Should proposed guidelines apply across the board to all (genetic) research or only selectively to certain procedures?

---

* The Lysenko affair in the Soviet Union which raged for nearly thirty years is frequently cited as the kind of danger which political interference poses for science. T. D. Lysenko rose from an obscure position in a far-flung agricultural experimental station in the late 1920s to become the President of the Lenin Academy of Agricultural Sciences in 1938 and Director of the Institute of Genetics of the Academy of Sciences in 1950. His claim to fame was based on a series of proposed panaceas for the grave agricultural problems of the Soviet Union derived from a kind of neo-Lamarckian biology in which species of winter wheat could be transformed into the spring variety by moistening and chilling the seeds—"vernalization" he called it. When Soviet geneticists challenged the scientific basis of this claim (vernalization was never proved experimentally but it did fit the Communist doctrine that controlling the environment, social or agricultural, can produce an ideal product), they were subjected to harassment and intimidation. Finally, in 1948, any Soviet geneticist who did not subscribe to "Lysenkoism" was absolutely denied the right to carry out research in genetics. The prohibition was reversed in 1952 and after another ten or so years, Soviet geneticists were again allowed to return to the mainstream of genetics. Bear in mind that these years were some of the most exciting in the field of genetics in the West. Lysenko's domination of Soviet genetics, carried out under the aegis of the state, effectively blocked a whole generation of genetic research in the Soviet Union. (See *The Rise and Fall of T. D. Lysenko*, by Zhores A. Medvedew, New York: Columbia University Press, 1971.)

2   If selectively, who is to decide which are permissible and which are prohibited?

3   What sort of controls should be developed? Can they be adopted or enforced?

4   What really are the social hazards inherent in scientific research and how can they be evaluated? (Regarding recombinant research, molecular biologist James Watson has said, "Our work with cancer tumors is many times more dangerous.")

Senator Edward Kennedy (D-Mass.), expressed his dissatisfaction with the Asilomar Conference in a public speech at Harvard in May of 1975:

> It was commendable that scientists attempted to think through the social consequences of their work. It was commendable, but it was inadequate. It was inadequate because scientists alone decided to impose the moratorium and scientists alone decided to lift it. Yet the factors under consideration extend far beyond their technical competence. In fact they were making public policy. And they were making it in private.

On a broader front what is posed here is a more fundamental issue, namely, is science a social institution like any other (e.g., banking), to be regulated in the public interest? Or is it a privileged establishment, like the church, where because of some transcending principle or objective, it can define its own goals and regulate itself?

The critics of science assert, whether scientists care to accept the judgment or not, that science is a social enterprise and because of this there is no distinction between science and any other occupation or profession. The medical profession presently is waging last-ditch warfare against external control for the apparent reason that self-regulation, self-interest, and public need are not always congruent. Can the basic scientist expect different treatment? In Harvey Wheeler's words:

> It is time for us all to realize that science is no more the private property of scientists than the economy is the private property of businessmen, as the government is the private property of politicians. Corruption occurs when scientists forget this.[23]

According to this view, self-policing is a nonviable option and must be rejected out of hand. A British report entitled "A Framework for Government Research and Development," released in November 1971, put it this way:

> However distinguished, intelligent and practical scientists may be, they cannot be so well qualified to decide what the needs of the nation are and their priorities, as those responsible for ensuring that those needs are met. (Rothschild Report)

Another defect seriously weakening the principle of self-regulation goes much closer to the point, namely, that neither individual experts nor their professional associations have generally shown the moral strength and distinterestedness to monitor their own activities. History repeatedly tells us that a body of specialists such as a learned society is too proud of its own expertise and too jealous of its privileges to admit to its own limitations. Committed to the advancement of its own branch of learning, science cannot at the same time guard the interests of laypersons who might be adversely affected thereby. The lack of anything more binding than conscience leaves open to doubt that self-regulation can ever be effective when those involved have a vested interest in the activities they are attempting to regulate (witness the now defunct Atomic Energy Commission and the "ailing" medical profession). Some younger scientists at the Asilomar Conference urged no, or only minimal, controls arguing they would function as needless constraints on research. Several instances of breaching the NIH guidelines by researchers have already been reported. The first occurred in early 1977 at the University of California, San Francisco, one of the leading research centers utilizing rDNA techniques. The episode involved the use of uncertified bacterial plasmids for experimental cloning of the gene for insulin. A second involved a Harvard researcher who also failed to obtain permission as stipulated in the guidelines. Although both issues posed no public health threat and subsequent investigations judged the experiments as "innocent errors," it does raise the question of reliability of the guidelines in policing research activities.[24]

Self-regulation to be effective must carry with it a mechanism for enforcement to coerce noncompliers and in this regard, one touches upon some very sensitive nerves when suggesting pressures to curb research in particular areas. For these reasons, self-regulation may rarely be workable; as some skeptics suggest, probably not even feasible."

A host of communities and states enacted or considered enacting legislation or regulations governing recombinant research in areas under their jurisdiction. New York, California, Illinois; Cambridge, Massachusetts; Madison, Wisconsin; Ann Arbor, Michigan are a few of the places where such action has been discussed or taken. Although these efforts at local legislation were compromised by subsequent events (see p. 124), they do indicate that even local communities are in a mood to regulate the activities of science.

Governmental regulation

It would seem that the new order of problems today suggests that controls beyond the profession are being called for. Increased regulation, including enforcement strategies from outside of science is probably inevitable and may be necessary. Since self-regulation by itself may not be the answer, the challenge is to invent a new form of control, a new form of justice appropriate for confronting the issues. The most likely resort is federal legislation.

Opponents to legislation insist that federal control of science will seriously impede research since, among other things, it will require vast and cumbersome bureaucracies through which the scientist must work. Others base their opposition on the observation that control legislation constitutes an infringement on First-Amendment freedoms of free speech and expression, extending the meaning of these to include the search for and publication of scientific knowledge. Still others fear that any kind of legislation, even for the most beneficial reasons, sets precedent for further federal interference leading to complete governmental control ("socialized science").

What will be the consequences of the state taking direct action through legislation? No one knows for sure for in our country, anyway, this is an action that heretofore is without precedent—at least at the federal level. Some experience, however, has been acquired at the state level, the Massachusetts law regulating fetal research, enacted in June 1974, for instance. This legislation may be representative of what is going on, or can be expected to go on in other states and at the national level if government intrudes itself into the activities of science. Although the Massachusetts law itself "restricts experimentation on live human fetuses," making it a *criminal* rather than a civil offense, it speaks to the larger issue of state control of science. Laws aimed at regulation inevitably alter the relationship of a scientist to his/her research by placing legal sanctions or prohibitions on courses of action that previously were theirs alone to determine. In the development and the writing of the Massachusetts law regulating fetal research there is a lesson to be learned. And here a bit of history may be in order.

The legislation as originally conceived would have banned all research on fetuses, living or dead, which were the subjects of planned abortion. (This law was enacted before the issuance of guidelines for fetal research by the National Commission for the Protection of Human Subjects—see Chapter 5, Section e.) However, there were a number of procedures, many in the experimental stage designed to diagnose and/or treat *in utero* certain fetal defects. Being experimental, they posed some risks to the fetus. If the original law was enacted, all fetal research would have been banned and the potential for developing new, *in utero* life-saving techniques and therapies would have been halted. Scientists conducting fetal research on the Harvard Medical School faculty objected to the original legislation on these grounds and, through much direct involvement with legislation, succeeded in modifying the bill to allow certain kinds of fetal research to continue. Although much time and effort had to be expended to gain this end—for involvement in controversial political issues is a full-time job—at least three salutary effects were thought to be realized. In the first place, the confrontation between scientists and law makers proved equally illuminating for both sides; scientists learned that "those of us in the statehouse do not have horns"; second, discussion between the two resulted in what was thought to be a much better law, satisfying those who saw sinister threats to life resulting from fetal experimentation (the lawmakers) but still permitting the necessary research to continue (the scientists); and third, a state advisory commission was set up to assist the legislature on bills that would influence future research.[25]

However, all that appears to end well may not necessarily be well and in this case we see the kinds of problems raised when legislation is aimed at regulating research. Since the bill was a product of compromise, researchers had difficulty in trying to figure out precisely what it allows and what it forbids. The author of the bill (William Delahunt) went to Harvard Medical School to answer questions. As reported in *Science* this was "quite a scene. . . . There they were, some of the biggest names at the Harvard Medical School standing up like schoolboys to describe their work and to ask: 'Please, Mr. Legislator, may I go on with what I'm doing?' "[26] Delahunt conceived the scenario of scientists carrying on fetal research as petitioner in which the researcher states in writing his/her contemplated research and some kind of board will advise the scientist about the research. In these petitions, Delahunt thought that emphasis should be placed on the researcher's *motives*, arguing from the position that throughout the experimental procedure nothing must substantially jeopardize the life or health of the fetus. This of course, rules out experimentation with fetuses scheduled for abortion. It is this prohibition, that significantly retarded research. As this law demonstrates, and as the real issue in the matter of legal regulation of science, the research community is in danger of losing control of its own destiny as it will be forced again and again to cope with the demands of people on the outside, many of whom may be uninformed as to procedures, benefits, or risks. For example, the Massachusetts statute produced unintended results.[27] Although the framers of the legislation submitted it as a "moderate and enlightened" law, designed to facilitate research, it amounted to a virtual ban on all fetal studies since so much uncertainty concerning permissible and prohibited research was generated. Perhaps the most ironic example of this is the result that the two Harvard researchers who fought the hardest to get scientifically satisfactory legislation have themselves had their research shut off. The overall effect of the law has been to stop all research out of fear or uncertainty of the consequences. A similar utterance was made by a Harvard molecular biologist in regard to the more recent concern over recombinant DNA legislation: "We are being hasseled out of existence for no reason at all."

Pressure for legislation designed to prevent or control aspects of scientific research will no doubt increase at all levels of government. The earlier described Bauman Amendment challenged the peer-review system of the National Science Foundation for evaluating research projects. Peer review is the process whereby scientists evaluate the work of other scientists in the awarding of government research funds. The heavy concentration of federally funded projects in a few locations and the staffing of review committees by "good buddies" suggest to some that the whole system is designed to perpetuate itself with only those judged to possess the proper credentials (or contacts) being allowed admittance. A number of senators and representatives (Senator Proxmire, Representatives Teague and Bauman, etc.) have expressed their suspicions of the peer-review system based on self-regulation followed up with demands that it be opened to public and/or Congressional scrutiny.

Advisory commission to public policy

George W. Ball, speaking at the 1977 annual meeting of the American Association for the Advancement of Sciences suggested that greater government intervention in research is inevitable. Further, he warns, if present trends continue, the point might be reached where the law would require bureaucratic review of almost every scientific research project to ascertain whether it meets some defined test of social desirability—a social-impact study modeled after environmental-impact studies now required of federal projects where the environment is threatened.[28] These and other actions of a like sort are matters of significance. As Philip Handler, director of the National Academy of Science, says: "The seed of distrust in the judgment-making apparatus is being firmly planted."[29] If reasonable lawmaking and the protection of scientific research is to be at all effective, scientists must assume roles in helping people acquire knowledge about matters scientific. The scientist's job must go beyond collecting, analyzing, and writing up information. It is perhaps the better part of wisdom for scientists to involve themselves in advising the decision-making process and to help determine what action is to be taken in scientific matters. One mechanism suggested for accomplishing this is through participation on advisory commissions similar to the one proposed in the Massachusetts statute governing fetal research.

It cannot be emphasized too strongly that any advisory board or commission cannot be subservient to political or commercial powers whom they are supposed to advise. The basic defect of such agencies presently in existence is just this: In practice their primary allegiance is to the parent agency. Advisory boards cannot have executive power, either, since that would usurp the authority of the state. They must be advisory only. Further, if they are not to be torn apart by ideological conflicts, they must have no special axe to grind or cause to promote. They must act on the premise that collective goodwill is needed. The only commodities, then, that such an agency can safely deal with are *information* and *informed opinion* about scientific matters, about government decisions, about human needs, and about ethical principles.

Although such a commission may sound idealistic, we are not without models. One approach is embodied in a proposed Science Court which would be concerned solely with questions of scientific fact. It would leave the social value questions, on which the ultimate policy decisions are based, to the normal decision-making apparatus of our society. The notion of a Science Court has been around for some time and more recently it has attracted a good deal of attention. The basic mechanism is this: An issue would be selected (such as nuclear reactor safety, fluoridation of drinking water, the question of whether fluorocarbons should be banned for fear of damage to the ozone layer, etc.); case managers would be chosen for each side of the issue; and these managers would compile the facts as their side views the issue and would argue their case in an adversary hearing before a panel of three scientific judges who had no involvement whatsoever with the issue. If the case managers were unable to narrow their areas of disagreement through mediation, then the scientific judges would write opinions on the contested statements.[30] The deliberations would in no way be binding on anyone, the sole objective of the Science Court is to bring the best judgments of the scientific community to bear on technical aspects of policy problems. This system will limit itself to expressing the state of scientific knowledge at a point in time, and to drawing a line between what is known and what is unknown.

One of the most fundamental criticisms of the Science Court has been the assertion that facts and values are inseparable when considering public policy issues.[31] Scientist Arthur Kantrowitz, the originator of the Science Court concept calls these "mixed decisions." Even matters of purest fact may be entangled with social and political suppositions. Moreover, controversies that do exist most often stem from uncertainties that allow for diverse and value-laden interpretations. The more controversial an issue, the greater the uncertainty (e.g., the value questions related to a plutonium economy). The effort to resolve factual questions apart from questions of value is exceptionally difficult, and for purposes of policy-making, may not even be possible for the point of disagreement seldom lies not with the facts but with the conception of values the uncertainties conjure up.

Other objections to the Science Court concept have been raised about the selection of judges, case managers, and referees. It will be a difficult matter to get scientifically competent people, who are willing to devote the time and risk their careers, and who have the necessary scientific credentials for recognition by both sides, who are able to maintain a strict sense of objectivity, and who can cut through the scientific obfuscation that will undoubtedly arise as adversaries confront one another in open debate. The very concept of adversary has been challenged as setting the basis for a "must-win" confrontation rather than a sincere search for facts and understanding. Polarization of the issues can result since advocates before a court are careful to introduce only facts that are clearly supportive of their position. Both sides will leave out evidence that might be between the two positions or might give advantage to the other side. And still another reservation is that the Science Court procedure, like any other social invention, may eventually be corrupted. Once it has been corrupted, its power could be dangerously authoritarian. Visions of a Plato's Republic of Science have been conjured up by some with "functions of canon court issuing pronouncements of scientific truth." Others have called it a "grand inquisition" and "a form of 1984 technocracy."[32]

Although the Science Court concept is still largely theoretical, its testing was suggested by the state of Minnesota. A proceeding of this type over the construction of a disputed high-voltage powerline in 1978 was the case in point. Because the contending parties were even unable to agree on a format for the hearing, however, it was never tried. This led some to the conclusion that the whole Science Court concept is completely unrealistic as a mechanism for reaching informed scientific judgment (see reference 55).

An alternative to the Science Court concept is the establishment of standing commissions which focus on controversial issues. A most relevant example here is the often-referred-to National Commission for the Protection of Human Subjects (see p. 255). Commissions patterned on this model could organize debates among informed people who hold conflicting views; they could create advisory panels to interpret and clarify differences in technical opinion to assist congressional leaders or federal agencies; they could hold public hearings where private citizens and interest groups would have a forum for expressing their views; and they could formulate guidelines to be submitted to agencies or groups responsible for regulating that aspect of public policy. The purpose of these procedures would be to draw into the debate of an issue the widest and most imaginative range of views and to subject them to a still broader dissemination to the general public. From there, public policy could be formulated.

The activities of the National Commission for the Protection of Human Subjects were terminated in October, 1978. An Ethics Advisory Board composed of fourteen members under the aegis of HEW assumed the advisory functions of the commission. Two problems have been assigned this Board for study and recommendation— in vitro fertilization and the regulation of clinical trials in medical research. Also, legislation has been introduced into Congress to establish a permanent Ethics Review Committee (Sen. Kennedy, D-Mass., Rep. Rodgers, D-Fla.) as a presidential commission. It is anticipated that this committee will function in similar fashion to the National Commission.

Citizens' rights to participation

In the matter of control, at least three different strategies have been considered. None of these are intended to be exclusive nor are they the only ways to approach the issue. Are any of these options moving in the right direction toward greater democracy in decision-making about science and technology? To adopt a diffident attitude about the debate is to fly in the face of reality for to repeat, increased regulation, at least in some areas, is certainly inevitable and probably necessary. Science can not continue to grow by closing its eyes to the political, legal, and moral consequences of its actions. If we are to prevent future abuses of and by science, scientists will have to become more involved. Wider public participation in science policy decision-making is being pushed by a number of nongovernmental and governmental agencies (e.g., Ralph Nader's citizen involvement program is representative of the first genre). Congress lately has become especially insistent in pressing for citizens' rights to participation. The notion that the public should have a voice in the formulation of science policy is a natural extension of a movement begun in the 1960s, when a number of groups insisted on a role for themselves in the establishment of policies and operation of programs (e.g., welfare groups, environmentalists, women's liberation movement, gay rights, etc.). It is not a very big step to go from these to the proposition that citizens have a right to be involved in science policy-making too. As a result, scientists in all disciplines are now confronted by public interest groups that want some say in the kind of research that is being done. They have an ally in Senator Edward Kennedy.

During the past couple of years, Senator Kennedy has actively pushed for a Science for Citizens program to be administered through the National Science Foundation. The purposes of the program are several:[33]

1. to improve public understanding of public policy issues;
2. to encourage scientists, engineers and students to participate in activities aimed at the resolution of public-policy issues;
3. to enable nonprofit citizens' public-interest groups to acquire technical expertise to assist them in dealing with scientific and technological aspects of public-policy issues.

Public hearings have been held around the country in an effort to round out the organization of such a program. One option considered might be the establishment of regional science centers designed to identify science-related issues of importance to the community and to provide expert information on them.

Opposition to the proposed Science for Citizens focuses especially on the third objective, namely, the provision which makes available to public interest groups the technical expertise to assist them in dealing with scientific and technological programs. This is interpreted by many to mean those programs to which they are opposed. Critics do not fancy the idea that the government ought to make professional help convenient to those opposed to government and/or commercial projects which have already been approved or are awaiting approval.[34] There seems to be a contradiction here. Senator Kennedy and some of his colleagues, however, are insistent that the program proceed and regardless of any foot-dragging, the government's aim to open up this aspect of science policy-making will come to fruition. Whatever emerges, it is fair to predict that the public participation in the science movement is clearly here to stay.

It can, of course, be argued that the suggestion of greater public participation is naive, impractical, or idealistic, for after all, how can laypersons even begin to understand the complexities of the issues involved? This is one of the more controversial areas. Clearly, the times are changing. There is a severe reaction against a purely technocratic mode of decision-making. Whether it is possible to have wide public participation in decision-making without a virtual paralysis of scientific activity and without the complete disappearance of any coherent plan for the future remains undetermined. In the past, public participation was used primarily as a strategy for stopping technology. It is difficult to think of a single instance where a technological project has been *advanced* by the participatory process. It is entirely possible that decisions by experts will be preferred over public participation for better defining the public interest if participatory activities serve only to further special interests or certain political ideologies determined to block certain scientific projects.[35]

There is another side to the issue of public participation that asks whether or not citizens can acquire the knowledge considered necessary to formulate an intelligent response. Can the public comprehend the science involved sufficiently well enough to make useful judgments about it? Paul Ehrlich submits that "any person with a high school education who is willing to put in some effort can learn enough of the pertinent science to make a sound judgment on most of the science-society issues of the day, if scientists are willing to explain the issues."[36] Lord Solly Zuckerman of the United Kingdom and former chief science adviser to Her Magesty's Government said, "a public which has little or no understanding of the significance of the letters DNA, nonetheless has no hesitation about the wisdom of encouraging or disallowing work in the field of genetic engineering."[37]

Senator Jacob Javits (R-N.Y.) put it in these terms:

The decisions with respect to the future of biomedical research, the determination of priorities, the weighing of the nonquantifiable social costs and benefits of medical technology—these decisions are in fact political because they involve the entire body politic including, of course, the research community itself. A scientist is no more trained to decide finally the moral and political implications of his or her work than the public—and its elected representatives—is trained to decide finally on scientific methodologies.[38]

In testimony before the Senate Subcommittee on Health, psychiatrist Willard Gaylin, president of the Institute of Society, Ethics and the Life Sciences (Hastings Center), defended the appropriateness of a public role in the regulation of scientific research. It is not necessary that the public possess a level of expertise comparable to that of the scientist in order to understand the ramifications involved in a proposed bit of scientific research. As Gaylin says:

There is probably not a member of Congress who completely understands the physics behind the creation of the atom bomb, and (furthermore) it is not necessary that they do. The decisions on whether to build bombs, how many should be built, and how and when, if ever, they should be used, requires a minimal knowledge of that technology. It would be appalling if this were deemed a problem in physics. The decisions are political and must rest with the people and their representatives.[39]

No doubt, though, there are enormous risks in arguing that decisions on such matters be influenced by popular opinion or even popular vote. In science, there is the particular danger of short-sightedness if the public and/or legislators are allowed to determine its course on this basis. The failure to understand the importance of speculative research priorities can be seriously questioned but since some level of intervention can no longer be avoided, channels must be created through which the interests and desires of the citizens can influence the work of the scientist. This requires that scientists explain their work and its consequences publicly and expose their views to the workings of the democratic process.

The national experience with public participation is very recent. Thus, participatory decision-making is still subject to considerable social learning. Those who advocate this position are not necessarily calling for communal *control* over science (for example, of the sort promulgated by Science for the People movement), but a good deal more public *influence* if only to keep the whole enterprise healthy.

Justification for public involvement can be argued from at least three perspectives:[40] First, it is now abundantly clear that the experts *do not* always know what is best (scientists have failed so often to see the many ill effects of their work that they have forfeited automatic respect—experts can be wrong or dishonest like anyone else); second, because of the huge outlay of public funds necessary for research and technology, people are simply going to demand to know much more about what scientists are up to and why; third, and probably most compelling, public involvement is a democratic right. Who but the citizens should decide between the many conflicts arising from science when the public sector is concerned? Numerous instances can be cited: Financial cost of scientific projects against benefits to be gained, for it is the public's money being spent; societal impact of a proposed piece of science, for it is their lives that will be affected; establishing priorities when all programs cannot be supported. (A case in point is the War on Cancer program where huge sums of money were devoted to cancer research, some of dubious quality. Specialists tell us that more than half of all cancer patients could be cured if the disease were diagnosed early and treated promptly. Would it not be wiser to devote more public money into diagnosis and treatment? The public has had little say in the matter, probably because the decision was made for political reasons.)

To emphasize again, the effort should not be aimed at communal control over science but at a good deal more public influence. This places considerable responsibility not only on the scientific community, but on the press and other media in interpreting science and discussing its social implications intelligently. Scientists have roles to play here in helping people acquire knowledge about scientific matters. This is as important as they themselves participating in debates on the issues. The public too, has a responsibility to involve itself in the matters of science, to be receptive to the new knowledge from whatever source it may come, and to help decide the importance of proposed scientific research in relation to all other pressing national needs. If the present trend afoot in the country continues, the message is quite clear—the practical applications of scientific discoveries and their moral and ethical consequences are matters that will need the collective wisdom of *all* society. To accomplish this, decision making about science will become more open to public assessment. In the words of Halstead Holman:

> The issue is not a struggle between science and antiscience or anti-intellectualism. It is a struggle to achieve a healthy relationship between science and citizens who support it and are affected by it. Science as a human endeavor, like medicine, can develop appropriately only with the consent and support of those whom it affects. Scientists, like physicians, should be partners of the public.[41]

This brings us back full-circle to where these discussions began at the outset of this text: The call for public discussion and participation concerning societal use of science and its technologies!

AN ETHOS OF SCIENCE

The moral responsibility of scientists

Society no longer recognizes the fundamental maxim on which basic research in modern science was formerly based: The search for knowledge is warranted wherever it may lead, no matter how prepared or unprepared the world may be to cope with the facts that scientists discover.[42] Scientific research today is being recognized for what it is, a social activity, and scientists can no longer isolate themselves in the laboratory. Questions previously kept out of the scientific domain now intrude with a personal immediacy:[43]

> Do scientists have any unique responsibility as scientists for what is happening and for changing what is happening?
>
> How can scientists ensure that their research will be used for worthwhile purposes?
>
> What is the covert relationship between science and society?

These are questions that must be faced squarely by the scientific community but to date general agreement as to what constitutes an adequate reponse is still lacking. A reason often given for this omission is the earlier discussed moral-neutrality proposition. Science is only a means for gaining knowledge, not of using it socially or politically. Use is beyond the power of scientists to monitor or control. A technology must necessarily intervene between the scientific laboratory and society and that is not part of the scientist's domain. If the scientist is to be held accountable for the results that neither he nor anyone else can know in advance, then all human actions, including any pursuit of knowledge, must also come under moral accountability. If that be so, then all human activity must be circumspect. Who, after all, could possibly know all the consequences of any human activity?

Although the logic sounds convincing, it has been challenged. Ethicist Daniel Callahan argues that "if we claim the right to act at all, and if we claim the right to make use in action of knowledge that will put *power* into our hands, we cannot simultaneously disclaim responsibility for what thereafter happens."[44] Our actions are causes which bring about events. We cannot deny our role in those events which can be traced back to our actions as causal agents. If our actions have moral consequences, then we must assume moral responsibility for them even if our action was one among many, even countless many other causes. Since scientific thoughts and activities set the stage for other thoughts and activities, then like any thoughts or actions that have consequences, the entry point for moral responsibility on the part of the scientist is established. Scientists then, do have special obligations to society. What are these?

At least two forms of scientific responsibility can be identified, responsibility to the scientific community and responsibility to society.[45] The first considers the scientist primarily as a scholar where the demands of honesty, clarity of thought, independence, energy, and dedication, and the sense of awe for the workings of the universe are undergirding characteristics. An abbreviated list of scientific virtues might include these: individual truthseeking; the striving after rational knowledge, objectivity in the conduct of research and its interpretation; open-mindedness and a willingness to change opinions when data warrant; and unselfish humility reflected in an open sharing of knowledge. In the real world, scientists of course are not necessarily always persons demonstrating these high virtues and in fact, they can be wrong or dishonest like anyone else. The pressure upon individual investigators has been increasing and personal integrity can often be stretched to the breaking point (see p. 415). This essay will not pursue this issue further. It is well, though, that internal scientific virtue be recognized as an integral part of moral responsibility of the scientist.

A second part of the responsibility to the scientific community entails not demeaning the community or diminishing the standing of other members by acting in ways inappropriate to the traditions of science (as described above). Improper actions are viewed as threats to the integrity of science and a defacing of its popular image to the detriment of all science.

One school of this view considers it irresponsible to make public statements concerning areas beyond the competence of the researcher (e.g., to enter into the political or social realm) or to make assertions that are imprecise or unprovable (e.g., statements of value). Likewise it is ethically questionable to ally oneself with nonscientists in social or political causes, to advocate certain public policies, or to campaign for such policies. But now that the implications of scientific research have moved toward the center of the world stage, many scientists have rejected this historical view, substituting for it the second and broader interpretation of scientific responsibility, namely, responsibility to society rather than solely to the scientific community. Tensions between the two views, however, continue to persist.

Social responsibility of scientists

What are the dimensions of social responsibility and how should they be exercised? Regarding the first, Paul Sieghart, a British lawyer and an activist in the science-society movement in his country, proposes the following set of social obligations for scientists:[46]

1. *Refusing to do work.* It is obvious that some experiments cannot or should not be performed either because of the potential harm emanating from them or because they are too expensive. No scientist, for example, would defend an experiment which entailed the certain death of even one person. Certain types of research do present stark "black-white" choices. On those occasions, the scientist must refuse participation as part of his or her obligation to society. Even if other scientists are not similarly morally inclined, and the effect of refusal may be infinitesimally small, the ethical scientist should so act for it will serve several purposes: (a) Will improve the moral climate in which science must operate, encouraging others to similar actions; and (b) By encouraging professional restraint and censure, others may refrain even though moral constraints may not be the motivating factor.

2. *Choosing to do work.* Research or development of a technology where there is an urgent social need for which the scientist has special expertise or knowledge should receive higher priority than work of lower social value even when the former brings a lesser reward in earnings or professional prestige.

3. *Influencing other scientists.* Through direct interaction with others in science, the scientist has the opportunity to directly express his/her concern

about the social responsibility of his and others' experimentation including those areas that should or should not be investigated. Over the past few years, scientists have organized themselves into interest groups concerned with problems of science and society and to actively promote their concerns among fellow scientists and the general public. The Federation of American Scientists (FAS) is a group of 7000 natural and social scientists and engineers who are licensed to lobby in the public interest and through their monthly publication *Public Interest Report*, communicate their concerns to others. The Scientists' Institute for Public Information (SIPI) and its publication *Environment*, or *The Bulletin of Atomic Scientists*, the Pugwash Conferences, and the like are representatives of this new wave of professional involvement. The force of moral disapproval by a group of eminent scientists may act as a powerful deterrent to experimentation by others.

4. *Thinking out consequences.* The social consequences of a particular piece of work or its application should be thought through in advance. To the extent possible, risk-benefit assessments should be made objectively; that is, available agents, experiences, data, or procedures should be employed which consider both beneficial and harmful effects. However, it should be recognized that all risks and benefits cannot be authoritatively assessed. It would seem essential then to include at some point in the review process the viewpoints of others, scientists and nonscientists who are not directly involved with the work. Thus, even if the assessment is not completely objective, it is at least not one-sided, nor carried out to protect vested-interests of individuals or groups.

5. *Informing the public.* This is no doubt one of the most sensitive social responsibilities of scientists. Modern science is venturing into much unknown territory. Many times it is faced with a conflict of values and the ethical principles involved are still in the process of formulation. Matters of life and death for society are, of course, everybody's business and especially the business of politicians; but they can hardly be solved without a deep involvement by many scientists, far more than the small group presently working on these problems. If the work being done in a particular area might have significant social impact, the concerned scientist has the responsibility to make the matter public. Society then will have time to work out an intelligent response in advance by initiating what needs to be done about likely consequences. As expressed by the Committee on Scientific Freedom and Responsibility of the American Association for the Advancement of Science, scientists can claim no special rights, other than those possessed by every citizen, except those necessary to fulfill the responsibilities that arise from the possession of special knowledge and the insight arising from that knowledge.

It follows from this that the scientific community cannot by itself make decisions about the social consequences of its work for if it did, it would be put into a position above even national governments. Decisions affecting a community at large must remain public decisions and must be made by those departments of government and the community charged with the specific responsibility. In the words of Nobel laureate biologist, Arthur Kornberg, "science is too important a matter to be left to scientists." Scientists must communicate with the laity and although there may be an intelligent laity with whom science can communicate and an uneducated one with which it cannot, the effort must be encouraged in as many ways as possible.

A central issue in public communication pertains to standards of ethical behavior. Scientists should abide by a higher ethical standard than that adhered to by others, for example, by politicians.[47] They should avoid dogmatism; make their assumptions as objective as they can; qualify themselves when judgments are involved; be willing to recognize and admit weaknesses in their positions; and be ready to reason with those who disagree. A statement by Harvey Brooks is highly relevant here:

> Scientists can no longer afford to be naive about the political effects of publicly stated scientific opinions. If the effect of their scientific views is politically potent, they have an obligation to declare their political or value assumptions and to try to be honest with themselves, their colleagues, and their audience about the degree to which their assumptions have affected their selection and interpretation of scientific evidence. Once scientific opinion enters into the public domain, the possibility of political neutrality disappears but this does not mean that objectivity should be thrown to the winds rather than being held up as an ideal to be achieved as closely as circumstances allow.[48]

Scientists who speak out should be willing to be judged by their scientific peers as well as by the general marketplace of ideas. Societal monitoring of the public debate will provide effective control to the scientific contribution just as it does other kinds of contributions from a variety of experts (e.g., economists, social scientists, etc.) A competitive intermingling of ideas will keep the discussions relatively honest.

Morally questionable research areas

In this discussion of social responsibility, the assumption was implied that not all research is inherently good and desirable. There may very well be strong reasons for declaring certain areas of research off limits or at the least, imposing strong restrictions on them. The most widely discussed in this category of forbidden or restricted areas is some kinds of research dealing with recombinant DNA. The historically unprecedented move declared certain experiments off limits because of their potential, though unproven, hazards to human health, even though these experiments are probably of great scientific interest (e.g., the transfer of genes for botulism toxin or known tumor genes).

Another area of research that some have suggested should be off limits for scientific investigation involves the role of genetics and environmental factors in determining certain behaviors.[49] One aspect of the debate focuses on I.Q. differences between whites and blacks and much bitterness has been engendered on all sides of the argument. Some have drawn the conclusion that differences between racial groups in I.Q. performance are due primarily to genetic factors. Other scientists have hotly disputed such claims, insisting that research done in this field serves only to enflame racism and that it should, therefore, be condemned by the scientific community.

The relationship between the chromosomal abnormality XYY and socially deviant behavior has been hotly contested and at least one research project aimed at what was hoped to be an objective evaluation of the hypothesis has been discontinued. Gerald and Walzer, of the Harvard Medical School, concluded their long-term study begun in 1969 because of outside pressure being exerted on them to stop, including professional criticism from other notable scientists.[50]

There is another area where extensive although far from clear-cut evidence indicates that adverse social and psychological factors in early childhood can exert a crippling influence on subsequent development. The problems of research in this area are appallingly difficult, raising grave ethical issues. It would, for example, be immoral to subject young children deliberately to conditions of deprivation, for example, malnutrition or social suffering, in order to observe their behavior when compared to a control group. Some studies similar to this have been done with animal subjects (e.g., H. F. Harlow at the University of Wisconsin Primate Laboratory) and have yielded valuable insights. But even the use of animals for these kinds of studies raises a whole new set of sensitive issues, which must consider carefully the suffering that might be inflicted on animal subjects in relation to the value of the experiment being performed. A small but active school of proponents insist that experiments with animals should be undertaken only for extraordinary reasons.[51]

Research involving human subjects inevitably raises serious questions concerning experimental protocol; we generally acknowledge today the absolute necessity of full and informed consent on the part of the subject before experimentation can proceed (see chapter 7). In some instances, such consent is difficult, if not impossible to obtain. Prisoners in penal institutions, experiments on young children, fetal experimentation, psychological experiments on "normal" subjects which may be morally degrading or psychologically damaging all place heavy responsibilities on both the investigator and the society which allows the experiment to be carried out. In the United States at least, human research is a desirable but not an essential activity. Since no person can be compelled to be a research subject, progress which is dependent upon human experimentation is an optional, not a necessary goal. It is well to bear in mind that central ethical axiom of human experimentation which insists that an experiment is ethical or not ethical at its inception and is not judged morally valid on the basis of results. The recent ban on some aspects of the fetal research exemplifies this concern.

Some studies involving deliberate ecological modification of regions of considerable size must also be carefully considered. In such cases, one must weigh the prospective value of the information that may be gained from the experiment against the harmful effects of possible damage to the region involved.

Robert Sinsheimer, a molecular biologist, would add several more to the list of questionable research areas.[52] These include attempts to contact presumed "extraterrestrial intelligence" (ETI), research on the predetermination of sex of children, and experimentation dealing indiscriminately with the aging process. The first he objects to because if ETI is discovered, its societal effect would be shattering, especially if the life discovered is more advanced than ours. Research resulting in the controlled determination of sex could result in an unsettling imbalance in the human sex ratio in the population at large. Research into the aging process, assuming it succeeds in keeping people young, has never been determined to result in overall societal good and, in fact, Sinsheimer contends that the few sociological analyses that have been done portend great problems.

In all of these areas where concern has been expressed, the point at issue is where is the balance between the search for new knowledge and the risks to participants and/or society attendant in the search? These are social and political questions. At present, there are powerful pressures in favor of safeguarding the public interest even if it means sacrificing the attainment of knowledge that may promise some potential future benefit. The issues are complex and they have no simple answers.

The future consequences of scientific research hold much uncertainty. It is obvious that no one has perfect knowledge of the future, hence, absolute predictability is not a human quality. Daniel Callahan submits the following moral propositions as points of consideration for the problem of consequences:[53]

1. "Individuals and groups are ordinarily responsible only for the consequences of those actions that are voluntary and intentional on their part."

   They may also be held responsible for the unintended consequences of their actions if, through negligence, they failed to take into account such consequences.

2. "Individuals and groups cannot be held responsible for those actions where the consequences are totally unknown and cannot be known."

   However, if they voluntarily undertake acts where consequences cannot be known in advance, they may be held responsible for outcomes unless there were serious reasons for undertaking the action in the first place. One cannot, without serious reason, just "play around" in the unknown while disclaiming responsibility for the results even though they cannot be known.

3. "When others may be affected by the actions and/or consequences, then 'the others' have a right to demand that their wishes and values be respected."

   This is especially so if the results may result in harm.

4. "Individuals, scientists, and groups are subject to the same norms of ethical responsibility as those of all other individuals and groups in society."

   Scientists have neither more responsibility, nor less; there is no special ethic of responsibility applying to scientists that does not apply to other professions, such as physicians, or lawyers. This rejects the principle that scientists are not morally or ethically responsible for the consequences of their work regardless of how it was used providing they had no role in its implementation.

How direct must be the causal sequence between the research (i.e., basic research as opposed to applied research) and subsequent applications? Is Mendel, for example, to be held responsible for the present I.Q.-race controversy? Or Madame Curie for the ravages of Hiroshima and Nagasaki? Clearly, the answer is no. There is no possible way that these early researchers could have foreseen the future consequences of their work. But this dissociation from guilt does not carry the same weight of moral persuasion today. We now know, in a way earlier generations could not know, how what is assumed to be innocent knowledge, can in other times and in other places, have harmful consequences. Historical experience in all areas of human activity, including science, increases over time and cannot be ignored. (The expression "he who ignores history is doomed to repeat it" has application here.) There is simply too much accumulated knowledge, especially in recent times, to discharge even basic research from responsibility for its outcomes. However hard it may be or however remote the possibility for harmful consequences, the researcher must carry the moral burden of responsibility, according to Callahan.

In cases of conflict where individuals are uncertain of the consequences of a piece of either basic or applied research, the matter should be decided by individual conscience. No person should act against his or her own moral principals. The *morally* responsible individual cannot disclaim liability unless he/she has rigorously examined the consequences and measured them against the simple but fundamental test: "Would I be satisfied to have these actions or consequences applied to me?" If the positive benefits outweigh the foreseeable harmful consequences, then a direction is suggested. The goal that must remain uppermost in research that may have both beneficial and harmful consequences to humans is what its effects will be on human welfare. Every scientific or technological undertaking must respect basic human rights and cherish human dignity. Every innovation must be judged by its contributions to the development of genuinely free and creative persons.[54] In cases of uncertainty or in those cases which are morally mixed, society has the right to consultation and the scientist is obliged to seek out that involvement. The issue must be brought out into the open and exposed to both the scientific community and to the public at large.

In dealing with uncertainty, a variety of options exists and several have already been described (e.g., the Science Court). One more—the worst-case scenario—will be mentioned here. The worst-case scenario may be used when consequences have the potential to effect major perturbations. Its underlying rationale is simply stated: If err we must, it is best to err on the side of safety. This scenario attempts to identify the worst conceivable outcome of an action that might occur. Callahan defines *worst* as that result which is judged to (a) threaten the welfare or the rights of individuals, or (b) threaten the general welfare. The burden of proof is on those seeking to advance scientific or technological innovations or particular projects, not on those advocating a slowdown or halting. These principles, if applied, question the notion that scientific progress is a cardinal goal; more realistically, scientific progress may merely be an optimal one. Absolute commitment to scientific progress is not, nor can it ever be, a part of the social contract between society and the scientific profession. Although knowledge may be good, it is not an absolute good. Human values ought to take precedence when conflict exists. However, many scientists have great difficulty with this proposition. Choosing the course of moral safety—by imagining the worst of all outcomes—is the morally responsible way to act in Callahan's view.

It is time to bring this discussion to a close. Undoubtedly it has raised far more problems than solutions. The air is still filled with rhetoric of "no regulation," and the counterrhetoric of "more regulation"; of the demand for an exercise of moral responsibility by practicing scientists, to the position that science is value-neutral. There exists at present no demonstrated way for dealing with these problems to the satisfaction of all. The task, if it is to be accomplished at all, is absolutely dependent upon dialogue within science among scientists and dialogue between the scientific community and the general public. Only then will it be possible to hope that major points of contention can be resolved. And that is the most imperative present need!

The following affirmation encapsulates some of the views expressed here and is an appropriate way to bring the discussion to a close.

OATH for scientists (similar to the Hippocratic oath in the medical profession) This is quoted from M. W. Thrings, *New Scientists,* January 7, 1971.

> I vow to strive to apply my professional skills only to projects which, after conscientious examination, I believe to contribute to the goal of co-existence of all human beings in peace, human dignity, and self-fulfillment.
>
> I believe that this goal requires the provision of an adequate supply of the necessities of life (good food, air, water, clothing, and housing, access to natural and man-made beauty), education, and opportunities to enable each person to work out for himself his life objectives and to develop creativeness and skill in the use of hands as well as head.
>
> I vow to struggle through my work to minimize danger; noise; strain, or invasion of privacy of the individual; pollution of earth, air, or water; destruction of natural beauty, mineral resources and wildlife.

Because of the mixed nature of this presentation, the section on values will not be included. The student is encouraged to develop a list of values that pertain.

REFERENCES

1   Roy O. Greep, "Science, politics and society," *Perspectives in Biology and Medicine* 18 (1975): 211–226.
2   Theodore Roszak, *Where the Wasteland Ends* (Garden City: Anchor, 1973), p. 207.
3   Robert J. Yaes, "The science establishment," *The Center Magazine* 8, 2 (1975): 55–66.
4   Harvey Wheeler, "Science's slippery slope," *The Center Magazine* 8, 1 (1975): 64–72.
5   Victor F. Weiskoff, cited in "Weiskoff on the frontiers and limits of science," *Science* 188 (1975): 721.
6   Harvey Wheeler (in Reference 4), p. 66.
7   Harvey Wheeler (in Reference 4), p. 68.
8   Barbara Yuncker, "The strange case of the painted mice," *Saturday Review,* (November 30, 1974), pp. 50–53.
9   Richard W. Roberts, cited in "Symposium scores misuse of scientific data," *Chemical and Engineering News* (February 10, 1975), pp. 17–18.
10   Barbara Yuncker (in Reference 8), p. 50.
11   Ernest Borek, "The twilight of integrity?" *Chemical and Engineering News* (March 17, 1975), p. 2.
12   Robert J. Yaes (in Reference 3), p. 62.
13   Donald Brown, "Quality and relevance," *Hastings Center Report* 5, 3 (1975): 8.
14   Albert F. Plant, "We're too quiet about research," *Chemical and Engineering News,* (August 25, 1975), p. 4.
15   Willard Gaylin, "Scientific research and public regulation," *Hastings Center Report* 5, 3 (1975): 5–7.
16   Robert Heilbronner, quoted in "Whither the NSF?—the higher derivative," by H. Guyford Stever, *Science* 189 (1975): 264–267.
17   Stephen Rose and Hilary Rose, "Can science be neutral?" *Perspectives in Biology and Medicine* 16, 4 (1973): 605–624.

18 Maurice B. Visscher, "Science and value," *Perspectives in Biology and Medicine* **18**, 3 (1975): 299–305.

19 Hans Jonas, "Freedom of scientific inquiry and the public interest," *Hastings Center Report* **6**, 4 (1976): 15–17.

20 Theodore Roszak (in Reference 2), p. 215.

21 James K. Glassman, "Harvard genetics researcher quits science for politics." *Science* **167** (1970): 963–964.

22 John Walsh, "The state of academic science: concern about the vital signs," *Science* **196** (1977): 1184–1185.

23 Harvey Wheeler, "The regulation of scientists," *The Center Magazine* **8**, 1 (1975): 73–77.

24 Nicholas Wade, "Recombinant DNA: NIH rules broken in insulin-gene project" *Science* **197** (1977): 1342–1345.

25 Barbara J. Culliton, "Fetal research: the case history of a Massachusetts law," *Science* **187** (1975): 237–241.

26 Barbara J. Culliton, "Fetal research (II): the nature of a Massachusetts law," *Science* **187** (1975): 411–413.

27 Barbara J. Culliton, "Fetal research (III): the impact of a Massachusetts law," *Science* **187** (1975): 1175–1176.

28 George Ball, cited in "AAAS grapples with scientific freedom issue," *Chemical and Engineering News*, (March 7, 1977), p. 19.

29 Philip Handler, cited in "Handler assesses federal science affairs," by Fred H. Zerkel, *Chemical and Engineering News*, (February 3, 1975): pp. 18–19.

30 Task Force of the Presidential Advisory Group on Anticipated Advances in Science and Technology, "The Science Court experiment: an interim report," *Science* **197** (1976): 653–656. "Science Court 'tried', cleared for test case," by E. M. Leeper, *Bioscience* **26**:11 (1976); "Experiment planned to test feasibility of a Science Court" by Philip M. Boffey, *Science* **193** (1976): 129.

31 Arthur Kantrowitz, "The Science Court experiment: criticisms and responses," *Bulletin of Atomic Scientists* **33**, 4 (1977): 43–50.

32 Dorothy Nelkin, "Thoughts on the proposed Science Court," *Newsletter on Science, Technology and Human Values* **19** (1977): 20–31.

33 Barbara J. Culliton, "NSF: trying to cope with congressional pressure for public participation," *Science* **191** (1976): 274–318.

34 Nicholas Wade, "Science for citizens," *Science* **194** (1976): 306.

35 Harvey Brooks, "Technology assessment in retrospect," *Newsletter on Science, Technology and Human Values* **17** (1976): 17–29.

36 Paul R. Ehrlich, "Ecologists, ethics, and the environment," *Bioscience* **27**, 4 (1977): 239.

37 Lord Solly Zuckerman (in Reference 28), p. 19.

38 Jacob Javits, cited in "The goals of science," by S. E. Luria, *Bulletin of Atomic Sciences* **33**, 5 (1977): 32.

39 Willard Gaylin (in Reference 15), p. 5.

40 Bernard Dixon, *What Is Science For?* (New York: Harper & Row, 1973).

41 Halstead Holman, "Scientists and citizens," *Hastings Center Report* **5**, 3 (1975): 8.

42 "Max Tishler on basic research," *Chemical and Engineering News* (March 28, 1977), p. 5.

43 Robert E. Filmer, "The Roots of Political Activism in British Science," *Bulletin of Atomic Scientists* **32**, 1 (1976): 25–29.

44 Daniel Callahan, "Ethical Responsibility in Science in the Face of Uncertain Conse-

quences," in *Ethical & Scientific Issues Posed by Human Uses of Molecular Genetics*, Marc Lappé and Robert S. Morrison (eds.) (New York: New York Academy of Sciences, 1976), pp. 1–12.

45 "To whom are public interest scientists responsible?" *F.A.S. Public Interest Report* **29**, 10 (1976): 1–2.

46 Paul Sieghart et al., "The social obligations of the scientist," *Hastings Center Study* **1**, 2 (1973): 7–16.

47 F.A.S. Public Interest Report, (in Reference 45), p. 1.

48 Harvey Brooks (in Reference 35), p. 22.

49 John T. Edsall, *Scientific Freedom & Responsibility*, (Washington, D.C.: American Association for the Advancement of Science, 1975), p. 12.

50 Richard Roblin, "The Boston XYY case," *Hastings Center Report* **5**, 4 (1975): 5–8.

51 Peter Singer, *Animal Liberation*, (New York: Random House, 1975), and Catherine Roberts, *The Scientific Conscience* (New York: George Braziller, 1967).

52 Robert Sinsheimer, "Inquiring into inquiry: two opposing views," *Hastings Center Report* **6**, 4 (1976): 18.

53 Daniel Callahan, (in Reference 44), p. 2.

54 "Mount Carmel declaration on technology and moral responsibility," *STPP News* (June, 1976).

55 Barry M. Casper and Paul David Wellstone, "The Science Court on trial in Minnesota." *Hastings Center Report* **8**, 4 (1978): 5–8.

BIBLIOGRAPHY

Baker, W. O., et al., "The making of modern science: biographical studies," *Daedalus* (Fall, 1970).

Bronowski, J., *The Ascent of Man* (Boston: Little, Brown, 1973).

Bronowski, J., *Science and Human Values* (New York: Harper & Row; 1956).

Bush, Vannevar, *Science is Not Enough*, (New York: William Morrow, 1967).

Brown, Martin, (ed.), *The Social Responsibility of the Scientist*, (New York: The Free Press, 1971).

Farson, Richard, (ed.), *Science and Human Affairs*, (Palo Alto: Science and Behavior Books, 1965).

Holton, Gerald, (ed.), *Science and Culture*, (Boston: Beacon, 1965).

Standen, Anthony, *Science is a Sacred Cow*, (New York: E. P. Dutton, 1950).

Schooler, Jr., Dean, *Science, Scientists and Public Policy*, (New York: The Free Press, 1971).

Zuckerman, Sir Solly, *Beyond The Ivory Tower* (New York: Taplinger, 1970).

AUTHOR INDEX

SUBJECT INDEX